D1483634

$D_1 : D_2$ Dopamine Receptor Interactions

edited by

J.L. Waddington

Department of Clinical Pharmacology
Royal College of Surgeons in Ireland
Dublin, Republic of Ireland

ACADEMIC PRESS
Harcourt Brace & Company, Publishers
London   San Diego   New York
Boston   Sydney   Tokyo   Toronto

ACADEMIC PRESS LIMITED
24/28 Oval Road,
London NW1 7DX

United States Edition published by
ACADEMIC PRESS INC.
San Diego, CA 92101

This book is printed on acid free paper

A catalogue record for this book
is available from the British Library

ISBN 0–12–729045–1

Typeset by P & R Typesetters Ltd, Salisbury, UK
Printed and bound in Great Britain
by TJ Press Ltd, Padstow, Cornwall

Contents

Contents

Contributors

Hessah A. Al-Naser Laboratory of Psychopharmacology, School of Psychology, University of Birmingham, Edgbaston, Birmingham B15 2TT, UK

Richard J. Beninger Department of Psychology, Queen's University, Kingston, K7L 3N6, Canada

Steven J. Cooper Laboratory of Psychopharmacology, School of Psychology, University of Birmingham, Edgbaston, Birmingham B15 2TT, UK

Siobhan A. Daly Department of Clinical Pharmacology, Royal College of Surgeons in Ireland, St Stephen's Green, Dublin 2, Ireland

Sara Goldsmith School of Medicine, Laboratory of Chemical Neuroanatomy, University of Pennsylvania, 127 Clinical Research Building, 422 Currie Boulevard, Philadelphia, PA 19104-6141, USA

Xiu-Ti Hu Neuropsychopharmacology Laboratory, University of Health Sciences/The Chicago Medical School, 3333 Green Bay Road, North Chicago, IL 60064, USA

Jeffrey N. Joyce School of Medicine, Laboratory of Chemical Neuroanatomy, University of Pennsylvania, 127 Clinical Research Building, 422 Currie Boulevard, Philadelphia, PA 19104-6141, USA

Frederick J. Monsma Jr Experimental Therapeutics Branch, National Institute of Neurological Disorders and Stroke, National Institutes of Health, Building 10, Room 5C-108, 9 Rockville Pike, Bethesda, Maryland, USA

Angela M. Murray School of Medicine, Laboratory of Chemical Neuroanatomy, University of Pennsylvania, 127 Clinical Research Building, 422 Currie Boulevard, Philadelphia, PA 19104-6141, USA

Erik B. Nielsen Department of CNS Pharmacology, CNS Division, Novo Nordisk A/S, Novo Nordisk Park, DK-2760 Måløv, Denmark

Ennio Ongini Schering-Plough SpA, Via Ripamonti 89, 20141 Milano, Italy

Yong Shen Experimental Therapeutics Branch, National Institute of Neurological Disorders and Stroke, National Institutes of Health, Building 10, Room 5C-108, 9 Rockville Pike, Bethesda, Maryland, USA

David R. Sibley Experimental Therapeutics Branch, National Institute of Neurological Disorders and Stroke, National Institutes of Health, Building 10, Room 5C-108, 9 Rockville Pike, Bethesda, Maryland, USA

Michael S. Starr Department of Pharmacology, School of Pharmacy, 29–39 Brunswick Square, London WC1N 1AX, UK

John L. Waddington Department of Clinical Pharmacology, Royal College of Surgeons in Ireland, St Stephens Green, Dublin 2, Ireland

Francis J. White Neuropsychopharmacology Laboratory, University of Health Sciences/The Chicago Medical School, 3333 Green Bay Road, North Chicago, IL 60064, USA

Series Preface

The driving force for the production of this series lies in my own inability to keep up with the advances occurring in those areas of neuroscience in which I am especially interested. So many times I have been frustrated by being unable to find a current review of an important research area. Even when I resort to bothering colleagues who are experts in a particular field, I am told, more often than not, that such an overview does not exist. In my own area of expertise I frequently send away empty handed students who have asked me to direct them to a definitive article on a well researched topic.

Although regrettable, perhaps this situation is not surprising since the neurosciences are one of the most diverse and rapidly advancing areas in the biological sphere. By definition, research in the neurosciences encompasses anatomy, pathology, biochemistry, physiology, pharmacology, molecular biology, genetics and therapeutics. Indeed, there are few individuals capable of maintaining a grasp of the literature in all these aspects of their own research interests let alone in other fields.

My answer was to establish *Neuroscience Perspectives* and to develop gradually a series of individual edited monographs dealing in depth with issues of current interest to those working in the neuroscience area. Each volume is being designed to bring a multidisciplinary approach to the subject matter by pursuing the topic from the laboratory to the clinic. As a consequence I have asked the editors of the individual volumes to produce a balanced critique of their topic which will be read, understood and enjoyed by as wide an audience as possible within the realm of neuroscience.

The choice of the topics for the series is a difficult matter. In the first instance these were largely dictated by my own interests or by my awareness of important and fundamental work being undertaken by colleagues. More recently, I have been recruiting subject matter and editors through attending a variety of diverse symposia in the neuroscience area. However, the choice of topics should reflect the needs of the audience reached by the series. So I invite you to let me know of areas which you feel are of importance and to give me suggestions for individuals who would be keen to edit a book for *Neuroscience Perspectives*.

Finally, it only remains to thank those individuals at Academic Press who have already worked for several years to develop *Neuroscience Perspectives*. In particular, Dr Carey Chapman who has the unenviable task of recruiting the editors that I suggest and then harassing them for the completed work. My hope is that the series will fill the gap that I perceive and provide for my colleagues in the neurosciences a collection of interesting books which will become reference volumes in their field. I hope you will enjoy *Neuroscience Perspectives*.

Peter Jenner

Preface

Few areas in contemporary neuroscience and psychopharmacology can have undergone no less than *three* important revisions over a time span so short as that separating recent insights into the nature and function of brain dopamine receptor subtypes. Subsequent to the presumed prepotence of the D_2 receptor in the context of the now classical D_1/D_2 nomenclature, the introduction of the first selective D_1 antagonist changed fundamentally that perspective: the D_1 receptor was recognized to exert a profound functional role. Thereafter, in response to a rapidly increasing body of otherwise paradoxical findings, evolved the concept and, ultimately, the substance of $D_1 : D_2$ interactions in the regulation of the totality of dopaminergic neurotransmission and of psychomotor behaviour. Very recently, we have witnessed in molecular biological studies the cloning, expression and preliminary characterization of what appear to be yet broader substrata of D_1 to D_5 subtypes that are conveniently accommodated within the original D_1/D_2 scheme as families of 'D_1-like' (D_{1A}, D_{1B}/D_5) and 'D_2-like' ($D_{2L/S}$, D_3, D_4) receptors.

The purpose of the present volume is to present up-to-date, comprehensive reviews, by appropriate authorities, of neuroscience research and theory on the fundamental interactions between those two families of dopamine receptor subtypes, at numerous levels of investigation: from molecular biology and neuroanatomy, through electrophysiology, to the psychopharmacology of multiple forms of behaviour, putative clinical significance and therapeutic potential. It is now clear that any individual dopamine receptor subtype can no longer be assumed to function in a manner independent of its counterpart subtypes; this volume of *Neuroscience Perspectives* seeks to stand as a reference source on the evolution of the concept of $D_1 : D_2$ interactions, and on their substrates and psychopharmacological roles and, in such a continually evolving field, to look to the future.

John L. Waddington

—————————— CHAPTER 1 ——————————

MOLECULAR NEUROBIOLOGY OF D$_1$ AND D$_2$ DOPAMINE RECEPTORS

David R. Sibley, Frederick J. Monsma Jr and Yong Shen

Experimental Therapeutics Branch, National Institute of Neurological Disorders and Stroke, National Institutes of Health, Building 10, Room 5C-108, 9000 Rockville Pike, Bethesda, Maryland, USA

Table of Contents

1.1 Introduction

Dopamine receptors belong to a large superfamily of neurotransmitter and hormone receptors which are coupled to their specific effector functions via guanine nucleotide regulatory (G) proteins. Historically, dopamine receptors have been divided into two major subtypes referred to as D$_1$ and D$_2$. D$_1$ receptors activate the enzyme adenylyl cyclase and increase intracellular levels of cAMP, whereas D$_2$ receptors exert an inhibitory influence on this enzyme (Andersen *et al.*, 1990). D$_2$ receptors may also be linked to additional second messenger systems including activation of K$^+$ channels and inhibition of Ca^{2+} channels and phosphatidylinositol turnover (Vallar and Meldolesi, 1989). With the advent of molecular cloning techniques, however, and their application to the dopamine

DOPAMINE RECEPTOR INTERACTIONS
ISBN 0–12–729045–1

receptor family, it has become clear that the D_1/D_2 classification scheme will need to undergo some revision. At the time of writing, five pharmacologically distinct dopamine receptors have been defined through molecular cloning methods. Two of these cloned receptors exhibit the functional and pharmacological properties expected for a classical D_1 receptor, while the other three receptors exhibit the pharmacological characteristics of a D_2 receptor. We thus have to now recognize that families of D_1 and D_2 receptors exist rather than singular receptor subtypes. In this chapter we will review the recent cloning work for the different dopamine receptor subtypes and the current state of knowledge concerning their molecular biological characteristics.

1.2 The D_1 receptor subfamily

1.2.1 The D_1/D_{1A} receptor

The D_1 receptor linked to the activation of adenylyl cyclase activity was first cloned in 1990 by four different groups working independently (Dearry et al., 1990; Monsma et al., 1990; Sunahara et al., 1990; Zhou et al., 1990). Three of the groups employed the polymerase chain reaction while one group used a probe derived from the previously cloned D_2 receptor for library screening. This approach enabled the isolation of D_1 receptor cDNAs and/or genes from either rat or human libraries. The translational start sites for the D_1 receptor clones are not entirely clear as there are two potential initiator methionines in the human sequence (Dearry et al., 1990; Sunahara et al., 1990; Zhou et al., 1990) and three in the rat (Monsma et al., 1990). Preliminary evidence from expression of the rat cDNA, however, suggests that the initial Met residue in this sequence is not used for initiation of translation (Sibley et al., unpublished observations). Assuming that translation begins at the first Met residue in the human and the second Met in the rat, then both receptors are 446 residues in length. Overall, the human and rat receptors exhibit 91% amino acid sequence identity. The D_1 receptor genes appear to lack introns, at least within the coding regions, with the human gene being localized to chromosome 5 (Sunahara et al., 1990). The subsequent cloning of another distinct D_1 receptor linked to stimulating adenylyl cyclase (see below) has now led to the designation of the initially cloned receptor as D_{1A}.

Figure 1 shows a diagram of the proposed membrane organization of the rat D_{1A} receptor. Hydropathy analysis of this protein predicts the presence of seven transmembrane domains where the N-terminus is localized to the extracellular surface and the C-terminus projects into the cytosol. This overall membrane typography has been suggested for all of the G protein-linked receptors that

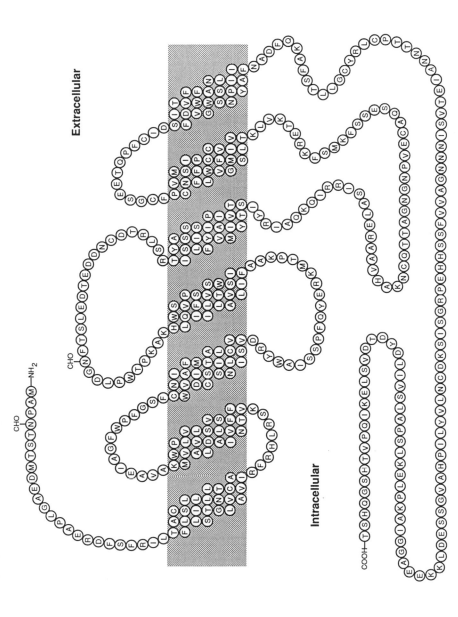

Figure 1 Proposed membrane topography of the rat D_{1A} dopamine receptor. Membrane-spanning domains are defined on the basis of hydropathy analysis. CHO: potential *N*-linked glycosylation sites.

have been cloned thus far (Strader *et al.*, 1989; Dohlman *et al.*, 1991). It should be emphasized, however, that biochemical evidence supporting this model has been generated for only two members of this family, namely rhodopsin and the β_2-adrenergic receptor (Strader *et al.*, 1989; Dohlman *et al.*, 1991). Several other structural features of the D_{1A} receptor are particularly noteworthy. First, there are two potential sites for *N*-linked glycosylation, one on the N-terminus and another on the second extracellular loop. Previous biochemical experimentation had, in fact, indicated that D_1 receptors are glycoproteins. The D_{1A} receptor also has a small third cytoplasmic loop and a long C terminus. This seems to be a characteristic of receptors which are coupled to G_s and activate adenylyl cyclase such as the β-adrenergic receptor (Strader *et al.*, 1989; Dohlman *et al.*, 1991). In addition, there is one consensus site for cAMP-dependent phosphorylation in the third cytoplasmic loop and a conserved Cys in the COOH tail, the latter of which may serve as a site for palmitoylation (Strader *et al.*, 1989; Dohlman *et al.*, 1991). The C-terminus also contains numerous Ser and Thr residues which may serve as additional sites of regulatory phosphorylation.

When expressed in various mammalian cells, the cloned rat and human D_{1A} receptors were shown to exhibit the pharmacological and functional characteristics expected for a D_1 receptor subtype. Saturable, high-affinity and pharmacologically specific binding of either $[^3H]SCH$ 23390 or $[^{125}I]SCH$ 23982, D_1-selective antagonist ligands, was demonstrated using transfected cell membranes (Dearry *et al.*, 1990; Monsma *et al.*, 1990; Sunahara *et al.*, 1990; Zhou *et al.*, 1990). The D_{1A} receptors were also shown to mediate dopaminergic stimulation of adenylyl cyclase activity with a pharmacology identical to that seen in endogenous receptor-expressing tissue systems (Dearry *et al.*, 1990; Monsma *et al.*, 1990; Sunahara *et al.*, 1990; Zhou *et al.*, 1990).

The tissue distribution of mRNA encoding the D_{1A} receptor has been determined by both Northern blot analysis and *in situ* hybridization histochemistry (Dearry *et al.*, 1990; Gerfen *et al.*, 1990; Monsma *et al.*, 1990; Sunahara *et al.*, 1990; Zhou *et al.*, 1990; Fremeau *et al.*, 1991; Le Moine *et al.*, 1991; Meador-Woodruff *et al.*, 1991; Mengod *et al.*, 1991; Weiner *et al.*, 1991). The localization of D_{1A} receptor mRNA correlates fairly well with previous information on the regional distribution of dopamine-stimulated adenylyl cyclase and/or D_1 receptor binding activities. The areas of highest expression include the caudate-putamen, nucleus accumbens and olfactory tubercle, with lower levels of mRNA being observed in the cerebral cortex, limbic system, hypothalamus and thalamus. Within the caudate-putamen, about 50% of the medium-sized neurones appear to exhibit labelling (Gerfen *et al.*, 1990; Meador-Woodruff *et al.*, 1991; Weiner *et al.*, 1991), although a small number of the large-sized neurones (presumably cholinergic interneurones) may also express low levels of D_{1A} mRNA (Le Moine *et al.*, 1991). Preliminary evidence indicates that the majority of the medium-sized neurones which express high levels of D_{1A} receptor mRNA belong to the striatonigral projection system and also express substance P (Gerfen *et al.*, 1990; Le Moine *et al.*, 1991).

1.2.2   The D_{1B}/D_5 receptor

A second member of the D_1 receptor subfamily, initially termed the 'D_5' receptor, has subsequently been isolated and cloned. Three different groups, using fragments of either the human D_{1A} dopamine or $5HT_{1A}$ serotonin receptor DNAs as probes, isolated from human genomic libraries a clone encoding a putative 477 amino acid protein exhibiting high homology to the D_{1A} receptor (Grandy et al., 1991; Sunahara et al., 1991; Weinshank et al., 1991). Hydropathy analysis suggests seven transmembrane domains in the protein with a membrane topography similar to that of the D_{1A} receptor. The level of homology is 50% between the D_{1A} and D_5 receptors, but the homology increases to about 80% within the transmembrane regions. Other similarities include consensus N-linked glycosylation sites in the N-terminus and second extracellular loops, a cAMP-dependent phosphorylation site in the third cytoplasmic loop, and a conserved Cys residue in the C-terminus. The coding region in this gene also lacks introns (Grandy et al., 1991; Sunahara et al., 1991; Weinshank et al., 1991). When expressed in mammalian cells, the D_5 receptor exhibits linkage to stimulating adenylyl cyclase activity with a D_1-like pharmacology (Grandy et al., 1991; Sunahara et al., 1991; Weinshank et al., 1991). More detailed pharmacological analysis using radioligand binding methods shows that various agonist and antagonist ligands exhibit similar affinities for the D_{1A} and D_5 receptors with the notable exception of dopamine, which is about 5–10-fold more potent at D_5 than D_{1A}. This has led to the hypothesis that the D_5 receptor may be important in maintaining dopaminergic tone and arousal.

Interestingly, two genomic sequences which apparently represent pseudogenes of the D_5 receptor have also been detected within the human genome (Grandy et al., 1991; Nguyen et al., 1991a, b; Weinshank et al., 1991). These pseudogenes, referred to as $D_{5\Psi1}$ and $D_{5\Psi2}$, are 98% homologous to each other at the nucleotide level and 95% homologous to the D_5 receptor genomic sequence (Grandy et al., 1991; Nguyen et al., 1991a, b; Weinshank et al., 1991). Relative to the D_5 sequence, both pseudogenes contain insertions and deletions resulting in in-frame stop codons, thus precluding the expression of functional receptors. Nevertheless, one of these pseudogenes ($D_{5\Psi1}$) appears to be transcriptionally active as mRNA for this gene is found in many of the regions (see below) which express D_5 receptor transcript (Nguyen et al., 1991b; Weinshank et al., 1991). Chromosomal analysis of these gene sequences has indicated that the D_5 gene is localized to chromosome 4 whereas the $D_{5\Psi1}$ and $D_{5\Psi2}$ pseudogenes are found on chromosomes 1 and 2 (Grandy et al., 1991; Nguyen et al., 1991a). It appears that the emergence of the D_5 pseudogenes is a recent event in mammalian evolution as the pseudogenes are not found in the African green monkey but at least one of them is present in the gorilla (Nguyen et al., 1991b). Interestingly, these findings represent the first demonstration of pseudogene sequences within the superfamily of G protein-coupled receptors.

The distribution of the D_5 receptor mRNA in the brain has been preliminarily

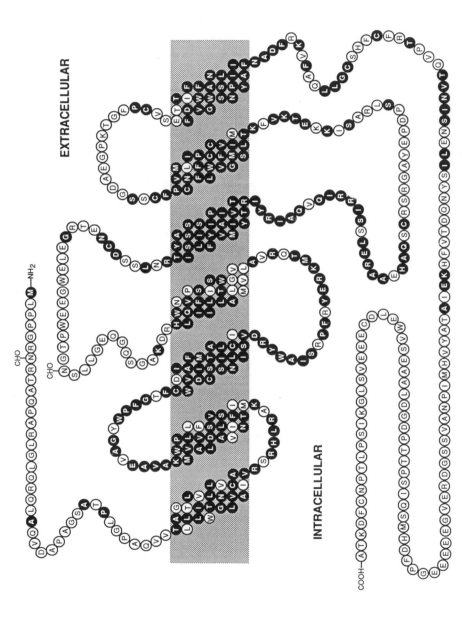

Figure 2 Proposed membrane topography of the rat D_{1B} dopamine receptor. Solid circles indicate amino acids which are identical in both the D_{1A} and D_{1B} receptors. CHO: potential N-linked glycosylation sites.

characterized by Northern blot analysis (Sunahara *et al.*, 1991; Weinshank *et al.*, 1991). The areas of highest expression are in the limbic system and include the hippocampus and hypothalamus, with lower amounts being found in the frontal and temporal cortices. Very low levels of D_5 transcript were observed in the striatum. In general, the D_5 receptor is expressed at lower levels and with a more restricted distribution in comparison to the D_{1A} receptor. This analysis is complicated somewhat by the fact that one of the D_5 pseudogenes is transcriptionally active (see above) and most probes for the D_5 receptor will recognize the pseudogene mRNA as well.

Two groups have recently cloned the rat homologue of the human D_5 receptor which they have termed D_{1B} (Monsma *et al.*, 1991; Tiberi *et al.*, 1991). Both groups used the polymerase chain reaction approach, using either genomic DNA (Tiberi *et al.*, 1991) or kidney mRNA (Monsma *et al.*, 1991) for initial amplification. The rat receptor is 475 amino acids in length and is 83% identical overall but 95% identical in the transmembrane regions in comparison with the human D_5 receptor (Figure 2). Expression of the rat D_{1B} receptor exhibits a similar pharmacology to the D_5 receptor, including a relatively high affinity for dopamine and linkage to stimulating adenylyl cyclase (Monsma *et al.*, 1991; Tiberi *et al.*, 1991). The regional distribution of the D_{1B} receptor mRNA also agrees well with that for the D_5, with the areas of highest expression seen in the hippocampus and hypothalamus and with little to no mRNA found in the striatum (Monsma *et al.*, 1991; Tiberi *et al.*, 1991). In addition, using *in situ* hybridization histochemistry, the D_{1B} receptor was demonstrated to be expressed in high levels in the mammillary and pretectal nuclei (Tiberi *et al.*, 1991).

Because of the extremely high structural, pharmacological and functional similarities between the D_1 and D_5 receptors, it is suggested that the D_{1A}/D_{1B} nomenclature developed for the rat receptor clones be extended to the corresponding receptors in humans as well as other species. The D_{1A} and D_{1B} receptors thus currently constitute the D_1 subfamily of dopamine receptors.

1.3 The D_2 receptor subfamily

1.3.1 The D_2 receptor

The first member of the dopamine receptor family to be cloned was actually the D_2 receptor. Using a probe derived from the β-adrenergic receptor gene, Bunzow *et al.* (1988) isolated clones encoding putatively novel receptors from a rat genomic library. One of these genomic clones was subsequently used to isolate a corresponding full-length cDNA from a rat brain library. The cDNA encoded a protein of 415 amino acids which, when expressed in mouse fibroblast cells, exhibited appropriate radioligand binding activity with the pharmacological characteristics expected for a D_2 receptor. Figure 3 shows a schematic diagram

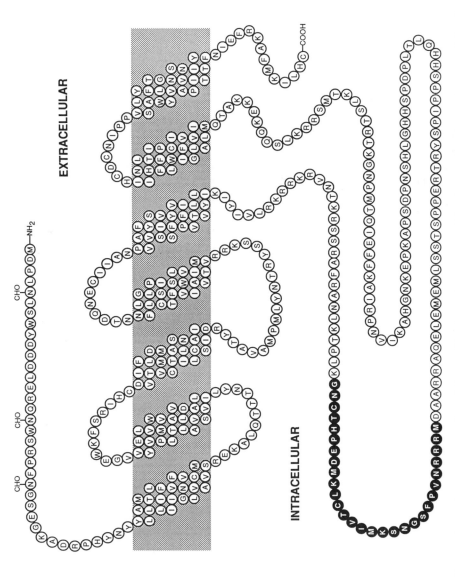

Figure 3 Proposed membrane topography of the rat D_2 dopamine receptor. Membrane-spanning regions are defined on the basis of hydropathy analysis. The filled circles indicate the alternatively spliced exon of the D_2 receptor. CHO: potential N-linked glycosylation sites.

of the D_2 receptor as it is believed to be organized in the plasma membrane. Notably, the N-terminus lacks an apparent signal sequence and contains consensus sequences for three potential N-linked glycosylation sites in keeping with previous data suggesting that the D_2 receptor is a glycoprotein. In contrast to the structures of the D_{1A} and D_{1B} receptors, the predicted size of the C-terminus of the D_2 receptor is rather small while the third cytoplasmic loop between transmembrane regions 5 and 6 is quite large. This feature of having a large third cytoplasmic loop and short C-terminus is a characteristic of many receptors which inhibit adenylyl cyclase activity. The human homologue of the rat D_2 receptor has been subsequently cloned and shown to be 96% identical to the rat receptor with one amino acid deletion (Dal Toso et al., 1989; Grandy et al., 1989b; Selbie et al., 1989; Stormann et al., 1990). Chromosomal analysis has indicated that the D_2 receptor gene is found on human chromosome 11 (Grandy et al., 1989a).

When expressed in stably transfected LtK$^-$ fibroblasts the D_2 receptor was shown to exhibit guanine nucleotide-sensitive agonist binding as well as pharmacologically specific inhibition of adenylyl cyclase activity (Neve et al., 1989). Interestingly, the D_2 receptor in these cells has also been reported to stimulate phosphoinositide hydrolysis and Ca^{2+} mobilization (Vallar et al., 1990), although these events have not previously been seen in tissues which endogenously express this receptor (Vallar and Meldolesi, 1989). When expressed in the GH_4C_1 pituitary cell line, the D_2 receptor was shown to inhibit adenylyl cyclase activity and prolactin release in addition to reducing Ca^{2+} levels and hyperpolarizing the cells (Albert et al., 1990). All of these events are known to occur in response to D_2 receptor stimulation in normal lactotroph cells (Vallar and Meldolesi, 1989). Interestingly, when expressed in Chinese hamster ovary (CHO) cells, the D_2 receptor also appears to potentiate ATP-mediated arachidonic acid release (Kanterman et al., 1991), a property now known for several receptors which are linked to their effector systems through G_i proteins (Felder et al., 1991). In these initial studies, the potentiation of arachidonic acid release by the D_2 and other receptors was shown to occur independently from changes in intracellular cAMP (Felder et al., 1991; Kanterman et al., 1991). A recent report has demonstrated a similar observation for the D_2 receptor; however, in this study, elevation of cAMP (either artificially or by D_{1A} receptor stimulation) was shown to augment the D_2 response (Piomelli et al., 1991). The D_{1A}-mediated augmentation of the D_2 response was hypothesized as a possible mechanism for $D_1:D_2$ receptor synergism (Piomelli et al., 1991). At present, it is not clear what is responsible for these discrepant findings.

The regional distribution of mRNA for the D_2 receptor has been determined by both Northern blot analysis and in situ hybridization histochemistry (Bunzow et al., 1988; Dal Toso et al., 1989; Meador-Woodruff et al., 1989, 1991; Mengod et al., 1989; Najlerahim et al., 1989; Weiner and Brann, 1989; Mansour et al., 1990; Stormann et al., 1990; Weiner et al., 1990). The D_2 receptor mRNA distribution correlates well with previous information on D_2 receptor distribution generated using receptor binding and autoradiography methods. The areas of highest expression in the brain include the caudate-putamen, nucleus accumbens and olfactory tubercle. Receptor mRNA is also found in dopaminergic cell bodies within the substantia nigra pars compacta and ventral tegmental areas, suggesting an additional presynaptic role for the D_2 receptor. Cellular localization of the D_2 receptor mRNA has also been investigated in the striatum, where about 50–75% of the medium-sized cells appear to express receptor mRNA (Gerfen et al., 1990; Weiner et al., 1990; Meador-Woodruff et al., 1991). Investigations using antibodies directed against the D_2 receptor protein have also indicated that about 50% of the medium-sized cells express the D_2 receptor protein (McVittie et al., 1991). Recent evidence indicates that most of the cells which express the D_2 receptor mRNA in high abundance are enkephalinergic neurones (Gerfen et al., 1990; Le Moine et al., 1990a). D_2 receptor mRNA has also been observed in large-diameter cells in the striatum, the majority of which appear to be cholinergic interneurones (Le Moine et al., 1990b).

Since there is a wealth of behavioural, physiological and biochemical evidence for 'D_1' and 'D_2' receptor interactions including both opposition and synergism (see other chapters in this volume), it will obviously be important to determine how many and which neurones may co-express the various members of the D_1 and D_2 receptor subfamilies. Preliminary experiments in this regard have thus far yielded conflicting results. Using in situ hybridization histochemistry techniques, Gerfen et al. (1990) have suggested that there are few, if any, cells in the striatum which co-express the D_{1A} and D_2 receptors, whereas Meador-Woodruff et al. (1991) have estimated that at least a third of all striatal cells contain mRNA for both of these receptor subtypes. Obviously, additional experiments using a variety of approaches, including direct cellular localization of the receptor proteins, will be necessary to resolve this controversy.

1.3.2 D_2 receptor isoforms

Shortly after the initial cloning of the D_2 receptor, it was determined that this receptor exists in two protein isoforms that differ in length by 29 amino acids and are derived from the same gene by alternative RNA splicing (Dal Toso et al., 1989; Eidne et al., 1989; Giros et al., 1989; Grandy et al., 1989b; Monsma et al., 1989; Selbie et al., 1989; Chio et al., 1990; Miller et al., 1990; O'Dowd et al., 1990; O'Malley et al., 1990; Rao et al., 1990; Gandelman et al., 1991; Mack et al., 1991; Montmayeur et al., 1991). The location of this splice variation occurs within the third cytoplasmic loop of the receptor protein, approximately 30 residues from the fifth transmembrane domain (Figure 3). Detailed investigation of the D_2 receptor gene has revealed the presence of at least eight exons, one of which codes for the 29 amino acid insert sequence (Dal Toso et al., 1989; Grandy et al., 1989b; O'Malley et al., 1990; Gandelman et al., 1991; Mack et al., 1991). Both D_2 receptor isoforms have been shown to be generated in human, rat, bovine and mouse tissues and both appear to be present in all tissues and regions where D_2 receptors are expressed. These two isoforms have been designated as D_{2S} (for short) and D_{2L} (for long).

Interestingly, the D_{2L} isoform appears to be expressed predominantly in all brain regions and tissues examined, although the exact ratio of these two isoforms can vary significantly (Dal Toso et al., 1989; Giros et al., 1989; Grandy et al., 1989b; Monsma et al., 1989; MacLennan et al., 1990; O'Malley et al., 1990; Gandelman et al., 1991; Le Moine and Bloch, 1991; Mack et al., 1991; Montmayeur et al., 1991; Neve et al., 1991; Snyder et al., 1991a). This latter observation might suggest some physiological relevance for the existence of two different receptor isoforms. It should be noted, however, that no pharmacological differences have been observed between these two isoforms (Dal Toso et al., 1989; Giros et al., 1989; Grandy et al., 1989b; Monsma et al., 1989). This is, perhaps, not that surprising as the location of the splice variation is in the third cytoplasmic loop whereas it is the transmembrane regions which are believed to constitute the ligand-binding domains in the G protein-coupled receptor (Strader et al., 1989; Dohlman et al., 1991). In contrast, mutagenesis studies with other catecholamine receptors have suggested that the third cytoplasmic loop is important for G protein coupling and effector regulation (Strader et al., 1989; Dohlman et al., 1991). Thus far, however, both of the D_2 receptor isoforms have been shown to inhibit adenylyl cyclase (Dal Toso et al., 1989; Rinaudo et al., 1990), active K^+ channels (Einhorn et al., 1990), potentiate arachidonic acid release (Kanterman et al., 1991) and undergo agonist-induced desensitization (Rinaudo et al., 1990) with approximately equal efficacy. Both isoforms have also been shown to mediate dopaminergic repression of the promotor of the rat prolactin gene (McChesney et al., 1991). In contrast, a recent report has claimed that the D_{2S} receptor isoform is more efficiently coupled to adenylyl cyclase inhibition in cells which were co-transfected with a reporter plasmid containing a cAMP-responsive element (Montmayeur and Borrelli, 1991). It should be pointed out, however, that cAMP levels were not actually measured in these experiments (Montmayeur and Borrelli, 1991). Additional experimentation will thus be required to determine what functional differences, if any, exist between the D_2 receptor isoforms.

1.3.3   The D_3 receptor

The second receptor within the D_2 subfamily to be cloned and characterized using molecular biological techniques has been the 'D_3' dopamine receptor (Sokoloff et al., 1990). The amino acid sequence, as well as the proposed membrane topography, of the D_3 receptor is very similar to that of the D_2 receptor (Figure 4). Both receptors exhibit relatively large third cytoplasmic loops and short C-termini. Overall, the D_3 receptor is 52% homologous with the D_2 receptor, however, this homology increases to about 75% within the transmembrane regions. As with the D_2 receptor, the D_3 receptor contains consensus sequences for N-linked glycosylation, two of which are in the

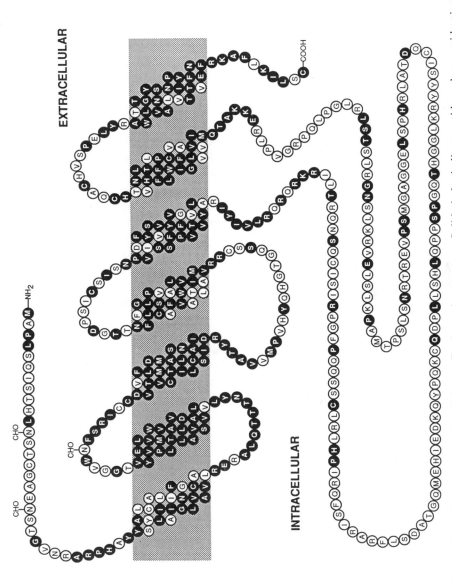

Figure 4 Proposed membrane topography of the rat D₃ dopamine receptor. Solid circles indicate residues that are identical in both the D₂ and D₃ receptors. CHO: potential *N*-linked glycosylation sites.

12

N-terminus and one in the first extracellular loop. Other similarities include a cAMP-dependent phos phorylation site in the third cytoplasmic loop and a conserved Cys residue at the C-terminus. The human gene and cDNAs for the D_3 receptor have also recently been characterized (Giros *et al.*, 1990). Surprisingly, the human receptor has 46 fewer amino acids in the third cytoplasmic loop, resulting in a protein of 400 residues in length. Excluding this deletion, the human receptor is 88% homologous overall and 97% homologous in the transmembrane domains when compared with the rat receptor. Chromosomal analysis of the human gene has assigned its location to chromosome 3.

Expression of the D_3 receptor in CHO cells indicates that its pharmacology is similar to that of the D_2 receptor (Sokoloff *et al.*, 1990). The only antagonists found to be selective for the D_3 receptor (but only by about four-fold), relative to the D_2 receptor, were the putative autoreceptor-selective agents AJ76 and UH232. Other antagonists examined were between 2- and 30-fold D_2 selective. Conversely, agonist ligands demonstrated either equal or greater affinity for the D_3 receptor. Given this information, it is interesting to note that a proposed characteristic of dopamine autoreceptors is a higher affinity for agonists compared to postsynaptic D_2 receptors. Curiously, agonist binding to the D_3 receptor expressed in the CHO cells was found to be guanine nucleotide insensitive (Sokoloff *et al.*, 1990). In addition, D_3 receptor activation was reported to have no effect on adenylyl cyclase activity. These observations would suggest the absence of appropriate G protein coupling in the CHO cells. Additional experimentation will thus be necessary to define the signal transduction pathway(s) associated with the D_3 receptor although, given its structural similarity to the D_2 receptor, inhibition of adenylyl cyclase activity is a distinct possibility.

Characterization of the gene for the D_3 receptor has indicated that, as in the D_2 receptor gene, the coding region is interrupted by multiple introns, four of which are in identical or similar locations in the two genes. Interestingly, the existence of two apparently non-functional RNA splice variants of the rat D_3 receptor gene has recently been described (Giros *et al.*, 1991; Snyder *et al.*, 1991b). One of these alternative transcripts is completely lacking exon 2, which encodes the first extracellular loop and the third transmembrane domain. This results in a shift of the open reading frame, introducing a downstream stop codon. The resulting putative protein would be truncated and possess only the first two transmembrane regions. The second RNA splice variant arises through the use of an alternative internal acceptor site within the fourth exon. This results in a deletion of most of the second extracellular loop and about a third of the fifth membrane-spanning domain, giving rise to a 428-residue protein. These two splice variants appear to comprise about 40% and 10%, respectively, of the total D_3 receptor mRNA in brain. Neither of these alternative transcripts appears to result in the expression of functional receptor (Giros *et al.*, 1991), presumably due to the lack of appropriate protein folding and/or insertion into the plasma membrane.

Regional analysis of D_3 receptor mRNA in the brain has indicated that it is much less abundant and more narrowly distributed than that for the D_2 receptor. In general, the D_3 receptor is expressed predominantly in telencephalic areas receiving dopaminergic inputs from the A10 cell group, including the nucleus accumbens, islands of Calleja, bed nucleus of the stria terminalis, and other limbic brain areas, including the olfactory tubercle, hippocampus, mammary nuclei as well as the hypothalamus (Sokoloff et al., 1990; Bouthenet et al., 1991). Some expression of mRNA is also observed in the caudate-putamen and certain cerebral cortical regions. This overall pattern of localization has suggested that the D_3 receptor may mediate dopaminergic control of cognitive and emotional functions and consequently may be relevant to antipsychotic therapy using dopaminergic antagonists. Importantly, the D_3 receptor also appears to be expressed in dopaminergic neurones within the substantia nigra, indicating that it may function presynaptically as an autoreceptor (Sokoloff et al., 1990). This observation would certainly be consistent with the preliminary pharmacological profile of the D_3 receptor (see above).

1.3.4 The D_4 receptor

The most recent receptor in the D_2 subfamily to be identified and cloned is the 'D_4' receptor. Van Tol et al. (1991) used the rat D_2 receptor cDNA as a probe to perform low-stringency screening of a human neuroblastoma cell cDNA library. One of the clones isolated contained a partial-length cDNA with an open reading frame consisting of protein sequences highly homologous to transmembrane regions 5, 6 and 7 of the D_2 receptor. This partial-length cDNA was subsequently used to isolate its corresponding gene from a human genomic library. The genomic clone isolated contained the cloned cDNA sequence which was preceded by DNA sequences encoding the putative N-terminus through the fourth transmembrane domain of the receptor. The putative coding region of this gene is interrupted by four introns in transmembrane regions, 1, 3 and 6, as well as the third cytoplasmic loop, all of which are in equivalent positions to intron sequences found in the D_2 and D_3 receptor genes. Chromosomal analysis has indicated that the gene encoding the D_4 receptor is located on human chromosome 11, as is the gene for the D_2 receptor.

Based on the genomic and cDNA sequences, the D_4 receptor would consist of a protein of 387 residues in length with seven putative membrane-spanning domains (Figure 5). The proposed membrane topography is similar to that for the D_2 and D_3 receptors, including the existence of a putative large third cytoplasmic loop and short C-terminus. The homology of the D_4 receptor to the D_2 and D_3 receptors is 41% and 39% overall, respectively, and about 56% for both D_2 and D_3 receptors within the membrane-spanning domains. There is one potential site for N-linked glycosylation in the N-terminus and one consensus cAMP-dependent phosphorylation site in the third cytoplasmic loop of the D_4

receptor. The C-terminal amino acid is a conserved Cys residue as with the D_2 and D_3 receptors (Figure 5).

Since a full-length D_4 receptor cDNA was unobtainable either from additional library screening or through the polymerase chain reaction, a hybrid gene–cDNA was constructed for expression in mammalian cells (Van Tol *et al.*, 1991). When transiently transfected into COS-7 cells, this construct imparted saturable and specific [³H]spiperone binding to the cell membranes with an affinity similar to that seen for D_2 and D_3 receptors. Characterization of the binding activity revealed a pharmacological profile which was also similar to those of the D_2 and D_3 receptors. The D_4 receptor displayed similar or lower affinities for both dopaminergic antagonists and agonists compared to the D_2 receptor. Importantly, however, the atypical antipsychotic clozapine, and its congener octoclothepin, exhibited about 10-fold higher affinity for the D_4 receptor. The affinity constant of clozapine, in fact, is close to the concentration of clozapine measured in blood when administered for antipsychotic therapy. This has led to the suggestion that clozapine might exert its antipsychotic activity primarily through blocking the D_4 receptor.

Using radioligand binding assays, the interaction of dopamine with the D_4 receptor was found to be sensitive to guanine nucleotides, suggesting effective receptor coupling to endogenous G proteins in the COS-7 cell membranes (Van Tol *et al.*, 1991). Unfortunately, however, functional activity of the D_4 receptor, such as regulation of adenylyl cyclase activity, was not examined in this study. The signal transduction mechanism of the D_4 receptor thus remains to be characterized, although, given its structural similarity to the D_2 receptor, it would not be suprising if inhibition of adenylyl cyclase activity is eventually observed.

Very recently, what appears to be the rat homologue of the D_4 receptor has been cloned (O'Malley *et al.*, 1991). The rat receptor is 385 amino acids in length and is 73% homologous overall with the human D_4 receptor, although this homology increases within the putative transmembrane domains. Preliminary pharmacological analysis suggests that the rat receptor also exhibits high affinity for clozapine.

The distribution of mRNA encoding the D_4 receptor in the brain was initially investigated by Northern blot analysis using either the partial-length human cDNA or a fragment of the human gene which contains the fifth exon as a probe (Van Tol *et al.*, 1991). As with the D_3 receptor, the D_4 receptor appears to be expressed at a lower level than the D_2 receptor. The areas of highest D_4 mRNA expression included the frontal cortex, midbrain, amygdala and medulla, with lower levels observed in the striatum and olfactory tubercle. This distribution profile in the central nervous system may partly explain the lack of extrapyramidal side-effects observed with clozapine treatment. Northern blot analysis using the rat D_1 receptor sequences as probes has confirmed the human data demonstrating that the frontal cortex, olfactory bulb and hypothalamus contain the highest levels of mRNA in the rat brain (O'Malley *et al.*, 1991).

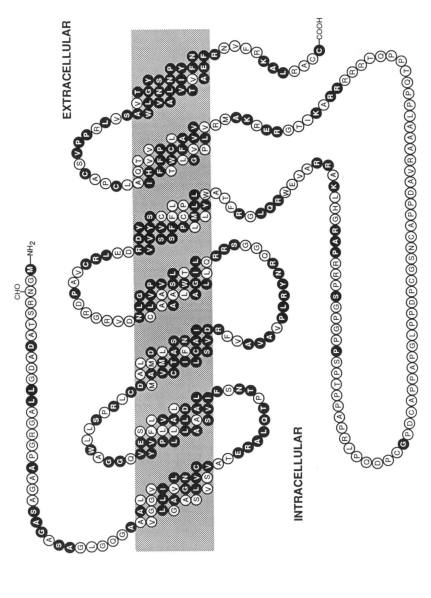

Figure 5 Proposed membrane topography of the human D₄ dopamine receptor. Solid circles indicate residues that are identical in both the D₂ and D₄ receptors. CHO: potential *N*-linked glycosylation site.

Surprisingly, a survey of peripheral tissues indicated that the rat heart contains a very high level of D_4 mRNA which is at least an order of magnitude greater than that seen in any brain region (O'Malley et al., 1991). Although the function of the D_4 receptor in the cardiovascular system remains to be determined, there have been reports of D_2-like agonists promoting bradycardia, hypotension and vasodilation.

1.4 Conclusions

Table 1 summarizes the properties of all of the dopamine receptors that have been cloned to date. Thus far, five different genes encoding pharmacologically distinct receptors have been identified and isolated. Two of these, the D_{1A} and D_{1B} (or D_1 and D_5), comprise the D_1 subfamily based on their structural, pharmacological and functional similarities. Similarly, the D_2, D_3 and D_4 receptors represent a D_2 subfamily whose members are also structurally and pharmacologically (and perhaps functionally) similar. In fact, given these considerations, it has been suggested that the D_2, D_3 and D_4 receptors be termed the D_{2A}, D_{2B} and D_{2C} receptors, respectively, in recognition of their D_2-like properties.

Given the unexpected heterogeneity of the dopaminergic receptor system, it is logical to ask if there are still other dopamine receptor subtypes remaining to be identified. This seems probable as the characteristics of the cloned subtypes do not match all of the properties of some dopamine receptors which have been previously investigated. For instance, there is extensive evidence that 'D_1-like' dopamine receptors exist which are linked to the activation of phospholipase C, phosphatidylinositol turnover and Ca^{2+} mobilization. Dopamine, as well as several 'D_1-selective' agonists, has been shown to stimulate phophatidylinositol turnover in both brain slices and kidney membranes (Felder et al., 1989; Undie and Friedman, 1990; Vyas et al., 1991) and injection of striatal mRNA into Xenopus oocytes leads to dopamine-stimulated phosphatidylinositol turnover and Ca^{2+} mobilization (Mahan et al., 1990). These dopamine receptors might be analogous to the α_1-adrenergic receptors which stimulate phospholipase C activity and might define a third distinct subfamily of dopamine receptors.

There is also evidence for additional members of the D_2 subfamily of receptors. Using gene transfer methods, a receptor with D_2-like pharmacology has been identified and expressed but not yet sequenced (Todd et al., 1989). Also, a D_2-related receptor has recently been characterized in kidney inner medulla membranes (Huo et al., 1991). It thus appears that we may only be in the middle of dopamine receptor cloning efforts, with perhaps a double of subtypes yet to come.

Table 1 Properties of dopamine receptor subtypes.

	D_{1A}	D_{1B}	D_{2S}/D_{2L}	D_3	D_4
Amino acids					
Human	446	477	414/443	400	387
Rat	446	475	415/444	446	385
Introns in gene	No	No	Yes	Yes	Yes
Human chromosome	5	4	11	3	11
Effector pathways	↑cAMP	↑cAMP	↓cAMP ↑K^+ channel ↓Ca^{2+} channel	↓cAMP? ?	↓cAMP? ?
mRNA distribution	Caudate-putamen Nucleus accumbens	Hippocampus Hypothalamus	Caudate-putamen Nucleus accumbens	Olfactory tubercle Hypothalamus	Frontal cortex Heart
Selective agonists	SK & F 38393 Fenoldopam	SK & F 38393 Fenoldopam	N-0437 Bromocriptine	Quinpirole	?
Selective antagonists	SCH 23390 SK & F 83566	SCH 23390 SK & F 83566	Spiperone Domperidone (−)Sulpiride	Spiperone (+)AJ76 (+)UH232	Spiperone Clozapine

References

Albert, P.R., Neve, K.A., Bunzow, J.R. & Civelli, O. (1990) *J. Biol. Chem.* **265**, 2098–2104.
Andersen, P.H., Gingrich, J.A., Bates, M.D., Dearry, A., Falardeau, P., Senogles, S.E. & Caron, M.G. (1990) *Trends Pharmacol. Sci.* **11**, 231–236.
Bouthenet, M.L., Souil, E., Martres, M.P., Sokoloff, P., Giros, B. & Schwartz, J.C. (1991) *Brain Res.* **564**, 203–219.
Bunzow, J.R., Van Tol, H.H.M., Grandy, D.K., Albert, P., Salon, J., Christie, M., Machida, C.A., Neve, K.A. & Civelli, O. (1988) *Nature* **336**, 783–787.
Chio, C.L., Hess, G.F., Graham, R.S. & Huff, R.M. (1990) *Nature* **343**, 266–269.
Dal Toso, R., Sommer, B., Ewert, M., Herb, A., Pritchett, D.B., Bach, A., Shivers, B.D. & Seeburg, P.H. (1989) *EMBO J.* **8**, 4025–4034.
Dearry, A., Gingrich, J.A., Falardeau, P., Fremeau, R.T. Jr, Bates, M.D. & Caron, M.G. (1990) *Nature* **347**, 72–76.
Dohlman, H.G., Thorner, J., Caron, M.G. & Lefkowitz, R.J. (1991) *Annu. Rev. Biochem.* **60**, 653–688.
Eidne, K.A., Taylor, P.L., Zabavnik, J., Saunders, P.T.K. & Inglis, J.D. (1989) *Nature* **342**, 865.
Einhorn, L.C., Falardeau, P., Caron, M.G. & Oxford, G.S. (1990) *Soc. Neurosci. Abstr.* **16**, 382.
Felder, R.A., Felder, C.C., Eisner, G.M. & Jose, P.A. (1989) *Am. J. Physiol.* **275**, F315–F327.
Felder, C.C., Williams, H.L. & Axelrod, J. (1991) *Proc. Natl Acad. Sci. USA* **88**, 6477–6480.
Fremeau, R.T., Duncan, G.E., Fornaretto, M.G., Dearry, A.E., Gingrich, J.A., Breese, G.R. & Caron, M.G. (1991) *Proc. Natl. Acad. Sci. USA* **88**, 3772–3776.
Gandelman, K.-Y., Harmon, S., Todd, R.D. & O'Malley, K.L. (1991) *J. Neurochem.* **56**, 1024–1029.
Gerfen, C.R., Engber, T.M., Susel, Z., Chase, T.N., Mahan, L.C., Monsma, F.J. Jr & Sibley, D.R. (1990) *Science* **250**, 1429–1432.
Giros, B., Sokoloff, P., Martres, M.P., Riou, J.F., Emorine, L.J. & Schwartz, J.C. (1989) *Nature* **342**, 923–926.
Giros, B., Martres, M.-P., Sokoloff, P. & Schwartz, J.-C. (1990) *C. R. Acad. Sci. Paris* **311**, 501–508.
Giros, B., Martres, M.-P., Pilon, C., Sokoloff, P. & Schwartz, J.-C. (1991) *Biochem. Biophys. Res. Commun.* **176**, 1584–1592.
Grandy, D.K., Litt, M., Allen, L., Bunzoe, J.R., Marchionni, M., Makan, H., Reed, L., Magenis, R.E. & Civelli, O. (1989a) *Am. J. Hum. Genet.* **45**, 778–785.
Grandy, D.K., Marchionni, M.A., Makan, H., Stofko, R.E., Alfano, M., Frothingham, L., Fischer, J.B., Burke-Howie, K.J., Bunzow, J.R., Server, A.C. & Civelli, O. (1989b) *Proc. Natl Acad. Sci. USA* **86**, 9762–9766.
Grandy, D.K., Zhang, Y., Bouvier, C., Zhou, Q.Y., Johnson, R.A., Allen, L., Buck, K., Bunzow, J.R., Salen, J. & Civelli, O. (1991) *Proc. Natl Acad. Sci. USA* **88**, 9175–9179.
Huo, T., Ye, M.Q. & Healy, D.P. (1991) *Proc. Natl Acad. Sci. USA* **88**, 3170–3174.
Kanterman, R.Y., Mahan, L.C., Briley, E.M., Monsma, F.J. Jr, Sibley, D.R., Axelrod, J. & Felder, C.C. (1991) *Mol. Pharmacol.* **39**, 364–369.
Le Moine, C. & Bloch, B. (1991) *Mol. Brain Res.* **10**, 283–289.
Le Moine, C., Normand, E., Guitteny, A.F., Fouque, B., Teoule, R. & Bloch, B. (1990a) *Proc. Natl. Acad. Sci. USA* **87**, 230–234.
Le Moine, C., Tison, F. & Bloch, B. (1990b) *Neurosci. Lett.* **117**, 248–252.
Le Moine, C., Normand, E. & Bloch, B. (1991) *Proc. Natl Acad. Sci. USA* **88**, 4205–4209.
Mack, K.J., Todd, R.D. & O'Malley, K.L. (1991) *J. Neurochem.* **57**, 795–801.

MacLennan, A.J., Frantz, G.D., Weatherwax, R.C., Tillakaratne, N.J.K. & Tobin, A.J. (1990) *Mol. Cell. Neurosci.* **1**, 151–160.
Mahan, L.C., Burch, R.M., Monsma, F.J. Jr & Sibley, D.R. (1990) *Proc. Natl Acad. Sci. USA* **87**, 2196–2200.
Mansour, A., Meador-Woodruff, J.H., Bunzow, J.R., Civelli, O., Akil, H. & Watson, S.J. (1990) *J. Neurosci.* **10**, 2587–2600.
McChesney, R., Sealfon, S.C., Tsutsumi, M., Dong, K., Roberts, J.L. & Bancroft, C. (1991) *Mol. Cell. Endocrinol.* **79**, R1–R7.
McVittie, L.D., Ariano, M.A. & Sibley, D.R. (1991) *Proc. Natl Acad. Sci. USA* **88**, 1441–1445.
Meador-Woodruff, J.H., Mansour, A., Bunzow, J.R., Van Tol, H.H.M., Watson, S.J. Jr & Civelli, O. (1989) *Proc. Natl Acad. Sci. USA* **86**, 7625–7628.
Meador-Woodruff, J.H., Mansour, A., Bunzow, J.R., Van Tol, H.H.M., Watson, S.J. Jr & Civelli, O. (1989) *Proc. Natl Acad. Sci. USA* **86**, 7625–7628.
Meador-Woodruff, J.H., Mansour, A., Healy, D.J., Kuehn, R., Zhou, Q.Y., Bunzow, J.R., Akil, H., Civelli, O. & Watson, S.J. Jr (1991) *Neuropsychopharmacol.* **5**, 231–242.
Mengod, G., Martinez-Mir, M.I., Vilaró, M.T. & Palacios, J.M. (1989) *Proc. Natl Acad. Sci. USA* **86**, 8560–8564.
Mengod, G., Vilaro, M.T., Niznik, H.B., Sunahara, R.K., Seeman, P., O'Dowd, B.F. & Palacios, J.M. (1991) *Mol. Brain Res.* **10**, 185–191.
Miller, J.C., Wang, Y., & Filer, D. (1990) *Biochem. Biophys. Res. Commun.* **166**, 109–112.
Monsma, F.J. Jr, McVittie, L.D., Gerfen, C.R., Mahan, L.C. & Sibley, D.R. (1989) *Nature* **342**, 926–929.
Monsma, F.J. Jr, Mahan, L.C., McVittie, L.D., Gerfen C.R. & Sibley, D.R. (1990) *Proc. Natl Acad. Sci. USA* **87**, 6723–6727.
Monsma, F.J. Jr, Shen, Y., Gerfen, C.R., Mahan, L.C., Jose, P.A., Mouradian, M.M. & Sibley, D.R. (1991) *Soc. Neurosci. Abstr.* **17**, 85.
Montmayeur, J.-P. & Borrelli, E. (1991) *Proc. Natl Acad. Sci. USA* **88**, 3135–3139.
Montmayeur, J.-P., Bausero, P., Amlaiky, N., Maroteaux, L., Hen, R. & Borrelli, E. (1991) *FEBS Lett.* **278**, 239–243.
Najlerahim, A., Barton, A.J.L., Harrison, P.J., Heffernan, J. & Pearson, R.C.A. (1989) *FEBS Lett.* **255**, 335–339.
Neve, K.A., Henningsen, R.A., Bunzow, J.R. & Civelli, O. (1989) *Mol. Pharmacol.* **36**, 446–451.
Neve, K.A., Neve, R.L., Fidel, S., Janowsky, A. & Higgins, G.A. (1991) *Proc. Natl Acad. Sci. USA* **88**, 2802–2806.
Nguyen, T., Bard, J., Jin, H., Taruscio, D., Ward, D.C., Kennedy, J.L., Weinshank, R., Seeman, P. & O'Dowd, B.F. (1991a) *Gene* **109**, 211–218.
Nguyen, T., Sunahara, R., Marchese, A., Van Tol, H.H.M., Seeman, P. & O'Dowd, B.F. (1991b) *Biochem. Biophys. Res. Commun.* **181**, 16–21.
O'Dowd, B.F., Nguyen, T., Tirpak, A., Jarvie, K.R., Israel, Y., Seeman, P. & Niznik, H.B. (1990) *FEBS Lett.* **262**, 8–12.
O'Malley, K.L., Mack, K.J., Gandelman, K.Y. & Todd, R.D. (1990) *Biochemistry* **29**, 1367–1371.
O'Malley, K.L., Harmon, S., Tang, L., Hans, S. & Todd, R.D. (1991) *Soc. Neurosci. Abstr.* **17**, 598.
Piomelli, D., Pilon, C., Giros, B., Sokoloff, P., Martres, M.P. & Schwartz, J.C. (1991) *Nature* **353**, 164–167.
Rao, D.D., McKelvy, J., Kebabian, J. & MacKenzie, R.G. (1990) *FEBS Lett.* **263**, 18–22.
Rinaudo, M.S., Monsma, F.J. Jr, Black, L.E., Mahan, L.C. & Sibley, D.R. (1990) *Soc. Neurosci. Abstr.* **16**, 209.
Selbie, L.A., Hayes, G. & Shine, J. (1989) *DNA* **8**, 683–689.
Snyder, L.A., Roberts, J.L. & Sealfon, S.C. (1991a) *Neurosci. Lett.* **122**, 37–40.

Snyder, L., Roberts, J.L. & Sealfon, S.C. (1991b) *Biochem. Biophys. Res. Comm.* **180**, 1031–1035.

Sokoloff, P., Giros, B., Martres, M.P., Bouthenet, M.L. & Schwartz, J.C. (1990) *Nature* **347**, 146–151.

Stormann, T.M., Gdula, D.C., Weiner, D.M. & Brann, M.R. (1990) *Mol. Pharmacol.* **37**, 1–6.

Strader, C., Sigal, I.S. & Dixon, R.A.F. (1989) *FASEB J.* **3**, 1825–1832.

Sunahara, R.K., Niznik, H.B., Weiner, D.M., Stormann, T.M., Brann, M.R., Kennedy, J.L., Gelernter, J.E., Rozmahel, R., Yang, Y., Israel, Y., Seeman, P. & O'Dowd, B.F. (1990) *Nature* **347**, 80–83.

Sunahara, R.K., Guan, H.C., O'Dowd, B.F., Seeman, P., Laurier, L.G., Ng, G., George, S.R., Torchia, J., Van Tol, H.H.M. & Niznik, H.B. (1991) *Nature* **350**, 614–619.

Tiberi, M., Jarvie, K.R., Silvia, C., Falardeau, P., Gingrich, J.A., Godinot, N., Bertrand, L., Yang-Feng, T.L., Fremeau, R.T. Jr & Caron, M.G. (1991) *Proc. Natl Acad. Sci. USA* **88**, 7491–7495.

Todd, R.D., Khurana, T.S., Sajovic, P., Stone, K.R. & O'Malley, K.L. (1989) *Proc. Natl Acad. Sci. USA* **86**, 10134–10138.

Undie, A.S. & Friedman, E. (1990) *J. Pharmacol. Exp. Ther.* **253**, 987–992.

Vallar, L. & Meldolesi, J. (1989) *Trends Pharmacol. Sci.* **10**, 74–77.

Vallar, L., Muca, C., Magni, M., Albert, P., Bunzow, J., Meldolesi, J. & Civelli, O. (1990) *J. Biol. Chem.* **265**, 10320–10326.

Van Tol, H.H.M., Bunzow, J.R., Guan, H.-C., Sunahara, R.K., Seeman, P., Niznik, H.B. & Civelli, O. (1991) *Nature* **350**, 610–614.

Vyas, S.J., Eichberg, J. & Lokhandwala, M.F. (1992) *J. Pharmacol. Exp. Ther.* **260**, 134–139.

Weiner, D.M. & Brann, M.R. (1989) *FEBS Lett.* **253**, 207–213.

Weiner, D.M., Levey, A.I. & Brann, M.R. (1990) *Proc. Natl Acad. Sci. USA* **87**, 7050–7054.

Weiner, D.M., Levey, A.I., Sunahara, R.K., Niznik, H.B., O'Dowd, B.F., Seeman, P. & Brann, M.R. (1991) *Proc. Natl Acad. Sci. USA* **88**, 1859–1863.

Weinshank, R.L., Adham, N., Macchi, M., Olsen, M.A., Branchek, T.A. & Hartig, P.R. (1991) *J. Biol. Chem.* **266**, 22427–22435.

Zhou, Q.Y., Grandy, D.R., Thambi, L., Kusher, J.A., Van Tol, H.H.M., Cone, R., Pribnow, D., Salon, J., Bunzow, J.R. & Civelli, O. (1990) *Nature* **347**, 76–80.

_____ CHAPTER 2 _____

NEUROANATOMICAL LOCALIZATION OF D_1 VERSUS D_2 RECEPTORS: SIMILAR ORGANIZATION IN THE BASAL GANGLIA OF THE RAT, CAT AND HUMAN AND DISPARATE ORGANIZATION IN THE CORTEX AND LIMBIC SYSTEM

Jeffrey N. Joyce, Sara Goldsmith and Angela Murray

Departments of Psychiatry and Pharmacology, University of Pennsylvania School of Medicine, Philadelphia, PA 19104-6141, USA

Table of Contents

DOPAMINE RECEPTOR INTERACTIONS
ISBN 0-12-729045-1

J.N. Joyce, S. Goldsmith and A. Murray

2.1 Background

While it was established in the 1950s that dopamine (DA) was a transmitter in the central nervous system, the mechanisms by which DA altered neuronal signalling in the nervous system lagged in understanding. This is because the development of methods for measuring and localizing DA preceded by two decades the development of methods for assaying receptors that responded to DA. However, the general strategies for development of anatomically discrete methods were similar. Thus, gas chromatography and fluorometric assays for estimating concentrations of the monoamines in brain were supplanted, in the 1960s, by the use of high-pressure liquid chromatography coupled with electrochemical detection to measure small quantities of monoamines and their metabolites in small tissue samples. These techniques, while quantitative, are limited by their level of anatomical resolution. The degree of anatomical specificity is determined by the tissue dissection technique and the sensitivity of the assay. A major advance in the ability to define transmitter pathways in the brain came with the improvements in fluorescence histochemistry for visualization of DA in the central nervous system (Falck et al., 1962) and the delineation of the DA pathways in rat brain (Dahlstrom and Fuxe, 1964a, b). More recently, immunocytochemical methods for visualization of antibodies directed against enzymes of the DA synthetic pathway (tyrosine hydroxylase, TH) or DA itself have been developed (Hökfelt et al., 1984). While these procedures allow for detailed analysis of the distribution of DA pathways, they are largely non-quantitative. There is no direct relationship between the concentration of the amine of interest and either the monoamine fluorophores or antibody reaction. Consequently, there has been a continual search for quantitative techniques that have a high degree of anatomical resolution. Application of autoradiographic techniques for visualizing and quantifying the dopaminergic innervation of brain regions has subsequently been accomplished. In this case, the principles derived in biological membranes for labelling of high-affinity transport sites for DA have been successfully applied to autoradiography (Joyce et al., 1991b).

A parallel development in the detection of the receptors responsive to DA occurred during the 1970s. In the early 1970s, the ability of DA to stimulate adenylyl cyclase activity in the tissues derived from the central nervous system was demonstrated in several laboratories (e.g. Kebabian et al., 1972). For example, tissue derived from rat striatum shows increased cAMP production to stimulation by DA which could be inhibited with dopaminergic blockers. Proof that DA-sensitive adenylyl cyclase is localized to neurones postsynaptic to DA terminals came from lesion experiments. Damage to DA afferents did not reduce DA-stimulated adenylyl cyclase but removal of intrinsic neurones with local injections of neurotoxins (e.g. kainic acid) did remove DA-stimulated adenylyl cyclase activity (e.g. McGeer et al., 1976). In subsequent experiments it was determined that several dopaminergic ergots that stimulated DA receptors in the anterior pituitary did not stimulate adenylyl cyclase in the striatum, but

24

inhibited DA-stimulated adenylyl cyclase activity (Kebabian *et al.*, 1977; Pierie *et al.*, 1978). Consequently, the concept of multiple DA receptors was proposed (Kebabian and Calne, 1979). However, it was not until the development of radioligand binding assays and the subsequent development of selective radioligands for subtypes of the DA receptor that the concept of multiple DA receptors could be firmly established. Thus, radiolabelled butyrophenones (spiroperidol, haloperidol) have been used to label the D_2 receptor and the benzazepine antagonist SCH 23390 has been used to label the D_1 receptor.

The concept of multiple subtypes of the DA receptor was extended by a series of developments. First, biochemical and pharmacological evidence was developed that supported the hypothesis that the physiological actions of DA were mediated by its interaction with two basic types of G protein-coupled receptors, D_1 and D_2, which stimulate and inhibit, respectively, the enzyme adenylyl cyclase (Stoof and Kebabian, 1984). Second, careful lesion experiments combined with the use of *in vivo* binding of selective radioligands provided strong evidence that the D_2 subtype was located at more than one synapse in the striatum, perhaps to both intrinsic neuropil and afferents arising from other brain regions (Theodorou *et al.*, 1981). Third, in the late 1970s, several groups reported that tissue sections could be radiolabelled with compounds that bound to receptors and visualized by dipping in emulsions or by placing against autoradiographic film (Kuhar *et al.*, 1978). Since these tissue sections retain their anatomical integrity and the autoradiographic images can be quantified, this technique has proven to be a powerful tool for imaging receptor systems. Evidence rapidly accumulated that the distributions of D_1 and D_2 receptors in rat brain were only partially overlapping (Boyson *et al.*, 1986; Dawson *et al.*, 1986b; Joyce *et al.*, 1985).

In recent years, additional subtypes of the DA receptor have been identified based on gene cloning strategies (Civelli *et al.*, 1991; Sokoloff *et al.*, 1990). There is significant homology for the sequences of the D_2, D_3 and D_4 receptors. Moreover, radioligands that selectively label the D_2 receptor have high affinity for the D_3 and D_4 receptors (Civelli *et al.*, 1991). Similarly, the sequences for the D_1 and D_5 receptors are highly homologous and are labelled with compounds classically used to label the D_1 receptor (Civelli *et al.*, 1991). Consequently, it is more appropriate to assume that the selective D_1 antagonist [^{3}H]SCH 23390 is labelling a D_1-like family of receptors and the D_2 antagonists [^{3}H]spiroperidol, [^{3}H]raclopride and [^{125}I]epidepride are labelling a family of D_2-like receptors. Nonetheless, a significant amount of information is available on the organization of the D_1 and D_2 receptors, based on receptor autoradiographic experiments. The recent *in situ* hybridization protocols that allow localization of mRNA coding for the various subtypes of the DA receptor have, however, added important additional information. In the following sections we will discuss the organization of DA receptors in different regions of the brain. That is because, as with the topography of DA itself (Berger *et al.*, 1991), the subcortical regions show a similar organization across species, but there are major species differences in the anatomy of DA receptor systems in cortical and limbic system regions.

2.2 Basal ganglia

DA levels and terminal density vary significantly between the structures that make up the basal ganglia (Fallon and Moore, 1978; Veening *et al.*, 1980; Voorn *et al.*, 1986). Thus, DA innervation is densest in the components of the striatum, the caudate-putamen (CPu), nucleus accumbens septi (NAS) and olfactory tubercle (Olf Tub), and less so in the globus pallidus (GP) and entopeduncular nucleus (EN). DA concentration is, of course, highest in the substantia nigra pars compacta (SNpc) and ventral tegmental area (VTA) but considerably lower in the substantia nigra pars reticulata (SNpr). These data are also consistent with the regional distribution of DA uptake sites (Javitch *et al.*, 1985). The only important exception is that there are regional variations in the number of high-affinity DA uptake sites within the striatum that are not matched by a similar heterogeneity in DA itself (Joyce *et al.*, 1985; Joyce, 1991a; Marshall *et al.*, 1990). Thus, DA uptake sites are higher in density in the dorsal and lateral CPu than more medially or ventrally in the striatal complex but DA concentration does not show dorso-ventral or mediolateral gradients.

2.2.1 Basal ganglia of the rat brain

The reported distribution of D_1 receptor sites observed in the adult rat when labelled with [^{125}I]SCH 23982 (Altar and Marien, 1987; Dawson *et al.*, 1986b; Rao *et al.*, 1991) is similar to that found when utilizing [^{3}H]SCH 23390 and/or [^{3}H]SK & F 83566 (Boyson *et al.*, 1986; Dawson *et al.*, 1986a). The density of D_1 receptors is highest in the striatum and lower in the efferents of the striatum. Within the striatum the density is somewhat lower in the NAS and Olf Tub than in the CPu. The density of D_1 receptors is higher in the EN than in the GP and greater in the SNpr than in the SNpc (Rao *et al.*, 1991). The latter difference has not been reported by all investigators (Aiso *et al.*, 1987; Altar and Marien, 1987; Dawson *et al.*, 1986a, b) and may reflect difficulties in discriminating SNpc from SNpr in autoradiographic images. In the adult, D_2 receptors labelled with iodinated benzamides, such as [^{125}I]IBZM or [^{125}I]iodosulpiride (Rao *et al.*, 1991; Matres *et al.*, 1985), or with [^{3}H]spiroperidol (Joyce *et al.*, 1985; Boyson *et al.*, 1986), are also highest in the striatum and lower in the other regions of the basal ganglia. Within the striatum the density of sites is highest in the lateral CPu and lowest in the nucleus accumbens (Boyson *et al.*, 1986; Joyce and Marshall, 1985; Joyce *et al.*, 1985). D_2 receptors are higher in the GP than in the EN and denser in the SNpc than in the SNpr.

The discordant distribution of D_1 and D_2 receptors in rat striatum (Boyson *et al.*, 1986; Joyce, 1991a), with a marked lateromedial gradient for the D_2 receptor but not for the D_1 receptor, has suggested that they are localized to different neuronal populations. The D_2 receptor appears enriched in density within the lateral CPu and in register with zones with a high density of cholinergic terminals (Joyce and Marshall, 1985; Loopjuit, 1989) and DA terminals (Joyce *et al.*, 1991a), whereas the D_1 receptor is more homogeneously distributed. This differential distribution of DA receptor is observed early in development of the striatum (Rao *et al.*, 1991); however, the relationship to DA terminals is reversed from that in the adult. D_1 receptors appear earlier in development than do D_2 receptors and their topography does not initially overlap with that of D_2 receptors (Rao *et al.*, 1991). The D_1 receptors are initially in register with the early formed 'patch-distributed' DA terminals (Murrin and Zeng, 1989; Rao *et al.*, 1991). It is only later in the postnatal development that the adult-like pattern of a homogeneous distribution of D_1 receptors and the reorganization of DA terminals to show a prominent lateromedial gradient of [^{3}H]mazindol sites occurs. In contrast, the development of D_2 receptors occurs in the lateromedial axis and remains organized along this axis in the adult (Rao *et al.*, 1991). Therefore, in the mature adult there is not a strong relationship between D_1 receptors and [^{3}H]mazindol-labelled DA terminals (Joyce, 1991a). However, there does exist a robust relationship between the topography of [^{3}H]mazindol-labelled DA terminals and D_2 receptors (Joyce, 1991a). This appears to be the case even though the gradient of [^{3}H]mazindol-labelled DA terminals is not matched by an equivalent gradient of DA levels (Joyce *et al.*, 1985; Marshall *et al.*, 1990). Initially the development of the D_2 receptor is not related to maturation of DA terminals. The development of D_2 receptors appears related to that of maturation of cholinergic interneurones, as both develop in a lateromedial gradient (Rao *et al.*, 1991). However, in the adult there is a significant correlation between the binding of [^{3}H]hemicholinium-3 ([^{3}H]HC-3) to cholinergic terminals, [^{3}H]mazindol to DA terminals and [^{3}H]spiroperidol to D_2 receptors in subregions of the striatal complex (Joyce, 1991a). These data are consistent with the DA denervation studies that suggest that the D_2 receptor system comes under the control of this DA system in the adult, but remains differentially regulated from the D_1 receptor system (Joyce, 1991a, b). [^{3}H]Mazindol-labelled DA terminals conform to the matrix-directed DA terminals (Lowenstein *et al.*, 1990) that arise from the dorsal tier of the SNpc (Gerfen *et al.*, 1987). This suggests that in the mature rat D_2 receptors are in register with this DA system but the D_1 receptor system less directly so.

Other evidence also suggests that D_1 and D_2 receptors are located at different synapses in the rat striatum and on distinct neurones. Lesion studies completed in the late 1970s and early 1980s suggested a differential localization of D_1 and D_2 receptors in the CPu. Injection of the axon-sparing neurotoxins kainic acid (KA) or quinolinic acid (QA) resulted in an almost complete loss of D_1 receptors (Barone *et al.*, 1987; Cross and Waddington, 1981) but not more than a 60% loss of D_2 receptors (Schwarcz *et al.*, 1978; Leff *et al.*, 1981; Cross and Waddington, 1981), as determined using *in vitro* membrane binding assays. Extensive ablation of the overlying neocortex produced 12–57% decreases in D_2 receptors in similar homogenate binding experiments, and in combination with KA lesion of the CPu an almost complete loss of D_2 sites could be obtained (Creese *et al.*, 1978; Schwarcz *et al.*, 1978). An enduring interpretation of these data is that D_2 receptors are localized to neurones intrinsic to the CPu and to corticostriatal axons, whereas D_1 receptors are localized almost exclusively to neurones intrinsic to the CPu. Since D_2 receptors are also thought to be the autoreceptors located on DA terminals in the striatum (Lehman et al., 1983), the hypothesis was that D_2 receptors in the striatum were localized to, at least three different neuropil (Creese, 1982).

More recent lesion studies that have utilized high-resolution autoradiography combined with careful histological reconstruction of the lesions have weakened the interpretation that D_2 receptors are located on corticostriatal axons (Joyce and Marshall, 1987; Trugman et al., 1986). Injection of QA into the striatum preferentially damages some neuronal populations while sparing others (Schwarcz et al., 1980; Schwarcz and Köhler, 1983; Joyce and Marshall, 1987). The spared population, predominantly the large cholinergic interneurones, could preferentially express the D_2 receptor and thus remain less affected by QA lesions. In addition, careful analysis of cortical ablation studies failed to replicate the earlier findings and did not support the evidence that D_2 receptors were located on corticostriatal axons (Joyce and Marshall, 1987; Trugman et al., 1986). Other studies have also provided support that D_2 receptors are expressed by the cholinergic interneurones (Joyce and Marshall, 1985; Dawson et al., 1988) but it was not until mRNA for the D_2 receptor was localized to the cholinergic neurones (LeMoine et al., 1990; Brene et al., 1990b) that the hypothesis that D_1 and D_2 receptors could be expressed in different neurones was substantiated. This was further confirmed with in situ histochemical studies that have demonstrated that D_2 mRNA is localized to more than one population of neurones in the striatum which only partially overlap with those expressing D_1 receptors (Gerfen et al., 1990; Weiner et al., 1990). Hence, D_1 receptor mRNA is expressed in medium-sized neurones that synthesize the neuropeptide substance P, whereas D_2 receptor mRNA is largely expressed in medium-sized neurones that display preproenkephalin mRNA and large neurones that express ChAT (Gerfen et al., 1990; LeMoine et al., 1990a, 1990b) (Figure 1). However, it should be noted that investigators using other techniques have found that D_1 and D_2 receptor-mediated actions can be mediated in individual striatal neurones (Bertorello et al., 1990; Uchimura and North, 1990), suggesting that many neurones should express both D_1 and D_2 mRNA. These potentially conflicting results have not been satisfactorily explained. The degree to which these neurones also express mRNAs that encode for D_3, D_4 and D_5 DA receptors is not known.

In many regions of the rat basal ganglia, the ratio of D_1 to D_2 receptors is high, particularly the GP and SN. D_1 mRNA is not found in these regions (Fremeau et al., 1991; Mansour et al., 1990). These data are consistent with evidence that D_1 receptors are transported in the axons of the striatal efferent neurones (Altar and Marien, 1987; Barone et al., 1987; Aiso et al., 1987). D_1 and D_2 receptors are visible in both the SNpr and SNpc, but here again they appear to have a different cellular localization to pre- and postsynaptic

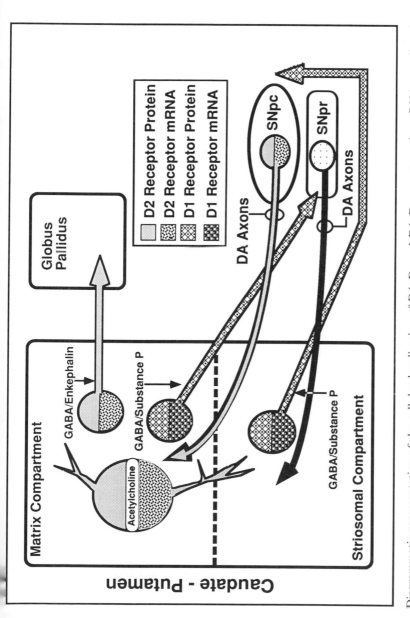

Figure 1 Diagrammatic representation of the cellular localization of DA D$_1$ and DA D$_2$ receptors, the mRNA encoding the receptors, and their localization to the striosomal or matrix compartments of the caudate-putamen (CPu). DA D$_2$ receptors are expressed by the large cholinergic interneurones of the CPu, the GABA efferent neurones of the CPu that project to the globus pallidus and contain enkephalin, and DA neurones of the substantia nigra pars compacta (SNpc) that give rise to the nigrostriatal pathway. DA D$_1$ receptors are expressed by the GABA efferent neurones that project to the entopeduncular nucleus and substantia nigra pars reticulata (SNpr) and contain substance P.

components of SN. D_2 receptors are expressed in higher numbers in the SNpc than in the SNpr, whereas the opposite is true for the D_1 receptor. Lesions of the striatonigral pathway result in a loss of D_1 but not D_2 receptors from the SNpr, whereas 6-hydroxydopamine-induced loss of DA neurones in the SN produces a loss of D_2 receptors in the SNpc (Filloux *et al.*, 1987; Savasta *et al.*, 1986). *In situ* studies have shown that neurones in the SNpc and VTA that express TH also express D_2 mRNA (Meador-Woodruff and Mansour, 1991; Le Moine and Bloch, 1991). Morover, 6-hydroxydopamine (6-OHDA) lesions of the medial forebrain bundle destroy the neurones in the SNpc that express mRNA for D_2 receptors and for TH (Meador-Woodruff and Mansour, 1991). These data support the hypothesis that D_1 receptors are located on terminals of the striatonigral and striatopallidal efferents but D_2 receptors in the midbrain are localized to DA-synthesizing neurones.

2.2.2 Basal ganglia of the carnivore and primate

The striatum of the primate and carnivore appears to be anatomically more differentiated than the rodent striatum. A particularly useful tool in exploring this differentiation is in the examination of a neurochemical organization intrinsic to the striatal complex, referred to as the striosome (patch) and matrix organization (Graybiel, 1984, 1990; Martin *et al.*, 1991). This neurochemical organization is not identical but is partially overlapping with that based on coticostriatal projection zones. One of the most obvious neurochemical heterogeneities is based on markers for the cholinergic system, including the histochemical demonstration of the cholinergic enzyme acetylcholinesterase (AChE) (Graybiel and Ragsdale, 1978) and the autoradiographic demonstration of the high-affinity uptake for choline with $[^3H]HC$-3 (Lowenstein *et al.*, 1990; Rhodes *et al.*, 1987). They are both enriched within the matrix compartment embedded within which are zones low in density referred to as striosomes or patches. Patterns of immunoreactivity for neuropeptides and the classic transmitters (e.g. the monoamines) also obey this organization, but differ in the dorsal and ventral striatum. Thus, in the dorsal striatum the striosomes are distinguished by their higher density of enkephalin, substance P and somatostatin immunoreactivity, and the matrix by calcium-binding protein and tyrosine hydroxylase immunoreactivities. The striosomes have also been shown to overlap with cytologically identified cell islands (Goldman-Rakic, 1982; Martin *et al.*, 1991) and with the autoradiographic mapping of μ opiate receptors (Herkenham and Pert, 1981). In the ventral striatum many of the neuropeptides show a higher density and their patterns are less distinct. In general, zones low in the amount of reaction product for tyrosine hydroxylase, substance P and leu-enkephalin are embedded in a matrix rich in these markers. However, some regions enriched in neurotensin immunoreactivity are spatially registered with zones low in tyrosine hydroxylase, low in substance P and enriched in

30

leu-enkephalin. This suggests that the chemoarchitectonic topography of the striatal compartments is different in the dorsal and ventral striatum.

There is also a marked heterogeneity in the organization of dopaminergic synapses of the striatum. First, distinct populations of dopaminergic neurones within the ventral mesencephalon innervate different territories of striatum (Fallon and Moore, 1978; Voorn et al., 1986; Langer and Graybiel, 1989) as well as, within these territories, the striosomal versus matrix compartments (Gerfen et al., 1987; Jimenez-Castellanos and Graybiel, 1987; Langer and Graybiel, 1989). Second, immunocytochemical and autoradiographic studies support the concept that high-affinity uptake sites for DA (Lowenstein et al., 1989, 1990) and tyrosine hydroxylase immunoreactivity (Graybiel et al., 1987) are higher in the extrastriosomal (matrix) compartment. In addition, high-affinity sites for DA (Marshall et al., 1990; Lowenstein et al., 1989) and tyrosine hydroxylase immunoreactivity (Graybiel et al., 1987; Martin et al., 1991) are higher in the dorsal than ventral striatum, even within the matrix compartment. In contrast, serotonin immunoreactivity (Lavoie and Parent, 1990) and high-affinity uptake sites for serotonin (Joyce et al., 1992) are higher in the matrix compartment of the ventral striatum. Thus, the monoaminergic projections to the dorsal striatum differ from those to the ventral striatum.

Not only do transmitters and their enzymatic markers for neurones differ between the striosome and matrix compartments, but so do receptors (Figure 2). There is a striosomal/matrix ordering to the subtypes of the DA receptor (Besson et al., 1988; Joyce et al., 1986b, 1991a). The selective D_1 antagonist [^{3}H]SCH23390 has been used to label the D_1 receptor in human and non-human primate brain (Cortes et al., 1989; De Keyser et al., 1988; Joyce et al., 1988; Joyce and Hurtig, 1990; Goldman-Rakic et al., 1990; Richfield et al., 1987, 1989; Besson et al., 1988). The D_2 receptor in the human and non-human primate brain has been labelled with the D_2 antagonists [^{3}H]spiroperidol (Camps et al., 1989; De Keyser et al., 1988; Joyce et al., 1986a, 1986b, 1988, 1990), [^{3}H]raclopride (Goldman-Rakic et al., 1990; Lidow et al., 1989) and [^{125}I]epidepride (Joyce et al., 1991a), as well as the agonist [^{3}H]CV 205-502 (Camps et al., 1989). In cats and primates, the DA D_1 receptor is present in higher density in the striosomal compartment of the caudate nucleus (Besson et al., 1986) whereas D_2 receptor density (Joyce et al., 1986a, b, 1991a), high-affinity uptake sites for DA (Lowenstein et al., 1990) and tyrosine hydroxylase immunoreactivity (Graybiel et al., 1987) are higher in the extrastriosomal compartment. Thus, in many respects, the D_1 and D_2 receptors show a complementary organization. However, high-affinity uptake sites for DA and D_2 receptors are lower in density in the ventral striatum, making these components less distinct in the matrix and striosomal compartments (Lowenstein et al., 1990; Joyce et al., 1986b). We have recently shown that D_3 receptors are expressed in the striosomal compartment of the ventral striatum (Murray et al., 1992). In addition, in the efferents of the striatum, D_2 receptors are higher in the globus pallidus external than in the globus pallidus internal, whereas D_1

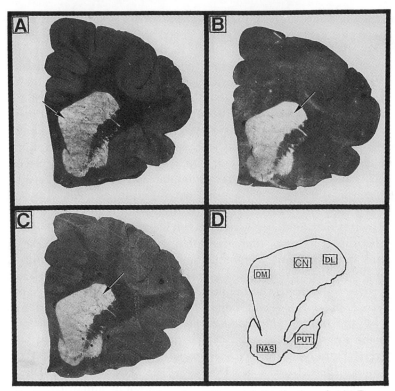

Figure 2 Within the cat striatum there is a differential distribution of: (A) D_1 receptors; (B) DA uptake sites; and (C) D_2 receptors. In the caudate nucleus (CN) the dorsolateral region (DL) shows higher [^{3}H]spiroperidol binding to D_2 receptors (arrow in C) and [^{3}H]mazindol binding to DA uptake sites (arrow in B) but lower binding of [^{3}H]SCH 23390 to D_1 receptors (arrow in A). In contrast, within the CN, [^{3}H]SCH 23390 binding to D_1 receptors is highest in the dorsomedial (DM) region. Even within the DL region microzones of high D_2 receptor density are complementary to microzones of less dense D_1 receptor density and within the DM region microzones of high D_1 receptor density are complementary to microzones of less dense D_2 receptor density. Higher densities of receptors are shown in darker grey tones.

receptors show the opposite pattern (Figure 3). Within the midbrain region containing DA-synthesizing neurones the microtopography of D_2 receptors correlates with the tyrosine hydroxylase-containing neurones (Joyce *et al.*, 1991a). D_1 receptors show a characteristic, heterogeneous distribution within the human ventral mesencephalon that is in accordance with a localization to substance P and dynorphin B immunoreactive terminals associated with striatonigral projections (Thibaut *et al.*, 1990). Consistent with that data is the information that mRNA encoding the human D_1 receptor is not localized to the GP_E, GP_I or SN where [^{3}H]SCH 23390 binding is found (Mengod *et al.*, 1991). Therefore, there is a high degree of similarity in the neuroanatomy of DA receptors and of DA itself in the basal ganglia of the rat, cat and primate (including the human).

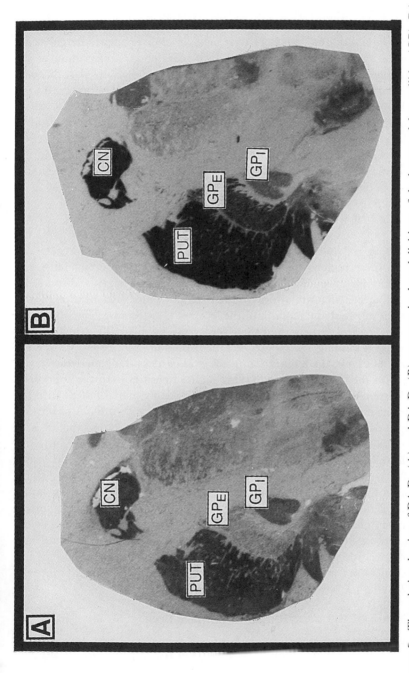

Figure 3 The relative density of DA D_1 (A) and DA D_2 (B) receptors in the subdivisions of the human globus pallidus (GP). DA D_1 and D_2 receptors are visible in the caudate nucleus (CN) and putamen (PUT). D_1 receptors are relatively higher in the GP internal (GP$_I$) than the GP external (GP$_E$), whereas the reverse holds for DA D_2 receptors (GP$_E$ greater than GP$_I$). Higher densities of receptors are shown in darker grey tones.

2.3 Cortex

DA innervations to the cortex of primates is significantly different both quantitatively and qualitatively from that of the rodent (reviews: Berger *et al.*, 1991; Lewis *et al.*, 1986). In the rodent, the dopaminergic innervation of the cortex is largely restricted to the prefrontal, anterior cingulate, insular, piriform and entorhinal regions. In the human, there is a more extended innervation of all cortical regions with a distinct laminar pattern (Gaspar *et al.*, 1989, 1991). Within most cortical regions the upper lamina has the densest number of fibres, the inner lamina slightly less and lamina IV the least (Lewis *et al.*, 1986; Gaspar *et al.*, 1989). Somatosensory and auditory cortex show the fewest fibres and the agranular cortical regions show the most. In addition, the motor and premotor cortices show a dense innervation across all laminae.

2.3.1 Cortex of the rat brain

DA receptors in rodent cortex are largely, but not exclusively, restricted in expression to those regions that have a dopaminergic innervation. Thus, the prefrontal, anterior cingulate, piriform and suprarhinal regions display D_1 receptor binding sites that are approximately one-fifth the concentration of sites in the CPu but substantially more than the levels of D_2 receptors. The superficial layers are labelled less densely than the deep layers, particularly layer 6, which shows the densest binding (Savasta *et al.*, 1986; Boyson *et al.*, 1986; Mansour *et al.*, 1991). In addition, the temporal and parietal cortices show moderate levels of binding with the deep layers displaying higher densities than the superficial layers. Expression of D_1 mRNA by neurones is relatively more limited, with the neurones in the deep layers of the neocortex expressing the D_1 mRNA (Mansour *et al.*, 1991; Fremeau *et al.*, 1991). The distribution of D_2 receptors labelled with [^{3}H]spiroperidol or [^{3}H]raclopride occurs in all neocortical regions, but with low densities and predominantly in the deep layers (Boyson *et al.*, 1986; Mansour *et al.*, 1990). Utilizing the compound [^{125}I]iodosulpiride, Matres *et al.* (1985) have reported that there is, in addition, light labelling in the superficial layers I–III of cingulate, somatosensory, temporal and parietal but not motor cortex. By comparison, relatively dense levels of D_2 receptor mRNA are detected in the superficial aspects of layer I and in layers II–III of the frontal, parietal and temporal cortex. Also, in the deeper layers of cingulate, frontal, parietal and temporal cortices are moderate to low levels of D_2 receptor mRNA (Mansour *et al.*, 1990; but see Mengod *et al.*, 1989).

2.3.2 Cortex of the carnivore and primate brain

There appears to be a more complex expression of DA receptors in the primate cortex. In the cortex of the monkey brain D_1 and D_2 receptors appear to show a complementary organization (Goldman-Rakic *et al.*, 1990; Lidow *et al.*, 1989,

1991). The relationship of D_2 to D_1 receptors has been difficult to ascertain in human cortex because of the low density of D_2 receptors; D_2 receptors may be as much as 10-fold lower in density than D_1 receptors in the frontal cortex (Cortes et al., 1989; Luabeya et al., 1984). In fact, some investigators are not able to identify D_2 receptors in human cortex with the radioligand [³H]spiperone (Camus et al., 1986; De Keyser et al., 1988). D_1 receptors show the greatest binding in the superficial layers (I, II, IIIa) of the frontal cortex, considerably less in the middle layers (IIIb and IV), and binding just slightly less than in the superficial layers in the deep layers V and VI (Goldman-Rakic et al., 1990; Richfield et al., 1989). There are lower numbers of D_1 sites in somatosensory and motor cortex with the highest labelling of D_1 receptors in superficial layers I, II and IIIa, with other layers containing much lower densities (Lidow et al., 1991). There have been no reports of the cortical distribution of neurones containing D_1 mRNA in primates. However, there is a report of the immunocytochemical distribution of DARP-32, which is thought to be associated with D_1 receptors in primate cortex (Berger et al., 1990). In the adult there are few neurones expressing DARP-32 in prefrontal, premotor, motor or visual cortices.

In the frontal cortex, D_2 receptors labelled with the selective compounds [³H]raclopride (Goldman-Rakic et al., 1990; Lidow et al., 1989) or [¹²⁵I]epidepride (Joyce et al., 1991a) show quite similar patterns. The D_2 receptor is low in density but with the highest density in the deep layers (layers V and VI) of both monkey and human cortex. This contrasts with reports using the less selective radioligand [³H]spiroperidol, wherein some groups have reported non-detectable densities in frontal cortex and others have reported that reasonably high densities are found in the external laminae (De Keyser et al., 1988; Camps et al., 1989; Richfield et al., 1989). Using the substituted benzamide [¹²⁵I]epidepride we have also shown that in the primary sensory cortices (somatosensory, auditory) D_2 receptors are almost undetectable whereas in agranular cortical regions (premotor and motor cortex) the binding is quite dense (Joyce et al., 1991a; Murray, Goldsmith, Neve and Joyce, unpublished findings). In the motor cortex, lamina IIIc shows the densest binding, with laminae V and VI showing lower binding and layer I none (Figure 4). The temporal cortex shows a three-fold higher density of binding than the frontal cortex and a trilaminar pattern predominates, binding is greater in the external (layers I and II) and internal layers than in the middle layers (III and IV).

The comparative distribution of DA, D_1 and D_2 receptors suggests interesting synaptic organizations in the human. In frontal cortex DA would interact with D_1 receptors in the upper laminae and both receptors in the inner laminae. Thus, neurones that give rise to cortico-cortico connections express D_1 receptors whereas those that give rise to subcortical efferents would have both D_1 and D_2 receptors. In primary somatosensory and auditory cortex, where the DA innervation is light, the D_1 receptor would almost entrely predominate. In contrast, in the promotor and motor cortex, DA innervation of D_1 and D_2 receptors would be

35

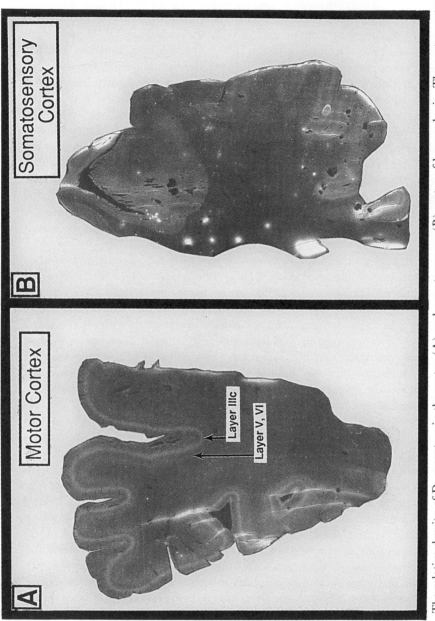

Figure 4 The relative density of D_2 receptors in the motor (A) and somatosensory (B) cortex of human brain. The motor cortex shows a highly laminated pattern of [^{125}I]epidepride binding to D_2 receptors with layer IIIc the highest, layer VI the next highest and layers I and II with almost no binding. The somatosensory cortex shows almost undetectable binding in all laminae. These dark-field photographs of [^{125}I]epidepride binding show regions of high binding as lighter than areas of sparse binding.

segregated by laminae. In the laminae of cortico-cortico connections the D_1 receptor would predominate, whereas in the laminae of thalamic input (IIIc) and the output (V, VI) the D_2 receptor would predominate. Interestingly, the corticostriatal efferents terminate in the matrix compartment of the putamen, a region of high expression of D_2 receptors and DA innervation. Consequently, the human brain would have at least two synapses in the motor loop where DA innervation and D_2 receptor expression are high. This might suggest that in neurodegenerative disorders affecting the DA system, such as Parkinson's disease, not only would the putamen be affected (Joyce and Hurtig, 1990) but also the motor cortex (Gaspar et al., 1991).

2.4 Limbic system

The limbic system includes the major cortical regions that project to the hippocampus and the major efferents of the hippocampus. Information from multimodal association areas of the cortex, including the temporal prefrontal, cingulate and insular regions, converges on the parahippocampal cortices (the entorhinal cortex in rats) and is transmitted to the hippocampal formation via the perforant pathway (Van Hoesen, 1982). Hippocampal efferent output is organized such that information from various subfields of the hippocampus is transmitted via intrahippocampal association pathways to the subicular complex before leaving the hippocampal complex. The subicular complex relays information back to the association cortices via the parahippocampal cortices and directly to the amygdala and ventral striatum (NAS, ventral CPu). DA innervation of the entorhinal cortex and amygdala, major components of the limbic system, is relatively dense in all species. Direct visualization of DA histofluorescence in the hippocampus has been difficult, suggesting that there was no dopaminergic innervation to this limbic region. In contrast, there have been biochemical (Bischoff et al., 1979; Saldate and Orrego, 1977), pharmacological (McCulloch et al., 1979) and anatomical (Simon et al., 1979; Swanson, 1982) data suggesting that DA did function in the hippocampal formation. Recent studies utilizing subtractive immunohistochemistry (comparing staining for tyrosine hydroxlyase to dopamine β-hydroxylase) have confimed the suspected dopaminergic innervation of the rat hippocampus, and revealed a different distribution in humans and other primates. In the rat brain DA fibres are observed in the subiculum, hilus of the dentate gyrus, strata radiatum and lacunosum-moleculare of CA3, with few reactive fibres in other strata of DG or CA3, and few in any region of CA1 (Milner and Bacon, 1989; Febvret et al., 1991). Berger et al. (1988) have reported that the superior and middle temporal gyri of the monkey exhibit the same bilaminar pattern of innervation seen in other granular cortical regions. Initial reports on the hippocampal dopaminergic innervation indicate differences between humans and non-human primates. In the human, CA4, CA3 and the presubiculum are more densely innervated, and CA1, the subiculum and the entorhinal cortex show sparser innervation (Torack and Morris, 1990). In the monkey, CA4 is densely innervated and the subiculum exhibits low, but significant, levels of DA innervation (Samson *et al.*, 1990)

2.4.1 Limbic system of the rat

In the rat, the amygdala exhibits a heterogeneous pattern of D_1 and D_2 receptors. D_1 receptors and D_1 receptor mRNA are evident but low in the basolateral, lateral and central nuclei. The number of binding sites and level of D_1 receptor mRNA are higher in the cortical and basomedial amygdaloid nuclei (Savasta *et al.*, 1986; Boyson *et al.*, 1986; Mansour *et al.*, 1991; Fremeau *et al.*, 1991). D_2 receptors are highest in number in the central nucleus, lower in basomedial and intercalated nuclei and lowest in the anterior and lateral areas (Boyson *et al.*, 1986; Matres *et al.*, 1985). D_2 receptor mRNA is expressed at low levels in the lateral and basolateral nuclei and at higher levels in the medial nucleus (Mansour *et al.*, 1990). The entorhinal cortex demonstrates moderate amounts of D_1 receptor binding in layers I, II, V and VI with low levels in the intermediate layers (Boyson *et al.*, 1986; Savasta *et al.*, 1986; Köhler *et al.*, 1990; Mansour *et al.*, 1991). Within the entorhinal cortex, neurones in layers II, V and VI exhibit D_1 mRNA labelling with none in layer I (Mansour *et al.*, 1991; Fremeau *et al.*, 1991). Entorhinal cortex shows some of the highest binding to D_2 receptor sites in the rat cortex, with layer I the densest, no binding in layer II and moderate levels in layer III (Boyson *et al.*, 1986; Köhler *et al.*, 1991; Mansour *et al.*, 1990). In comparison, layers II−III and superficial cells within layer I demonstrate dense levels of D_2 receptor mRNA (Mansour *et al.*, 1990; but see Mengod *et al.*, 1989). In the hippocampus quite low levels of D_1 receptor binding are observed in the molecular layer of the dentate gyrus and in the stratum moleculare of subfields CA1−CA3 (Dawson *et al.*, 1986a, b; Mansour *et al.*, 1991). D_1 receptor mRNA has been reported to be localized exclusively to the granule cells of the dentate gyrus (Mansour *et al.*, 1991) but another laboratory (Fremeau *et al.*, 1991) has reported that in the ventral hippocampus prominent labelling of the subicular complex was observed, pyramidal cells of subfields CA1−CA3 showed D_1 mRNA and rarely the granule neurones of the dentate gyrus. D_2 receptors are apparent in the stratum lacunosum moleculare of the dorsal hippocampus with the highest binding in the CA1 and least in the CA3 subfields and in the subiculum (Matres *et al.*, 1985; Mansour *et al.*, 1990). D_2 receptor mRNA is visualized in the pyramidal cell layer of the subfields and in the granule cells of the dentate gyrus. These studies suggest that there is little overlap of amygdaloid nuclei, laminae of the entorhinal cortex or regions of the hippocampus that express both D_1 and D_2 receptors. In addition, the correlation between DA innervation and DA receptor is better for D_1 receptors in the amygdala and entorhinal cortex but poor for hippocampus.

2.4.2 Limbic system of the carnivore and primate

In the amygdala of the human, D_1 and D_2 receptors are organized in complement with each other, with the density of D_1 receptors greatest in the medial aspect of the nucleus lateralis and least in cortical nucleus and basal nucleus (Cortés *et al.*, 1989). In contrast, the density of D_2 receptors is highest in the cortical and basal nuclei and lowest in accessory nucleus and lateral nucleus (Figure 5).

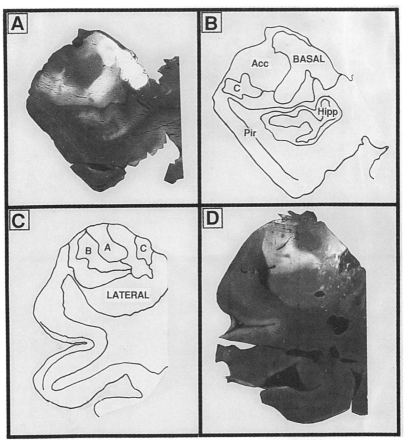

Figure 5 The relative density of D_2 receptors in the nuclei of the amygdala of human brain. The amygdala shows a heterogeneous pattern of $[^{125}I]$epidepride binding to D_2 receptors in the caudal amygdala (A) and rostral amygdala (D). The cortical and basal nuclei show the highest binding, and accessory and lateral nuclei have very low binding. These dark-field photographs of $[^{125}I]$epidepride binding show regions of high binding as lighter than areas of sparse binding. The diagram in (B) depicts the regions shown in (A) with accessory (Acc), basal (BASAL) and cortical (C) nuclei of the amygdala, the hippocampus (Hipp), and piriform (Pir) cortex shown. The diagram in (C) depicts the regions shown in (D) with accessory (Acc), basal (BASAL), cortical (C) and lateral (LATERAL) nuclei of the amygdala shown.

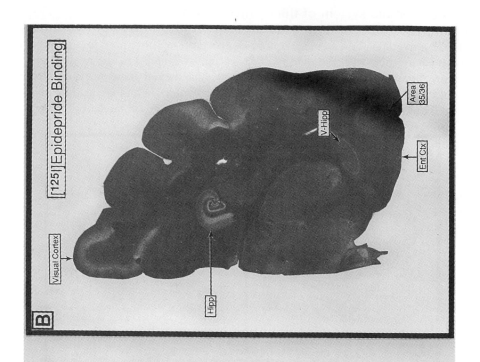

[¹²⁵I]Epidepride Binding

B

Visual Cortex

Hipp

V-Hipp

Ent Ctx

Area 35/36

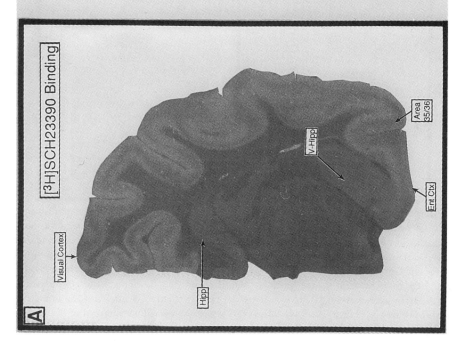

[³H]SCH23390 Binding

A

Visual Cortex

Hipp

V-Hipp

Ent Ctx

Area 35/36

In the temporal cortex D_1 receptor patterning appears to be similar to that in the frontal cortex, with the superficial layers exhibiting the highest binding, the deep layers less and the intermediate layers the least (Lidow *et al.*, 1991; Richfield *et al.*, 1989). The localization of DARP-32-positive neurones to pyramidal neurones in layer Va and in layers II–III of the inferior temporal gyrus of the adult monkey suggests that the D_1 receptors localized in this region are synthesized by intrinsic neurones (Berger *et al.*, 1990). In the parahippocampal gyrus the densest binding to D_1 receptors occurs in the superficial layers of the entorhinal cortex and CA1 of the hippocampus (Cortés *et al.*, 1989; Richfield *et al.*, 1989). In the entorhinal cortex DARP-32-positive neurones were observed in clusters in layers II and III with their apical dendrites visible in layer I, whereas DARP-32-positive neurones in layer VI had apical dendrites in layer III (Berger *et al.*, 1990).

Published (Joyce *et al.*, 1991a) and unpublished (Goldsmith *et al.*, 1991; Joyce, 1991c) work from this laboratory suggests that the complex patterned expression of D_2 receptors in the parahippocampal complex and the hippocampus of the cat and human predominates over the D_1 receptor. In the cat D_1 receptors are expressed in higher amounts in the cortex than hippocampal regions (Figure 6), with the typical trilaminar pattern of the carnivore and primate. The expression of D_1 receptors in the hippocampus and subiculum is negligible. However, binding is observed in the entorhinal cortex. In the cat (Figure 6) and human parahippocampus (Figure 7) there is a higher binding in areas 35/36, immediately adjacent to the entorhinal cortex, than in the entorhinal cortex. In the cat, as in the human, within the lateral occipitotemporal cortex binding is densest in layers I–III and very low in layers IV–VI with binding almost non-existent in the adjacent entorhinal cortex. In the cat, binding in dorsal hippocampus is highest in the molecular layer of the dentate gyrus (facia dentata) and lacunosum radiatum of CA1–CA3 subfields. The band of binding in the lacunosum radiatum shows increasing density from CA3 through the subiculum. Binding in the ventral hippocampus is two to three times lower than

---

Figure 6 The relative density of D_1 and D_2 receptors in the nuclei of the cat brain at the level of the hippocampus (low magnification) (A) D_1 receptors labelled with [^{3}H]SCH 23390 are much higher in number within the cortex than in the hippocampal regions. Almost all cortical regions show binding in the superficial and deep laminae, except in the entorhinal cortex (Ent. Ctx), which shows binding in deep laminae only. The visual cortex shows the densest binding of all cortical regions. The dorsal hippocampus (Hipp) and ventral hippocampus (V-Hipp) show negligible binding. (B) The heterogeneous pattern of [^{125}I]epideprine binding to D_2 receptors is highest in the dorsal hippocampus (Hipp), visible in the visual cortex, and present at lower densities in the ventral hippocampus (V-Hipp) and in area 35/36. Binding is not observed in the entorhinal cortex (Ent Ctx). The dark-field photographs of [^{3}H]SCH 23390 and [^{125}I]epidepride binding show regions of high binding as ligher than areas of sparse binding.

41

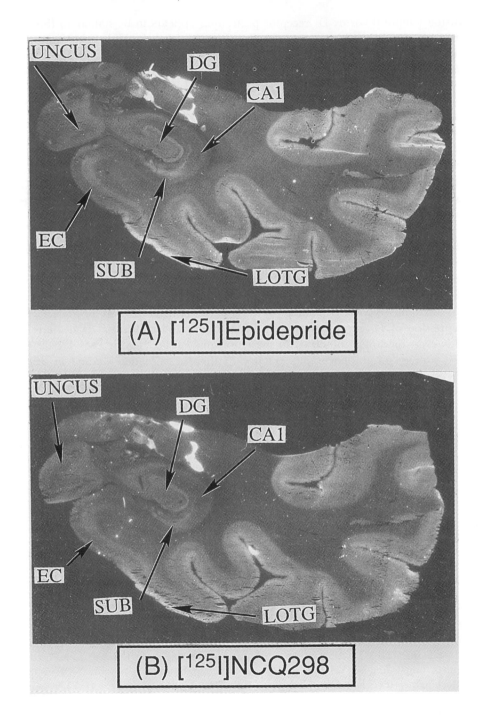

in dorsal hippocampus. The cortex lateral to the entorhinal cortex, lateral occipitotemporal gyrus (LOTG), shows a trilaminar pattern of binding with highest levels in the internal layers, middle layers the least, and external layers less than the internal laminae. The Timm's histochemical demonstration of the mossy fibres reveals an intriguing complementary pattern to the D$_2$ receptors in cat and human, but not in rat (Figure 8). In the cat, the hippocampal mossy fibre system is composed of the axons of the granule cells of the dentate gyrus which synapse with pyramidal cells of the CA3 subfield. The Timm's staining is observed in the dentate gyrus extending through CA3 in the mossy fibre zone, ending obliquely at the CA3–CA2 border. Binding to D$_2$ receptors is seen in the facia dentata, the lamina of the dendrites of the dentate granule cells complementary to the Timm's staining over the granule cell layer. The Timm's staining is intense throughout the hilus, but the D$_2$ binding is low in external hilus and higher in a circumscribed region where the mossy fibres leave the hilus. The Timm's staining in human tissue is suggestive of a similar relationship to that seen in the cat. Thus, it is unlikely that the D$_2$ receptors in the dentate gyrus are synthesized by the granule cells, but they may reside on the axons terminating in this region from the entorhinal cortex or LOTG.

The pattern of D$_2$ and D$_1$ receptors in the parahippocampal gyrus may be unique to mammals with cortices that are predominantly for visual functions. D$_1$ and D$_2$ receptors show a complex pattern of organization in the visual cortex of the monkey (Lidow et al., 1991), cat (Figure 6) and human brain (Cortes et al., 1989). Secondary visual cortical regions show a predominance of D$_2$ receptors in cat (Figure 6) and human (Figure 7) (Joyce et al., 1991a), which send efferents to the lateral occipitotemporal cortex (area 35/36). The entorhinal cortex and adjacent lateral occipitotemporal cortex are the major relay stations for cortical input to the hippocampus and represent sites of action for DA in limbic cortex. These regions, and the subfields of the hippocampus, show a reciprocal organization of D$_1$ and D$_2$ receptors that is not observed in the rat. D$_1$ receptors predominate in the EC, particularly in layers that give rise to the perforant pathway that innervates the dentate gyrus. D$_2$ receptors predominate in the LOTG, also in layers that give rise to an innervation of the molecular layer of the dentate gyrus (DG). The DG in turn gives rise to the mossy fibre input to the CA3 subfield, both of which predominate in D$_2$ receptor expression. The CA3 subfield in turn provides the Schaeffer collateral system input to the CA1

Figure 7 The heterogeneous pattern of [^{125}I] epidepride binding (A) and [^{125}I] NCQ298 binding (B) to D$_2$ receptors in the medial temporal lobe of the human brain. The pattern is similar with both radioligands. Highest binding in the hippocampus is in the dentate gyrus (DG) and subiculum (SUB). As in the cat there is a notable absence of binding in the entorhinal cortex (EC), with the distinct trilaminar pattern in the lateral occipitotemporal gyrus (LOTG). Binding in inferior and middle temporal gyrus also showed the trilaminar pattern but is less distinct.

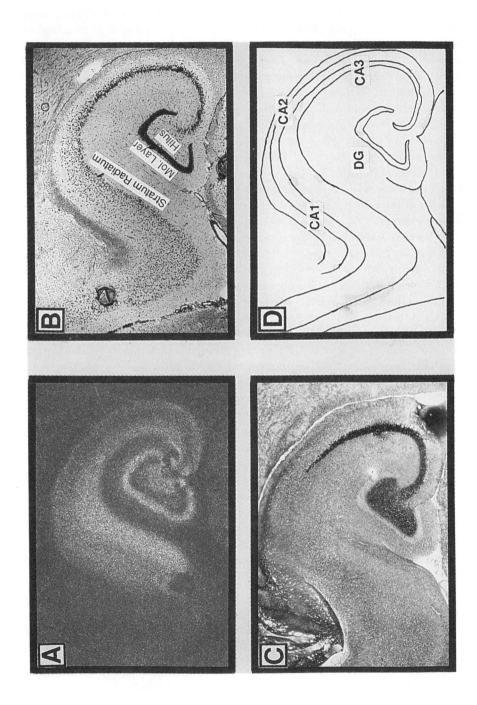

subfield, which expresses D_1 receptors and few D_2 receptors. The CA1 projects predominantly to the subiculum, which is enriched in D_2 receptors, and the subiculum gives rise to the major efferents of the hippocampal complex. Thus, D_1 and D_2 receptor synapses could modify signal processing into, within and exiting the hippocampal complex. Given the important roles that the LOTG (Lüders *et al.*, 1991), entorhinal cortex (Van Hoesen, 1982) and hippocampus (Friedman and Goldman-Rakic, 1988) play in memory, it is likely that DA can modify memory functions in humans.

2.5 Conclusions

The neuroanatomical organization of DA receptors may provide important clues as to the functional interactions that can occur. In the striatum of all mammals the DA receptors and DA innervation respect the patch (striosome) and matrix organization. Additionally, there appears to be a separation of the types of neurones that express the subtypes of the D_1 and D_2 receptors. Consequently, models of D_1 and D_2 interactions must take into account the fact that neural systems within the basal ganglia are predominantly subserved by D_1 or D_2 receptor-linked synapses. Moreover, alterations in such interactions that occur with removal of DA may relate to the altered neural expression of the DA receptors. For example, following adult 6-OHDA lesions to the mesostriatal DA system there are altered D_1 and D_2 interactions that may arise from opposing

---

Figure 8 The pattern of D_2 receptors in the cat hippocampus (A) is compared with the distribution of cell bodies (B) and the mossy fibres (C) in this same region. The heterogeneous pattern of $[^{125}I]$epidepride binding to D_2 receptors revealed an intriguing complementary pattern with the histochemical demonstration of the mossy fibres. In cat, Timm's histochemical staining of the mossy fibres was observed in the dentate gyrus (DG) extending through CA3 in the mossy fibre zone, ending obliquely at the CA3–CA2 border (D). $[^{125}I]$Epidepride binding to D_2 receptors was clearly observed in the molecular layer of the dentate gyrus (facia dentata), the lamina of the dendrites of the DG granule cells, whereas the zinc histochemistry is denser over the granule cell layer. The binding of $[^{125}I]$epidepride to D_2 receptors is also denser in the subiculum and lacunosum radiatum of CA1 than in CA3. The Timm's histochemical staining of the mossy fibres is intense throughout the hilus and in the CA3 subfield, but the D_2 receptors are low in the external hilus and higher in a circumscribed region where the mossy fibres leave the hilus. The dark-field photograph of $[^{125}I]$epidepride binding show regions of high binding as lighter than areas of sparse binding (A), bright-field photograph of the histochemical demonstration of cell bodies with cresyl violet (B), bright-field photograph of the histochemical demonstration of mossy fibres with the Timm's stain (C), the diagrammatic demonstration of regions of the hippocampus and perirhinal region shown in the other figures (D).

changes in the expression of D_1 and D_2 receptors in the matrix-related striatal efferents and interneurones (Gerfen *et al.*, 1991; Joyce, 1991a, b). In contrast, 6-OHDA lesions in the neonate produce a more selective loss of the DA system innervating the patch compartment of the striatum, a loss of D_1 receptors in the patch compartment, no change in the expression of D_2 receptors and a D_1 receptor-mediated behavioural supersensitivity (Neal and Joyce, 1991, 1992).

To a significant degree the possibility that D_1 and D_2 interactions could occur outside the basal ganglia has been ignored. This is due, in part, to the relative importance placed on the rat as a model of the anatomy of DA systems. However, it is clear that the carnivore and primate differ in the expression of D_1 and D_2 receptors, as well as the DA afferents, within the cortex. There may well be complex interactions between neuronal systems that predominantly express these subtypes of the DA receptor. There are at least three regions where the interactions might be teased apart: the predominance of D_1-mediated effects in the frontal cortex and on its functions (e.g. Goldman-Rakic *et al.*, 1990; Lidow *et al.*, 1991); a predominance of D_2-mediated effects in the motor cortex (see above); and a complex interaction of DA with D_1 and D_2 receptors within the hippocampal complex (e.g. Joyce *et al.*, 1991b; Joyce, 1991c) that may reflect the differential contribution of input from the frontal cortex (D_1-mediated) and inferior temporal cortex (D_2-mediated; language and visual association memory). To test these hypotheses, non-rodent models will need to be developed.

References

Aiso, M., Potter, W.Z. & Saavedra, J.M. (1987) *Brain Res.* **426**, 392–396.

Altar, C.A. & Marien, M.R. (1987) *J. Neurosci.* **7**, 213–222.

Barone, P.I., Tucci, S.A., Parashos, S.A. & Chase, T.N. (1987) *Eur. J. Pharmacol.* **138**, 141–145.

Berger, B., Trottier, S., Verney, C., Gaspar, P. & Avarez, C. (1988) *J. Comp. Neurol.* **273**, 99–119.

Berger, B., Febvret, A., Greengard, P. & Goldman-Rakic, P.S. (1990) *J. Comp. Neurol.* **299**, 327–348.

Berger, B., Gaspar, P. & Verney, C. (1991) *Trends Neurosci.* **14**, 21–27.

Bertorello, A.M., Hopfield, J.F., Aperia, A.A. & Greengard, P. (1990) *Nature* **347**, 386–388.

Besson, M.-J., Graybiel, A.M. & Nastuk, M.A. (1988) *Neuroscience* **26**, 101–119.

Bischoff, S., Satton, B. & Korf, J. (1979) *Brain Res.* **165**, 161–165.

Boyson, S.J., McGonigle, P. & Molinoff, P.B. (1986) *J. Neurosci.* **6**, 31177–31188.

Brene, S., Lindefors, N., Herrera-Marschitz, M. & Persson, H. (1990) *Exp. Brain Res.* **83**, 96–104.

Camps, M., Cortes, R., Gueye, B., Probst, A. & Palacios, J.M. (1989) *Neuroscience* **28**, 275–290.

Camus, A., Javoy-Agid, F., Dubois, A. & Scatton, B. (1986) *Brain Res.* **375**, 135–149.

Civelli, O., Bunzow, J.R., Grandy, D.K., Zhou, Q.-Y. & Van Tol, H.H.M. (1991) *Eur. J. Pharmacol.* **207**, 277–286.

Cortés, R., Gueye, B., Pazos, A., Probst, A. & Palacios, J.M. (1989) *Neuroscience* **28**, 263–273.

Creese, I. (1982) *TINS* **5**, 40–43.

Creese, I., Prosser, T. & Snyder, S.H. (1978) *Life Sci.* **23**, 405–500.

Cross, A.J. & Waddington, J.L. (1981) *Eur. J. Pharmacol.* **71**, 327–332.

Dahlstrom, A. & Fuxe, K. (1964a) *Acta Physiol. Scand.* **60**, 293.

Dahlstrom, A. & Fuxe, K. (1964b) *Acta Physiol. Scand.* **62** (supplement 232), 1.

Dawson, T.M., Gehlert, D.R., McCabe, R.T., Barnett, A. & Wamsley, J.K. (1968a) *J. Neurosci.* **6**, 2352–2365.

Dawson, T.M., Barone, P., Sidhu, A., Wamsley, J.K. & Chase, T.N. (1986b) *Neurosci. Lett.* **68**, 261–266.

Dawson, V.L., Dawson, T.M., Filloux, F.M. & Wamsley, J.K. (1988) *Life Sci.* **42**, 1933–1939.

De Keyser, J., Claeys, A., De Backer, J.-P., Ebinger, G., Roels, F. & Vauquelin, G. (1988) *Neurosci. Lett.* **91**, 142–147.

Falck, B., Hillarp, N.A., Thieme, G. & Torp, A. (1962)*J. Histochem. Cytochem.* **10**, 348.

Fallon, J.H. & Moore, R.Y. (1978) *J. Comp. Neurol.* **180**, 545–580.

Febvret, A., Berger, B., Gaspar, P. & Verney, C. (1991) *Brain Res.* **547**, 37–52.

Filloux, F.M., Wamsley, J.K. & Dawson, T.M. (1987) *Eur. J. Pharmacol.* **138**, 61–68.

Fremeau, R.T., Duncan, G.E., Fornaretto, M.-G., Dearry, A., Gingrich, J.A., Breese, G.R. & Caron, M.G. (1991) *Proc. Natl Acad. Sci. USA*, **88**, 3772–3776.

Friedman, H.R. & Goldman-Rakic, P.S. (1988) *J. Neurosci.* **8**, 4693–4706.

Gaspar, P., Berger, B., Febvret, A., Vigny, A. & Henry, J.P. (1989) *Comp. Neurol.* **279**, 249–271.

Gaspar, P., Duyckaerts, C., Alvarez, C., Javoy-Agid, F. & Berger, B. (1991) *Ann. Neurol.* **30**, 365–374.

Gerfen, C.R., Herkenham, M. & Thiabault, J. (1987) *J. Neurosci.* **7**, 3915–3934.

Gerfen, C.R., Engber, T.M., Mahan, L.C., Susel, Z., Chase, T.N., Monsma, F.J. Jr & Sibley, D.R. (1990) *Science* **250**, 1429–1432.

Goldman-Rakic, P.S. (1982) *J. Comp. Neurol.* **205**, 398–413.

Goldman-Rakic, P.A., Lidow, M.S. & Gallager, D.W. (1990) *J. Neurosci.* **10**, 2125–2138.

Goldsmith, S., Frohna, P.A. & Joyce, J.N. (1991) *Soc. Neurosci. Abstr.* **17**, 414.

Graybiel, A.M. & Ragsdale, C.W. (1978) *Proc. Natl Acad. Sci. USA* **75**, 5723–5726.

Graybiel, A.M., Hirsch, E.C. & Agid, Y.A. (1987) *Proc. Natl Acad. Sci. USA* **84**, 303–307.

Graybiel, A.M. (1986) In: *Neuropeptides in Neurologic and Psychiatric Disease* (eds Martin, J.B. & Barchas, J.D.) pp 135–161. Raven Press, New York.

Graybiel, A.M. (1990) *Trends in Neurosci.* **13**, 244–254.

Herkenham, M. & Pert, C.B. (1981) *Nature* **291**, 415–417.

Hökfelt, T., Johansson, O. & Goldstein, M. (1985) In *Handbook of Chemical Neuroanatomy*, vol. 2 (eds Bjorklun, A. & Hökfelt, T.), p 157. Amsterdam, Elsevier.

Javitch, J.A., Strittmatter, S.M. & Snyder, S.H. (1985) *J. Neurosci.* **5**, 1513–1521.

Jimenez-Castellanos, J. & Graybiel, A.M. (1987) *Neurosci.* **23**, 223–242.

Joyce, J.N. (1991a) *Exp. Neurol.* **113**, 261–276.

Joyce, J.N. (1991b) *Exp. Neurol.* **113**, 277–290.

Joyce, J.N. (1991c) *Soc. Neurosci. Abstr.* **17**, 415

Joyce, J.N. & Hurtig, H. (1990) *Prog. Brain Res.* **82**, 699–706.

Joyce, J.N. & Marshall, J.F. (1985) *Neurosci. Lett.* **53**, 127–131.

Joyce, J.N. & Marshall, J.F. (1987) *Neuroscience* **20**, 773–795.

Joyce, J.N., Lexow, N., Bird, E. & Winokur, A. (1988) *Synapse* **2**, 546–557.

Joyce, J.N., Loeschen, S. & Marshall, J.F. (1985) *Brain Res.* **338**, 209–218.

Joyce, J.N., Marshall, J.F., Bankiewicz, K.S., Kopin, I.J. & Jacobowitz, D.M. (1986a) *Brain Res.* **382**, 360–364.

Joyce, J.N., Sapp, D.W. & Marshall, J.F. (1986b) *Proc. Natl Acad. Sci. USA* **83**, 8002–8006.

Joyce, J.N., Janowski, A. & Neve, K.A. (1991a) *J. Pharmacol. Exp. Ther.* **253**, 1253–1263.

Joyce, J.N., Hensler, J.G. & Tejani-Butt, S.M. (1991b) In *Methods in Neurosciences*, vol. 7 (ed. Conn, P.M.), pp 216–240. San Diego, CA, Academic Press.

Joyce, J.N., Lexow, N., Kim, S.J., Artymysh, R., Lawrence, D., Cassanova, M., Kleinman, J., Bird, E. & Winokur, A. (1992) *Synapse* **10**, 228–246.

Kebabian, J.W. & Calne, D.B. (1979) *Nature* **277**, 93–96.

Kebabian, J.W., Petzold, G.L. & Greengard, P.L. (1972) *Proc. Natl Acad. Sci. USA* **69**, 2145–2149.

Kebabian, J.W., Calne, D.B. & Kebabian, P.R. (1977) *Commun. Psychopharmacol.* **1**, 311–318.

Köhler, C., Ericson, H. & Radesäter, A.-C. (1991) *Neurosci. Lett.* **126**, 107–109.

Kuhar, M.J., Murrin, C.L., Malouf, A.T. & Klemm, N. (1978) *Life Sci.* **22**, 203–210.

Langer, L.F. & Graybiel, A.M. (1989) *Brain Res.* **498**, 344–350.

Lavoie, B. & Parent, A. (1990) *J. Comp. Neurol.* **299**, 1–16.

Leff, S., Adams, L., Hyttel, J. & Creese, I. (1981) *Eur. J. Pharmacol.* **70**, 71–75.

Lehman, J., Briley, M. & Langer, S.Z. (1983) *Eur. J. Pharmacol.* **88**, 11–26.

LeMoine, C. & Bloch, B. (1991) *Mol. Brain Res.* **10**, 283–289.

LeMoine, C., Normand, E., Guitteny, A.F., Fouque, B., Teoule, R. & Bloch, B. (1990a) *Proc. Natl Acad. Sci. USA* **87**, 230–234.

LeMoine, C., Tison, F. & Bloch, B. (1990b) *Neurosci. Lett.* **117**, 248–252.

Lewis, D.A., Campbell, M.J., Foote, S.L. & Morrison, J.H. (1986) *Hum. Neurobiol.* **5**, 181–188.

Lidow, M.S., Goldman-Rakic, P.S., Rakic, P. & Innis, R.B. (1989) *Proc. Natl Acad. Sci. USA* **86**, 6412–6416.

Lidow, M.S., Goldman-Rakic, P.S., Gallager, D.W. & Rakic, P. (1991) *Neuroscience* **40**, 657–671.

Loopuijt, L.D. (1989) *Brain Res. Bull.* **22**, 805–817.

Lowenstein, P.R., Slesinger, P.A., Singer, H.S., Walkder, L.C., Casanova, M.F., Raskin, L.S., Price, D.L. & Coyle, J.T. (1989) *J. Comp. Neurol* **288**, 428–446.

Lowenstein, P.R., Joyce, J.N., Coyle, J.T. & Marshall, J.F. (1990) *Brain Res.* **510**, 122–126.

Luabeya, M.K., Maloteaux, J.-M. & Laduron, P.M. (1984) *J. Neurochem.* **43**, 1068–1071.

Lüders, H., Lesser, R.P., Hahn, L., Dinner, D.S., Morris, H.H., Wyllie, E. & Godoy, J. (1991) *Brain* **114**, 743–754.

Mansour, A., Meador-Woodruff, J.H., Bunzow, J.R., Civelli, O., Akil, H. & Watson, S.J. (1990) *J. Neurosci.* **10**, 2587–2600.

Mansour, A., Meador-Woodruff, J.H., Ahou, Q.-Y., Civelli, O., Akil, H. & Watson, S.J. (1991) *Neuroscience*, **45**, 359–371.

Marshall, J.F., O'Dell, S.J., Navarrete, R. & Rosenstein, A.J. (1990) *Neuroscience* **37**, 11–21.

Martin, L.J., Hadfield, M.G., Dellovade, T.L. & Price, D.L. (1991) *Neuroscience* **43**, 397–417.

Matres, M.-P., Bouthenet, M.-L., Sales, N., Sokoloff, P. & Schwartz, J.-C. (1985) *Science* **228**, 752–755.

McCulloch, J., Savaki, H.E., McCulloch, M.C. & Sokoloff, L. (1979) *Nature* **282**, 303–305.

McGeer, E.G., Innanen, V.T. & McGeer, P.L. (1976) *Brain Res.* **118**, 356–358.

Meador-Woodruff, J.H. & Mansour, A. (1991) *Biol. Psychiatry*, **30**, 985–1007.

Mengod, G., Martinez-Mir, M.I., Vilaro, M.T. & Palacios, J.M. (1989) *Proc. Natl Acad. Sci. USA* **86**, 8560–8564.

Mengod, G., Vilaro, M.T., Niznik, H.B., Sunahara, R.K., Seeman, P., O'Dowd, B.F. & Palacios, J.M. (1991) *Mol. Brain Res.* **10**, 185–191.

Milner, T.A. & Bacon, C.E. (1989) *J. Comp. Neurol.* **281**, 479–495.

Murray, A.M., Roo, H. & Joyce, J. (1992) *Eur. J. Pharmacol. Mol. Pharmacol. Sect.* **227**, 443–445.

Murrin, L.C. & Zeng, W. (1989) *Brain Res.* **480**, 170–177.

Neal, B.S. & Joyce, J.N. (1991) *Dev. Brain Res.* **60**, 105–113.

Neal, B.S. & Joyce, J.N. (1992) *Synapse* **11**, 35–46.

Pierei, L., Keller, H.H., Burkard, W. & Da Prada, M. (1978) *Nature,* **272**, 278–280.

Rao, P., Molinoff, P.B. & Joyce, J.N. (1991) *Dev. Brain Res.* **60**, 161–177.

Richfield, E.K., Young, A.B. & Penney, J.B. (1987) *J. Comp. Neurol.* **262**, 446–463.

Richfield, E.K., Young, A.B. & Penney, J.B. (1989) *J. Comp. Neurol.* **286**, 409–426.

Rhodes, K.J., Joyce, J.N., Sapp, D.W. & Marshall, J.F. (1987) *Brain Res.* **412**, 400–404.

Ruberg, M., Bokobza, B., Javoy-Agid, F., Montfort, J.C. & Agid, Y. (1984) *Eur. J. Pharmacol.* **99**, 159–165.

Saldate, M.C. & Orrego, F. (1977) *Brain Res.* **130**, 483–494.

Samson, Y., Wu, J.J., Friedman, A.H. & Davis, J.N. (1990) *J. Comp. Neurol.* **298**, 250–263.

Savasta, M., Dubois, A., Benavides, J. & Scatton, B. (1986) *Neurosci. Lett.* **72**, 265–271.

Schwarcz, R. & Köhler, C. (1983) *Neurosci. Lett.* **38**, 85–90.

Schwarcz, R., Creese, I., Coyle, J.R. & Snyder, S.H. (1978) *Nature* **271**, 766–768.

Schwarcz, R., Fuxe, K., Hökfelt, T., Terenius, L. & Goldstein, M. (1980) *J. Neurochem.* **34**, 772–778.

Simon, H., LeMoal, M. & Calas, A. (1979) *Brain Res.* **178**, 17–40.

Sokoloff, P., Giros, B., Matres, M.-P., Bouthenet, M.-L. & Schwartz, J.-C. (1990) *Nature* **347**, 146–151.

Stoof, T.C. & Kebabian, J.W. (1984) *Life Sci.* **35**, 2281–2296.

Swanson, L.W. (1982) *Brain Res. Bull.* **9**, 321–353.

Theodorou, A., Reavill, C., Jenner, P. & Marsden, C.D. (1981) *J. Pharm. Pharmacol.* **33**, 439–444.

Thibaut, F., Hirsch, E.C., Raisman, R., Javoy-Agid, F. & Agid, Y. (1990) *Neuroscience,* **37**, 387–398.

Torack, R.M. & Morris, J.C. (1990) *Neurosci. Lett.* **116**, 75–80.

Trugman, J.M., Geary, W.A. & Wooten, G.F. (1986) *Nature* **323**, 267–269.

Uchimura, N. & North, R.A. (1990) *Br. J. Pharmacol.* **99**, 736–740.

Van Hoesen, G.W. (1982) *Trends Neurosci.* **5**, 345–350.

Veening, J.G., Cornelissen, F.M. & Lieven, P.A.J.M. (1980) *Neuroscience* **5**, 1253–1268.

Voorn, P., Jorritsma-Byham, C., Van Dkjk & Buijs, R.M. (1986) *J. Comp. Neurol.* **251**, 84–89.

Weiner, D.M., Levey, A.I. & Brann, M.R. (1990) *Proc. Natl. Acad. Sci. U.S.A.* **87**, 7050–7054.

————————————— CHAPTER 3 —————————————

REGULATION OF UNCONDITIONED MOTOR BEHAVIOUR BY $D_1 : D_2$ INTERACTIONS

John L. Waddington and Siobhan A. Daly

Department of Clinical Pharmacology, Royal College of Surgeons in Ireland, St Stephen's Green, Dublin 2, Ireland

Table of Contents

DOPAMINE RECEPTOR INTERACTIONS
ISBN 0–12–729045–1

3.1 Evolution of the concept of $D_1:D_2$ interactions

3.1.1 The era of presumed D_2 prepotence

That dopamine (DA) plays a fundamental role in regulating a broad range of unconditioned, conditioned consummatory and other psychomotor behaviours has been, and remains, one of the most widely recognized facts in contemporary neuroscience and psychopharmacology. However, while more than 30 years of research (Carlsson, 1987) has sustained and elaborated this general concept, studies over the past 15 years have progressively engendered alternating cycles of insight and conjecture as to the precise nature of the behavioural processes and neuronal mechanisms involved.

At the level of unconditioned motor behaviour, the action of the classical DAergic drugs apomorphine and amphetamine in inducing syndromes of hyperactivity and stereotyped behaviour, which were sensitive to antagonism by DA receptor-blocking neuroleptic agents, was the basis of much early work seeking to clarify these issues. Though DA receptors were conceptualized initially as an essentially homogeneous entity, a number of subsequent functional considerations have led to several distinct proposals that there exist more than one form of DA receptor; however, none of these behaviourally based schemas for their subtyping has stood the test of time (Waddington and O'Boyle, 1989). Rather, the schema that was to dominate contemporary perspectives of DA receptor multiplicity, the D_1/D_2 classification of Kebabian and Calne (1979), had its origins in neurochemical and neuroanatomical considerations (Spano *et al.*, 1978); as a further complicating factor, at least in relation to putative functional dissociations, this classification emerged in the absence of any agent known to block the D_1 receptor selectively, and with only initial indications that a selective D_1 partial agonist might be available.

In the classical peripheral receptor systems we readily accept (and even expect) the phenomenon of double dissociation, such as the antagonism of a physiological response to a histaminergic H_2 agonist by a H_2 blocker but not by a H_1 blocker and vice versa. During this period, such a double dissociation strategy was simply not possible in relation to central DAergic function in the absence of any compound known to block D_1 receptors selectively. Behavioural distinctions between D_1 and D_2 receptors could, therefore, be probed only by two indirect methods: *correlational analysis,* whereby the pharmacological potencies of DA agonists and antagonists are compared with their affinities for D_1 and D_2 receptors, as determined usually in *in vitro* neurochemical or radioligand binding studies; or the *subtraction strategy,* whereby the pharmacological actions of selective D_2 agonists and antagonists are contrasted with those of drugs acting non-selectively at both D_1 and D_2 receptors. On the basis of (i) strong correlations between the behavioural potencies of both DA agonists and antagonists and their affinities for D_2 but not for D_1 receptors, and (ii) the ability of apparently selective D_2 agonists and antagonists to reproduce many of the actions of non-selective compounds, the D_2 receptor was ascribed a virtually exclusive role in the regulation of typical DAergic behaviours; additionally, the failure of the only available selective D_1 agent, the partial agonist SK & F 38393, to reproduce in the whole animal the actions of a classical non-selective agonist such as apomorphine (Setler et al., 1978) seemed to support the indirect corollary of D_2 prepotence, namely that the D_1 receptor had no known behavioural role (Seeman, 1980; Creese et al., 1983).

By further analogy with the classical peripheral receptor systems, this view would predict that these 'D_2-mediated' behaviours should show double dissociation in terms of insensitivity to selective D_1 antagonists, were they to be identified. With the introduction in 1983–1984 of SCH 23390 and R-SK & F 83566 as the first selective D_1 antagonists (Waddington, 1986), it rapidly became all too apparent that behavioural processes in intact adult animals are unexpectedly and powerfully influenced by these agents.

3.1.2 Recognition of the role of the D_1 receptor, and the anomalous findings

Initial studies with the selective D_1 antagonists SCH 23390 and R-SK & F 83566 surprisingly revealed that they readily reproduced the effects both of typical non-selective DA antagonists and of selective D_2 antagonists in a wide variety of typical behavioural paradigms in the whole animal: inhibition of stereotypy, hyperlocomotion and climbing induced not just by non-selective but also by D_2-selective agonists; induction of catalepsy; inhibition of spontaneous activity; inhibition of conditioned avoidance; inhibition of the discriminative stimulus properties of amphetamine; inhibition of intracranial self-stimulation. In contrast, the selective D_1 partial agonist SK & F 38393, especially its active R-enantiomer, failed to reproduce the behavioural effects of typical non-selective or D_2-selective agonists but induced fragmented episodes of non-stereotyped normal behaviours, including a particularly prominent grooming response; however, this profile of responses appeared sensitive to attenuation by D_2 as well as D_1 antagonists. The explanation offered (Molloy and Waddington, 1984; Christensen et al., 1984; Waddington, 1986) was that such similar and overlapping effects of D_1 and D_2 antagonists in the intact adult animal arise through functional interactions between D_1 and D_2 receptor systems.

However, in animals in whom the function of DA neurones had been eliminated by 6-hydroxydopamine (6-OHDA) lesions (unilateral or bilateral) or chronically interrupted by reserpine/α-methyl-p-tyrosine (αMPT), this profile appeared to be changed in at least two major respects: firstly, responses to selective D_1 agonists were more typical and similar to those of their D_2 counterparts, but were blocked only by selective D_1 antagonists. Thus, in animals chronically deprived of tonic DAergic activity, D_1 and D_2 receptor systems appeared to be no longer functionally linked to the same extent, but acted more as separate systems that could be independently manipulated with their respective agonists and antagonists. Furthermore, just as a selective D_1 antagonist could, in intact animals, block responses to a selective D_2 agonist, so a selective D_1 agonist (or D_1 receptor upregulation) was found to potentiate in a synergistic manner such D_2 agonist responses; temporary, *acute* interruption of tonic DAergic activity could only be fully overcome by concurrent stimulation of both D_1 and D_2 receptors. Collectively, these two patterns of results indicated the importance of both tonic and phasic D_1 receptor activation (as an 'enabling' or 'permissive' function) for the expression of behaviour(s) initiated through D_2 receptor stimulation; it should be noted that it is difficult to induce classical compulsive stereotyped behaviour with selective D_2 agonists, though it is readily induced by non-selective agonists such as apomorphine. The ability of selective D_2 antagonists to influence responses to a selective D_1 agonist in intact animals illustrated a possible reciprocity in the effects of endogenous and pharmacological stimulation of D_1 and D_2 receptors in the regulation of typical motor behaviours. The issue of the extent to which there exists synergism between D_1 and D_2 agonists in rats with unilateral 6-OHDA lesions or reserpine/α-MPT pretreatment is less straightforward (see Section 3.3.3) though, as previously discussed, the actions of selective antagonists were evident only against their respective selective agonists in such preparations. This suggested a somewhat complex relationship between endogenous DAergic function, its *acute* attenuation, and more *chronic* interruption perhaps sufficient to invoke adaptive (supersensitive?) responses, in determining the presence and the nature of cooperative/synergistic functional interactions between D_1 and D_2 systems in terms of typical motor behaviours. The multiple studies whose results are summarized above have been documented in a series of extensive reviews (Waddington, 1986; Breese and Creese, 1986; Waddington and O'Boyle, 1987; Arnt, 1987; Clark and White, 1987).

3.2 Elaboration of the concept of cooperative/synergistic $D_1 : D_2$ interactions

3.2.1 Scope, nature and sites of $D_1 : D_2$ interactions

In substantial measure, subsequent data have offered sustenance to and elaboration of such concepts (though, as in most areas of scientific enquiry, the picture that emerges ultimately is not always as clear as that initially envisaged; see Sections 3.3 and 3.4). A large number of studies have confirmed these *basic* notions of putative $D_1 : D_2$ interactions as outlined above, almost exclusively in laboratory rats and mice; a number of these in the second half of the 1980s have been reviewed previously (Waddington, 1989; Waddington and O'Boyle, 1989), and additional studies have continued to report generally similar phenomena in terms of typical D_1 (usually SK & F 38393) and D_2 (usually quinpirole or RU 24213) agonist-driven motor paradigms (Moore and Axton, 1988; Vasse et al., 1988; Ross et al., 1988, 1989; Pierce and Rebec, 1990; Abbott et al., 1991; Zarrindast and Naghashi, 1991), motor paradigms involving synergism between D_1 and D_2 antagonists (Parashos et al., 1989a; Dall'Olio et al., 1989; Wanibuchi and Usuda, 1990; Chandler et al., 1990a), or novel motor paradigms (Arnt and Hyttel, 1989; Giorgi and Biggio, 1990). Furthermore, there is a preliminary report of apparently indistinguishable $D_1:D_2$ interactions in the regulation of bladder motility (Kontani et al., 1990). In summary, studies in intact, adult rats and mice (and chicks; Zarrindast and Amin (1992)) indicate that the level of D_1 tone appears to exert important qualitative and quantitative cooperative/synergistic control of D_2-stimulated motor activity and 'enables' or 'permits' the full expression of such DA-dependent behaviour; more controversially, the level of D_2 tone may exert some influence in the same direction on the expression of certain D_1-stimulated motor behaviours (Section 3.5.3). Furthermore, the consequence of temporary, acute interruption of tonic DAergic activity can only be fully overcome by concurrent stimulation of both D_1 and D_2 receptors and, after short reserpinization, residual responses to D_1 and D_2 agonists are sensitive to antagonists acting selectively at either site; however, after prolonged reserpinization, responses to D_1 and D_2 agonists are heightened and sensitive only to their respective antagonists. This latter profile is similar to that evident after 6-OHDA lesions, and suggests a functional dissociation of striatal D_1 and D_2 receptors in such circumstances, at least in terms of antagonist sensitivity.

As initially conceived, such apparent $D_1:D_2$ interactions in the regulation of unconditioned motor behaviours were without mechanistic support. However, a prominent feature of the immediate subsequent period was the emergence of a body of electrophysiological data which indicated generally comparable profiles of cooperative/synergistic $D_1:D_2$ interaction in the regulation of cell firing in the striatum, nucleus accumbens and globus pallidus (Waddington and O'Boyle, 1987, 1989; Clark and White, 1987; Walters et al., 1987; Wachtel et al., 1989). Correspondingly, in terms of the anatomical regulation of individual motor phenomena or motor syndromes, intracerebral injection studies have indicated local synergistic/cooperative $D_1:D_2$ interactions within: (i) the striatum, particularly its ventral rather than dorsal extent, in the mediation of stereotyped sniffing and head-weaving (Starr, 1988), stereotyped sniffing and self-directed oral activity (Bordi and Meller, 1989; Delfs and Kelley, 1990) and rotational behaviour in unlesioned animals (Koshikawa et al., 1990a; Konitsiotis and Kafetzopoulos, 1990); (ii) the striatum and nucleus accumbens, in the mediation of locomotion (Starr, 1988; Dreher and Jackson, 1989; Plaznik et al., 1989); (iii) the ventral striatum, nucleus accumbens and globus pallidus, in the mediation of stereotyped jaw movements (Koshikawa et al., 1989, 1990b). To complement these behavioural and electrophysiological findings, counterpart cooperative/synergistic $D_1:D_2$ interactions have recently been identified in the regulation of neurochemical processes as diverse as striatal Na^+/K^+-ATPase activity (Bertorello *et al.*, 1990), release of ascorbic acid (Pierce and Rebec, 1990), and release of archidonic acid (Piomelli *et al.*, 1991).

It must be noted that other authors have argued for such interactions having their basis in D_1 and D_2 receptors that are located in anatomically distinct sites; thus, Robertson and Robertson (1987) and LaHoste and Marshall (1990) have offered evidence that typical $D_1:D_2$ synergism involves D_1 receptors located in the substantia nigra and D_2 receptors located in the striatum. However, neuroanatomical studies on the extent to which D_1 and D_2 receptors are or are not located on distinct populations of striatonigral and striatopallidal neurones that constitute non-overlapping efferent systems (Gerfen, 1992), together with functional studies on the extent to which such efferents do or do not subserve distinct D_1- and D_2-mediated behavioural processes (Fletcher and Starr, 1987, 1989; Ogren and Fuxe, 1988; Starr, 1988), are not conclusive on this issue; furthermore, the studies reviewed above constitute a substantial (though also not conclusive) body of evidence consistent with the alternative perspective. There remains the fundamental question of the extent to which D_1 and D_2 receptors are or are not expressed within the same cell and thus do or do not demonstrate co-localization in the same membrane (Section 3.5.2).

3.2.2   'Autoreceptor-selective' D_2 agonists and $D_1:D_2$ interactions

The ability of very low doses of DA agonists such as apomorphine to induce hypomotility, with yawning and inhibition of exploratory activity, has long been presumed to involve their action in stimulating D_2 (cell body and presynaptic terminal) autoreceptors which mediate the inhibition of DAergic cell firing and of the synthesis and release of DA; the inhibitory electrophysiological effects of low doses of D_2 agonist drugs at these sites, together with their behavioural actions in inducing hypomotility, were insensitive to D_1 antagonists, and thus suggested that D_2 autoreceptor effects were not regulated by $D_1:D_2$ interactions (Waddington and O'Boyle, 1989; Wachtel *et al.*, 1989; Lappalainen *et al.*, 1990).

However, yawning induced by low doses of D_2 agonists did appear sensitive to blockade by selective D_1 as well as selective D_2 antagonists, while reserpinization attenuated the yawning response and resulted in a loss of such sensitivity to D_1 antagonists; this profile was much more consistent with a basis in stimulation of postsynaptic rather than presynaptic D_2 receptors. Furthermore, drugs such as B-HT 920, which were initially proposed to be selective presynaptic D_2 agonists essentially devoid of action at stimulatory postsynaptic D_2 receptors when given alone to the whole animal, were noted to induce hyperactivity and stereotyped behaviour when given in combination with a selective D_1 agonist; this suggested the 'unmasking' by the D_1 agonist of covert postsynaptic activity through $D_1:D_2$ synergism (Waddington and O'Boyle, 1989). Subsequent behavioural studies (Arnt *et al.*, 1988a; Jackson *et al.*, 1989a, b; Anden and Grabowska-Anden, 1988, 1990; Arnt and Hyttel, 1990) have confirmed these findings and have elaborated the schema whereby such putative D_2

'autoreceptor-selective' agonists appear devoid of postsynaptic effects in the whole animal due to inhibition of DA release that would normally be available to tonically activate D_1 receptors but now cannot 'enable' their postsynaptic D_2 effects via synergistic $D_1:D_2$ interactions; electrophysiological data support such a schema (Johansen *et al.*, 1988).

These data and interpretations thereof comprise one element in a greater body of evidence which now questions the existence of D_2 'autoreceptor-selective' drugs (Drukarch and Stoof, 1990); it has been proposed that effects such as yawning and inhibition of exploratory behaviour induced by such putative agents are in fact mediated by one or more population(s) of a postsynaptic D_2 receptor that appears distinct from those involved in classical DAergic behavioural syndromes such as stereotypy, at least in the absence of concurrent stimulation of D_1 receptors (Yamada *et al.*, 1990; Stahle, 1992).

3.3 Complexities in cooperative/synergistic $D_1:D_2$ interactions

Though the extensive evidence marshalled above is clearly supportive of the general notion of cooperative/synergistic $D_1:D_2$ interactions, items of detail now indicate this scheme to be potentially more complex than envisaged originally.

3.3.1 Complexities in acute treatment paradigms

There is some evidence that selective D_1 and D_2 agonists administered together by a peripheral route do not necessarily act synergistically to induce a syndrome of typical stereotyped behaviour indistinguishable from that induced by classical non-selective DA agonists such as apomorphine; for example, they may act synergistically in the induction of sniffing but not of oral activity, at least in some rat strains (Meller *et al.*, 1988) and, when evident, oral behaviours induced by co-stimulation of D_1 and D_2 receptors can be qualitatively as well as quantitatively different from that induced by stimulation of either receptor alone (Koshikawa *et al.*, 1991). Furthermore, intracerebral injection studies suggest that the 'D_2-enabling' effect of striatal D_1 receptor activation may not regulate all elements of stereotypy that are usually associated with striatal DAergic hyperfunction; there can be synergism in relation to sniffing and self-directed oral activity, but this may not extend to typical biting, licking and gnawing stereotypies (Starr, 1988; Bordi and Meller, 1989). At the level of striatal electrophysiology, concurrent iontophoretic application of D_1 and D_2 agonists has been noted to give an additive rather than a synergistic effect, though synergism was evident in the striatum following intravenous co-administration (Hu and Wang, 1988; but see Wachtel *et al.*, 1989). Thus, it is possible that the action of classical DA agonists such as apomorphine in inducing compulsive stereotyped behaviour involves mechanism(s) additional to co-stimulation of D_1 and D_2 receptors, and/or that peripherally administered D_1 and D_2 agonists act synergistically via the integration of co-stimulatory effects in more than one DAergically innervated target area.

An alternative level of complexity related to the adoption of differing interpretations and terminologies for what appear to be comparable behavioural profiles. For example, the co-administration of increasing doses of a D_1 agonist with a D_2 agonist can initially transform the expansive D_2 locomotor response to a perseverative one confined to the perimeter of the test arena (an indicator of locomotor stereotypy (Schiorring 1979)) while, at higher doses, locomotion can cease and be replaced by fixation sniffing, licking and biting (Eilam *et al.*, 1991, 1992); these authors interpret such loss of locomotion as indicating an inhibitory effect of D_2 stimulation on this D_2 response, while others would regard it as a stage in the transition from one phase to another of the synergistic potentiation of stereotypy.

On the basis of a bimodal (enhancement then inhibition) effect of the selective D_2 antagonist sulpiride on locomotor responses to the non-selective DA agonist pergolide after αMPT pretreatment, and of an inverse bimodal (inhibition then enhancement) effect of quinpirole on the locomotor response to SK & F 38393 after reserpinization (to remove the potential confounding effects of tonic release of DA), Rubinstein *et al.* (1988a, b) have suggested that there may exist two different populations of D_2 receptor, either located on the same cell or with differing functional topographies, which in some circumstances mediate opposite functions. This profile has not proved entirely replicable in another laboratory (Starr and Starr, 1989); however, these investigators have presented evidence suggesting that sulpiride and its related selective D_2 antagonist metoclopramide may occlude differing populations of D_2 receptors in interaction studies with SCH 23390 (Chandler *et al.*, 1990a) and may reveal locomotor-stimulating and locomotor-inhibiting D_2 receptors in interaction studies with SK & F 38393, the latter also being facilitated by concurrent D_1 receptor activation (Chandler *et al.*, 1990b).

Though selective inactivation of D_2 receptors (using N-ethoxycarbonyl-2-ethoxy-1,2-dihydroquinoline (EEDQ) and protection of D_1 receptors with SCH 23390) decreases typical behavioural responses both to apomorphine and to quinpirole, the extent to which selective inactivation of D_1 receptors (using EEDQ and protection of D_2 receptors with raclopride) decreases these same responses is less clear; there may be a significant D_1 receptor reserve in cooperative $D_1 : D_2$ interactions (Arnt *et al.*, 1989b; Double and Crocker, 1990). Whether selective inactivation of D_2 receptors can decrease characteristic behavioural responses to D_1 agonists such as SK & F 38393 relates to further complexities and current issues to be considered below (Sections 3.4.2 and 3.5.3). Furthermore, there is preliminary evidence that EEDQ may only destabilize the D_1 receptor *in vivo*, with inactivation occurring only during *in vitro* preparation of tissue for subsequent neurochemical analyses (Andersen, 1988).

3.3.2 Complexities in chronic treatment paradigms

Repeated treatment with SCH 23390 results in the selective upregulation of D_1 but not of D_2 receptors, while repeated treatment with preferential or selective D_2 antagonists upregulates D_2 but not D_1 receptors, and there has been considerable interest in the behavioural consequences thereof in relation to $D_1 : D_2$ interactions (Waddington and O'Boyle, 1989). In one study, repeated treatment with the selective D_2 antagonist YM 09151 heightened both apomorphine stereotypy and quinpirole-induced motility, but not SK & F 38393-induced grooming while repeated treatment with SCH 23390 heightened apomorphine stereotypy and the extent of synergism produced by co-administration of the selective agonists, but not the consequences of their individual administration; one interpretation offered was that the behavioural expression of D_1 receptor supersensitivity requires the simultaneous activation of both D_1 and D_2 receptors (Gandolfi *et al.*, 1988; Dall'Olio *et al.*, 1988). However, Parashos *et al.* (1990) have recently reported that repeated treatment with SCH 23390 *can* heighten SK & F 38393-induced grooming, while repeated treatment with haloperidol attenuated this response; additionally, repeated co-administration of both antagonists failed to influence the grooming response to SK & F 38393. This latter finding could be a functional counterpart of earlier reports that repeated haloperidol or sulpiride co-administration reduces the ability of repeated SCH 23390 to upregulate D_1 receptor binding in most brain regions (Parashos *et al.*, 1987; McGonigle *et al.*, 1989). Furthermore, haloperidol- and SCH 23390-induced DAergic hypersensitivities to apomorphine appear similar but not additive (Parashos *et al.*, 1989b), while repeated co-treatment with sulpiride and a low dose of SCH 23390 gives synergistic blockade of the apomorphine response during such treatment but no evidence of supersensitivity thereafter (Dall'Olio *et al.*, 1990). Such interactive effects in chronic antagonist paradigms, and elsewhere (Cameron and Crocker, 1988), indicate an additional level of difficulty in specifying the totality of $D_1 : D_2$ interactions in behavioural terms.

In chronic agonist paradigms, the paradoxical phenomenon of behavioural sensitization, as reflected in the enhanced effects on repeated administration of DAergic agonists such as apomorphine, is well recognized but of uncertain mechanistic basis, and provides further fertile ground for the study of $D_1 : D_2$ interactions. Repeated treatment with SK & F 38393 can induce supersensitivity both in its own grooming response and in apomorphine stereotypy, while repeated treatment with quinpirole resulted in subsensitivity to apomorphine but was otherwise without prominent effect; these findings (Braun and Chase, 1988) were interpreted in terms of chronic D_1 receptor stimulation being pivotal in the development of DA agonist-induced behavioural sensitization (see also Mattingly *et al.* (1991)), with chronic D_2 receptor stimulation tending to have an opposite effect. Contemporaneously, Martin-Iverson *et al.* (1988) have reported tolerance to the motor-stimulant effects of the selective D_2 agonist PHNO that could be reversed by co-administration of SK & F 38393, suggesting that such tolerance may result from a loss of synergistic activation of D_1 receptors by endogenous DA. Subsequent studies have produced contradictory data as to whether repeated administration of SK & F 38393 does (White *et al.*, 1990) or does not (Neisewander *et al.*, 1991) result in an enhanced grooming response: in the former study, chronic SK & F 38393 enhanced not only grooming but also quinpirole-induced stereotypy, in general accordance with D_1 synergism of D_2-stimulated responses, and also enhanced the electrophysiological actions of both SK & F 38393 and quinpirole in the striatum; in the latter study, chronic SK & F 38393 not only failed to enhance grooming (though there was some enhancement of tongue protrusion) but also failed to influence either D_1 or D_2 receptor binding in relevant brain regions. As a counterpoint to these studies, it has recently been reported (Kelland *et al.*, 1991) that repeated administration of SK & F 38393 appears to produce electrophysiological densensitization of striatal D_1 receptors before withdrawal but sensitization thereafter; it is notable that White *et al.* (1990) did while Neisewander *et al.* (1991) did not utilize a withdrawal period, and thus their superficially discrepant results might be at least in part reconcilable in such terms.

3.3.3   Complexities in denervation paradigms

It is now well established that denervation of striatal DA receptors following 6-OHDA lesions results not only in the functional supersensitivity of both D_1 and D_2 receptors, but also in some functional uncoupling of these receptors; thus, after unilateral 6-OHDA lesions both D_1 and D_2 agonists induce rotational behaviour, but these responses are sensitive to blockade only by an antagonist of the receptor for the relevant agonist (Waddington and O'Boyle, 1989). This apparent functional uncoupling, under conditions of denervation and super-sensitivity, of at least these aspects of $D_1 : D_2$ interactions has a ready counterpart in the comparable effects of such lesions on the electrophysiological responses of striatal (Hu *et al.*, 1990) and globus pallidal (Carlson *et al.*, 1990) neurones to similar drug combinations.

However, there is evidence that after 6-OHDA lesions, other aspects of $D_1 : D_2$ interactions appear to endure; in particular, the ability of co-administered D_1 and D_2 agonists to act synergistically in the induction of rotational behaviour after unilateral 6-OHDA lesions has been reported in several studies (Robertson and Robertson, 1986; Sonsalla *et al.*, 1988), and such post-lesion synergism may be more sensitive to antagonism by sulpiride than by SCH 23390 (Rouillard and Bedard, 1988). Electrophysiological correlates of these particular effects at the level of the striatum are less clear, as the available evidence (Hu *et al.*, 1990) indicates that 6-OHDA lesions abolish the synergism normally evident on concurrent application of SK & F 38393 and quinpirole in this region; yet synergistic agonist interactions after 6-OHDA lesions can be seen at a more integrative level, e.g. in the substantia nigra, and indeed synergism may be evident in the nigra *only* following such lesions (Weick and Walters, 1987a, b).

Whether this represents the recruitment of alternative neuronal circuits to maintain these aspects of $D_1:D_2$ synergism after lesioning with 6-OHDA remains to be clarified. Furthermore, there remains the issue of specifying the mechanism(s) by which those functional $D_1:D_2$ interactions reflected in antagonist sensitivity appear decoupled while those reflected in agonist synergism appear considerably more resistant to such uncoupling in the same circumstances.

It should be noted that the action of SK & F 38393 in potentiating rotational responses to bromocriptine following unilateral 6-OHDA lesions increases with repeated administration of the D_1 agonist, suggesting that D_1 receptor activation can contribute to behavioural sensitization (Section 3.3.2) under conditions of denervation and resultant supersensitivity; in that process, it appears to downregulate D_2 receptors (Rouillard et al., 1988). At the electrophysiological level, repeated administration of quinpirole temporarily prevented the development of D_2 receptor supersensitivity after 6-OHDA lesions but did not prevent the associated loss of synergism, while repeated administration of SK & F 38393 temporarily prevented the development not only of both D_1 and D_2 supersensitivity but also of such synergism (Hu and White, 1992); this finding must be juxtaposed with the action of a co-administered D_2 antagonist in preventing D_1 receptor upregulation induced by repeated treatment with a D_1 antagonist (Section 3.3.2), and thus it is difficult to examine in detail the extent to which upregulation of both D_1 and D_2 receptors might result in uncoupling of $D_1:D_2$ interactions when there is integrity of presynaptic terminals.

3.3.4 Complexities in relation to other neurotransmitter systems

The ability of SK & F 38393 to act synergistically with and thus unmask the latent postsynaptic activity of the putative 'autoreceptor-selective' D_2 agonist B-HT 920 has already been discussed (see Section 3.2.2). It has been reported that the α_2-antagonists idazoxan, piperoxan and (at low doses) yohimbine exert a similar synergizing action; furthermore, idazoxan was able to additionally potentiate the response to the co-administration of SK & F 38393 and B-HT 920, to a level indistinguishable from that induced by co-administration of SK & F 38393 and quinpirole, though it did not potentiate the response to quinpirole alone (Johansen et al., 1988; Meltzer et al., 1989). The explanation offered for these findings was that the additional and potent α_2-agonist activity of B-HT 920 contributes in some way to masking its postsynaptic D_2 activity. However, Anden and Grabowska-Anden (1989) have reported that B-HT 958 acts synergistically with SK & F 38393, following reserpinization, in a manner similar to B-HT 920; as the pharmacology of B-HT 958 is very similar to that of B-HT 920, with the exception of it having α_2-antagonist rather than agonist activity, this would appear inconsistent with the above formulation. Also, B-HT 958 induces yawning in a manner similar to B-HT 920 (Ferrari et al., 1992), but the effect of D_1 receptor manipulation on this B-HT 958 response has yet to be examined.

On the basis of co-administering B-HT 920 and SK & F 38393 after reserpinization, Pichler and Pifl (1989) reported data that confirmed the action of co-stimulation of postsynaptic D_1 and D_2 receptors in eliciting motor activity in such animals, but came to the additional, indirect conclusion that endogenous noradrenaline (NA) might play a modulatory role. In a similar manner, NA receptor stimulation with clonidine was proposed as an alternative to D_1 stimulation in obtaining D_2-dependent motor responses in both normosensitive and supersensitive conditions; the blockade of such NA–DA synergism by prazosin indicated a basis in an α_1 mechanism (Rubinstein *et al.*, 1989). Similarly, prazosin blocked the locomotor stimulation (particularly biting, licking and grooming) induced by co-administration of SK & F 38393 and quinpirole (Singh and Jackson, 1990), while that induced by clonidine and quinpirole was blocked by prazosin and by raclopride, but not by idazoxane, yohimbine or SCH 23390 (Eshel *et al.*, 1990); it was thus suggested that α_1 activity may undergo synergism with D_2 stimulation at a location downstream from that at which D_1 stimulation can exert similar effects.

There is an emerging body of evidence that DA and glutamate act in functional opposition to regulate basal ganglia function, and that MK 801, a non-competitive antagonist of glutamate at the N-methyl-D-aspartate (NMDA) receptor, can greatly facilitate the locomotor-stimulatory properties of other pharmacological agents, including DAergic drugs (Carlsson and Carlsson, 1990). It has been reported that MK 801 potentiates D_1 but attenuates D_2 agonist-induced rotational behaviour in animals with unilateral 6-OHDA lesions (Morelli *et al.*, 1991a); similarly, MK 801 potentiates D_1-dependent but tends to inhibit D_2-dependent locomotion following reserpinization (Goodwin *et al.*, 1992). Such data suggest that there exists a role for α_1 (plus α_2?) NAergic and NMDA glutamatergic functions in processes known to be regulated by $D_1 : D_2$ interactions, and that α_1 and NMDA receptors may share a particular functional intimacy with D_2 and D_1 receptors, respectively.

3.4   The concept of oppositional $D_1 : D_2$ interactions

3.4.1   Regulation of atypical 'jerking' behaviour

As described by Grabowska-Anden and Anden (1983), both apomorphine and particularly B-HT 920 induced in reserpinized animals a syndrome of jerks of the head and upper trunk, during which the forepaws were usually lifted from the ground or, when very strong, the animals were propelled upwards using all four legs; this atypical response was blocked by D_2 antagonists but not by prazosin (selective D_1 antagonists were not then available), and was readily induced by injection of apomorphine or B-HT 920 into the nucleus accumbens but less so by their injection into the striatum. Such jerking was not seen after administration of these same drugs to intact animals, and it was speculated that endogenous DA might act at a population of DA receptors which was both distinct from that stimulated by B-HT 920 and inhibitory on the promotion of this behaviour.

Subsequently, such atypical jerking was reported to occur in response to apomorphine and particularly to D_2 agonists following pretreatment with SCH 23390 and (enantioselectively) with R- but not S-SK & F 83566, and to be inhibited by SK & F 38393 (Waddington et al., 1986; Grabowska-Anden and Anden, 1987; Murray and Waddington, 1989a). The apparent explanation was that endogenous DAergic activity through D_1 receptors exerts an inhibitory influence on the genesis of this behaviour in D_2 receptor stimulation, such that jerking is only evident when D_1 tone is blocked with a selective D_1 antagonist or removed by reserpinization; thus, this behaviour appears to be regulated by an oppositional D_1 : D_2 interaction. Recent studies have indicated such jerking to be induced by RU 24213 following pretreatment not just with SCH 23390 but with each of a range of new, chemically distinct selective D_1 antagonists (SCH 39166, NNC 756, A 69024 and BW 737C) to an extent proportional to their affinities and selectivities as D_1 antagonists; furthermore, since pretreatment with the selective D_2 antagonist YM 09151 (like SCH 23390, SCH 39166, NNC 756, A 69024 and BW 737C) reduced typical sniffing and locomotor responses to RU 24213, but *without* releasing jerking, release thereof does not occur through simple attenuation of competing behaviours (Daly and Waddington, 1982a, b). As selective D_1 antagonists release atypical jerking in response to a D_2 agonist while attenuating typical D_2 agonist-induced sniffing and locomotor responses, it appears that oppositional D_1 : D_2 interactions can be manifested contemporaneously with cooperative/ synergistic D_1 : D_2 interactions in the regulation of distinct elements of atypical and typical DAergic behaviours, respectively.

3.4.2 Regulation of atypical 'oral dyskinesia/vacuous chewing' behaviour

Rosengarten et al. (1983) reported the induction by acute SK & F 38393 administration of a syndrome of atypical oral dyskinesia characterized by repetitive opening and closing of the mouth and high-frequency clonic jaw movements; the same response was also induced by acute treatment with sulpiride or spiperone, and both D_2 antagonism and other decrements in D_2 function potentiated this response to SK & F 38393 while it was antagonized by a high, supramaximal dose of SCH 23390 (Rosengarten et al., 1986). This would be consistent with such atypical oral dyskinesia having its origin in (tonic or phasic) D_1 receptor stimulation but being regulated in an inhibitory manner by D_2 function. Oral movements (vacuous chewing) potentially similar to those reported by Rosengarten et al. (1983, 1986) as being induced by SK & F 38393 have been noted in some (e.g. Cameron et al., 1988) but not other (e.g.

Arnt *et al.*, 1987; Molloy and Waddington, 1987a; Murray and Waddington, 1989b) studies, while Neisewander *et al.* (1991) reported only tongue protrusions. Two other apparently positive reports (Johansson *et al.*, 1987; Glenthoj *et al.*, 1990) utilized a specific restraining system which renders most other motor behaviours impossible, and this may influence critically whether any such response to SK & F 38393 is or is not evident (Levin *et al.*, 1989); furthermore, another report found vacuous chewing to be induced not only by SK & F 38393 but also by D_2 agonists, D_2 antagonists and, paradoxically, by a high dose of SCH 23390 (Collins *et al.*, 1991). We have consistently failed to induce any such behaviour using a wide range of new D_1 agonist analogues of SK & F 38393 (SK & F 75670, SK & F 77434, SK & F 81297, SK & F 82958 and SK & F 83189) given alone (Murray and Waddington, 1989b; Daly and Waddington, 1992c), but do note that they induce vacuous chewing when D_2 receptors are contemporaneously blocked (Murray and Waddington, 1989b); this would be consistent with such atypical behaviour being regulated by an oppositional $D_1 : D_2$ interaction, in which D_2-mediated inhibition can be prepotent over D_1-mediated stimulation in its genesis.

When induced by SK & F 38393 given as sole treatment, repetitive jaw movements have been noted to endure even when the normal complement of striatal D_1 receptors has been reduced by 70% with EEDQ (Rosengarten *et al.*, 1989), indicating a substantial reserve thereof in the mediation of such behaviour; this would be consistent with evidence of a similarly large reserve in those striatal D_1 receptors involved in cooperative/synergistic $D_1 : D_2$ interactions (Arnt *et al.*, 1989b; Double and Crocker, 1990). These phenomena may have some origin in the dorsal striatum, where intracerebral injection of YM 09151 increased the frequency of apomorphine-induced jaw movements, an effect prevented by co-injection of SCH 23390, while quinpirole and SK & F 38393 inhibited and increased this response, respectively (Koshikawa *et al.*, 1990c); though no such oppositional $D_1 : D_2$ interaction was evident in the ventral striatum, where a cooperative/synergistic interaction predominated in the regulation of this response (Koshikawa *et al.*, 1989, 1990b), it is not always clear that these various studies are examining phenomenologically or physiologically equivalent behaviours.

3.4.3 Regulation of typical motor behaviours

There are a number of individual reports that suggest (or have been interpreted as suggesting) an oppositional $D_1 : D_2$ interaction in the regulation of more typical motor behaviours which the greater bulk of evidence has indicated to be regulated by a cooperative/synergistic $D_1 : D_2$ interaction: restoration of reserpine-induced akinesia (Rubinstein *et al.*, 1988b); catalepsy (Klemm and Block, 1988); rotational behaviour (Karlsson *et al.*, 1988; see also Morelli *et al.*, 1991b); and stereotyped behaviour (Mandel *et al.*, 1990; see also Eilam *et al.*, 1992). In the presence of such individual findings, and in view of difficulties over whether oppositional versus cooperative/synergistic interactions might be evident at differing drug dosages or might reflect differing uses of terminology, it is not yet possible to integrate them readily with those findings constituting either Sections 3.3.1 and 3.3.3 or Sections 3.4.1 and 3.4.2.

3.4.4   The nature of oppositional $D_1 : D_2$ interactions

While early proposals for cooperative/synergistic $D_1:D_2$ interactions were initially without mechanistic support, until the emergence of the substantial body of evidence as reviewed previously (Section 3.2.1), the *first* interaction identified between D_1 and D_2 receptors was their opposing roles in the stimulation and inhibition of adenylyl cyclase activity; though this phenomenon was evident in the striatum but was not initially apparent in the nucleus accumbens (Waddington and O'Boyle, 1989), subsequent evidence has suggested that such an oppositional process may be present in terms of the regulation of accumbal cAMP-dependent protein kinase and phosphorylation of the D_1-associated phosphoprotein DARPP-32 (Szmigielski and Zalewska-Kaszubska, 1991). The question is whether these oppositional $D_1:D_2$ interaction(s) might be a neurochemical counterpart of some of the apparently oppositional interactions that appear to regulate, in particular, the atypical DAergic behaviours considered above, and whether such oppositional interactions might be evident at other levels of neuronal function.

A reciprocal interaction between DA and acetylcholine (ACh) in the regulation of striatal function has long been recognized and accepted, but studies seeking to delineate the relative roles of D_1 and D_2 receptors in these processes did not produce consistent results (Waddington and O'Boyle, 1989). More recently, several reports have reaffirmed an oppositional role for D_1 and D_2 receptors in, respectively, the stimulation and inhibition of striatal ACh release (Bertorelli and Consolo, 1990; Friedman *et al.*, 1990; Damsma *et al.*, 1990); however, others have either not found such an effect (Ajima *et al.*, 1990; Dolezal *et al.*, 1992) or have noted that such an interaction apparently involves D_1 receptors located *outside* of the striatum (Damsma *et al.*, 1991) or depends critically upon methodological factors (De Boer *et al.*, 1992).

Oppositional $D_1:D_2$ interactions have been noted variably at some other levels of DAergic function (Waddington and O'Boyle, 1989), and this now extends to the attenuation of D_1 antagonist-induced upregulation of striatal and other D_1 receptors by concomitant D_2 antagonism (Parashos *et al.*, 1987; McGonigle *et al.*, 1989), and reciprocal control of cGMP levels (Altar *et al.*, 1990) and of GABA synthesis (Steulet *et al.*, 1990). However, this is very much a 'mixed bag' of individual oppositional $D_1:D_2$ interactions which, to date, lacks the detailed parallelism with atypical DAergic behavioural phenomena that is evident between other neuronal processes and more typical behavioural phenomena apparently regulated by cooperative/synergistic $D_1:D_2$ interaction (Sections 3.2.1 and 3.2.2). One of the most potentially significant of recent findings is evidence that though D_1 and D_2 receptors are well known to interact in a cooperative/synergistic manner in the regulation of cell firing in the (dorsal) globus pallidus (Walters *et al.*, 1987), they appear to interact in an oppositional manner in the regulation of cell firing in the ventral pallidum/substantia innominata (Maslowski and Napier, 1991).

3.5 Current issues in interactions between 'D_1-like' and 'D_2-like' receptors

3.5.1 The roles of new substrata of 'D_1-like' and 'D_2-like' receptors

Perhaps the most prominent development in the area of DAergic neuroscience over recent years has been an explosion in the breadth and depth of molecular biological studies indicating that the number of DA receptors appears much larger than initially conceived. We have moved rapidly from a period of questioning the prevailing D_1/D_2 classification (Waddington and O'Boyle, 1989; Waddington, 1989; Andersen *et al.*, 1990), through one of recognizing the importance of the cloning both of established and of some novel DA receptors (Civelli *et al.*, 1991), to the 'current' situation (perhaps already out of date) which encompasses at least six DA receptor sequences; on the basis of their known pharmacological characteristics, these might best be placed into two *families*, of 'D_1-like' (D_{1A}, D_{1B}/D_5) and 'D_2-like' ($D_{2L/S}$, D_3, D_4) receptors (Sibley and Monsma, 1992). As there exist essentially no agents able to discriminate within the individual members of either family, yet there exist numerous agents able to distinguish between these two families, the concept of $D_1:D_2$ interactions elaborated so far is by no means made irrelevant or redundant; on the contrary, it should be recast to emphasize more correctly the apparent existence of 'D_1-like':'D_2-like' receptor interactions. Delineation of the relative roles in such interactions of the various individual members of any one family with those of the other family awaits the identification of a range of new, selective agonist and antagonist compounds of appropriate discriminative capacity.

However, while the new molecular biology of DA receptors holds centre stage, it should not be overlooked that proposals for the further subtyping of DA receptors beyond the initial D_1/D_2 schema had their origins in considerably earlier findings; these were based primarily on the apparent heterogeneity of second messenger/transduction mechanisms by which events at DA receptor recognition sites are effected. For example, the notion that there exist 'D_1-like' receptors both independent of, and linked to, the stimulation of adenylyl cyclase (Mailman *et al.*, 1986; Waddington, 1989; Waddington and O'Boyle, 1989; Andersen *et al.*, 1990) has been followed by recent evidence for the linkage of some 'D_1-like' receptors to the stimulation of phosphatidylinositol turnover (Undie and Friedman, 1990; Mahan *et al.*, 1990). At the behavioural level, the ability of a wide range of benzazepine selective D_1 agonists to induce grooming and other typical motor responses, including synergism with a selective D_2 agonist, appears unrelated to their ability to stimulate adenylyl cyclase (Arnt *et al.*, 1988a, 1992; Murray and Waddington, 1989b; Daly and Waddington, 1992c); similarly, at the electrophysiological level, the ability of benzazepine D_1 agonists both to inhibit the firing of nucleus accumbens neurones and to act synergistically with quinpirole in such inhibition after αMPT treatment also appeared unrelated to their ability to stimulate this enzyme system (Johansen *et al.*, 1991). Unless such data simply have their basis in a substantial D_1 receptor reserve (Section 3.3.1), they suggest mediation via 'D_1-like' receptors which are linked to transduction mechanisms other than, or additional to, adenylyl cyclase. The question remains which of these putative 'D_1-like' receptors participate in cooperative/synergistic interactions with D_2 receptors; incomplete as the data are, at so early a stage in our understanding of D_1 receptor subtyping, they are consistent with the involvement of non-cyclase-linked 'D_1-like' receptors in such interactions as reflected in the regulation of typical DAergic motor behaviours.

It must be emphasized that the great majority of our knowledge of D_1 receptor function in relation to $D_1:D_2$ interaction derives from the use of a single chemical class of selective D_1 agonist, the 1-phenyl-1H-3-benzazepines (Waddington and O'Boyle, 1989). Some putative non-benzazepine D_1 agonists have become available but, for a variety of reasons, they have not been used extensively in pharmacological investigations (Daly and Waddington, 1992c). Only recently has the first behaviourally active, full-efficacy, non-benzazepine selective D_1 agonist become available, the isochroman A 68930 (DeNinno *et al.*, 1991), and some of the initial results obtained therewith have been unexpected. While A 68930 is an extremely potent inducer of intense grooming, it is the first D_1 agonist which we have found to also induce vacuous chewing when given as sole treatment (Daly and Waddington, 1991). This vacuous chewing response was enhanced by pretreatment with the selective D_2 antagonist YM 09151, consistent with it being regulated by oppositional $D_1:D_2$ interactions (Section 3.4.2); however, it could not be blocked with either of the benzazepine selective D_1 antagonists SCH 23390 (which actually induced some vacuous chewing when given alone) or NNC 756 but *was* blocked with the isoquinoline-selective D_1 antagonist BW 737C, while grooming was blocked by each of these antagonists (Daly and Waddington, 1992d). These data (Table 1) suggest that the receptor mediating vacuous chewing is relatively insensitive to the benzazepine D_1 agonists and antagonists but sensitive to the isochroman and isoquinoline D_1 agonist and antagonist; thus, grooming and vacuous chewing may be mediated by distinct subtypes of 'D_1-like' receptor, with that mediating vacuous chewing participating in oppositional $D_1:D_2$ interactions. How these subtypes of 'D_1-like' receptor apparent in such behavioural studies might or might not equate with any of those subtypes as defined either by molecular cloning or by transduction mechanism remains to be determined.

Table 1 Effects of the selective D_2 antagonist YM 09151 and of the selective D_1 antagonists SCH 23390, NNC 756 and BW 737C on intense grooming and vacuous chewing responses to the selective D_1 agonist A 68930.

Drug(s)	mg/kg	Behavioural counts	
		Intense grooming	Vacuous chewing
Vehicle	—	0.4 ± 0.1	0.8 ± 0.2
YM 09151	0.05	0.0 ± 0.0	0.8 ± 0.4
A 68930	0.25	$6.1 \pm 0.5**$	$3.7 \pm 0.6**$
+ YM 09151	0.005	$4.8 \pm 0.9**$	$4.8 \pm 1.4**$
	0.05	1.1 ± 0.4^a	6.4 ± 0.7^b
	0.5	1.5 ± 0.3^a	$5.8 \pm 1.2**$
SCH 23390	0.1	0.0 ± 0.0	$2.0 \pm 0.7**$
A 68930	0.25	$6.1 \pm 0.5**$	$3.7 \pm 0.6**$
+ SCH 23390	0.01	3.3 ± 1.3^b	$2.4 \pm 0.8**$
	0.1	1.0 ± 0.5^a	$3.6 \pm 1.4**$
	1.0	0.0 ± 0.0^a	$2.6 \pm 0.6**$
NNC 756	0.1	0.0 ± 0.0	1.0 ± 0.6
A 68930	0.25	$6.1 \pm 0.5**$	$3.7 \pm 0.6**$
+ NNC 756	0.01	2.6 ± 0.5^a	$1.9 \pm 0.4*$
	0.1	0.6 ± 0.2^a	$3.1 \pm 1.0**$
	1.0	0.2 ± 0.1^a	$2.0 \pm 0.7*$
Vehicle	—	0.4 ± 0.2	1.3 ± 0.6
BW 737C	1.0	0.0 ± 0.0	1.0 ± 0.5
A 68930	0.25	$5.4 \pm 1.3**$	$5.5 \pm 1.2**$
+ BW 737C	0.2	1.4 ± 0.5^b	3.1 ± 0.8
	1.0	0.1 ± 0.1^a	$3.3 \pm 0.7*$
	5.0	0.0 ± 0.0^a	1.4 ± 0.6^a

Means $\pm$ SEM, $n = 8$–56 per group. $**$ $p < 0.01$, $*$ $P \leqslant 0.05$ vs vehicle; ^{a} $P < 0.01$, ^{b} $P \leqslant 0.05$ vs A 68930. Data modified from Daly and Waddington (1992d); methods as described by Daly and Waddington (1992b, c).

Furthermore, the notion that there exist 'D$_2$-like' receptors both independent of, as well as linked to, the inhibition of adenylyl cyclase (Waddington and O'Boyle, 1989; Vallar and Meldolesi, 1989) has been followed by recent evidence for the linkage of cyclase-independent 'D$_2$-like' receptors to other transduction mechanisms (Andersen et al., 1990). In particular, there is evidence that such receptors might be subdivided into those linked to the inhibition of adenylyl cyclase and those linked to activation of voltage-dependent K$^+$ channels; while quinpirole exhibits little selectivity between these putative entities, the azepine derivative B-HT 920 (once considered an autoreceptor-selective D_2 agonist; Section 3.2.2) now appears to selectively activate voltage-dependent K^+ channels without inhibiting the activity of adenylyl cyclase (Pizzi et al., 1990). We have recently found that B-HT 920, when given as sole treatment, attenuates spontaneous activities without stimulating typical DAergic behaviours at high doses, yet induces episodes of atypical jerking behaviour (Section 3.4.1) at those same high doses; however, following pretreatment with BW 737C, B-HT 920 induced a heightened level of jerking behaviour similar to that induced by prototype selective D_2 agonists such as RU 24213 (Table 2). These data suggest that autoreceptor stimulation by B-HT 920 can reduce DA release and associated tonic DAergic activity through D_1 receptors so as both to 'dis-enable' typical postsynaptic D_2 receptor-mediated behaviours that are regulated by cooperative/synergistic $D_1 : D_2$ interactions and to 'release' atypical jerking behaviour that is regulated by oppositional interactions; pretreatment with BW 737C then blocks residual D_1-mediated DAergic tone and further heightens the release of jerking. On this basis, such jerking behaviour would seem to involve oppositional $D_1 : D_2$ interactions, the D_2 component of which may include 'D_2-like' receptors linked not to inhibition of adenylyl cyclase but to activation of voltage-dependent K^+ channels. As with 'D_1-like' receptors, how those subtypes of 'D_2-like' receptor apparent in such behavioural and neurochemical studies might or might not equate with any of those subtypes as defined by molecular cloning remains to be determined. These are nascent concepts, derived from preliminary data, whose substance and significance can be clarified only by much more extensive investigation, ideally, using a further generation of selective agents better able to discriminate between members of these new families of 'D_1-like' and 'D_2-like'

Table 2 Effects of the selective D_1 antagonist BW 737C on sniffing and jerking responses to the selective D_2 agonists RU 24213 and B-HT 920.

Drug(s)	mg/kg	Behavioural counts	
		Sniffing	Jerking
Vehicle	—	6.8 ± 1.7	0.0 ± 0.0
RU 24213	15.0	$30.0 \pm 0.0^{**}$	0.0 ± 0.0
+ BW 737C	5.0	22.1 ± 1.8^{a}	6.6 ± 2.7^{b}
Vehicle	—	6.5 ± 1.7	0.0 ± 0.0
B-HT 920	10.0	6.6 ± 1.7	$1.0 \pm 0.4^{*}$
+ BW 737C	5.0	5.5 ± 1.4	3.6 ± 1.0^{b}

Means $\pm$ SEM, $n = 8$ per group. [**] $P < 0.01$, [*] $P \leqslant 0.05$ vs vehicle; [a] $P < 0.01$, [b] $P \leqslant 0.05$ vs agonist alone. Methods as described by Daly and Waddington (1992b, c) receptors and to probe 'D$_1$-like': 'D$_2$-like' interactions at various levels of function.

3.5.2 Do 'D$_1$-like' and 'D$_2$-like' receptors co-localize on the same neurones?

Subsequent to initial proposals, increasing recognition of such functional interactions has prompted a debate as to whether they derive from 'D$_1$-like' and 'D$_2$-like' receptors that (i) reside intimately on the membrane of the same neurones, and thus give rise to interactions directly via a unitary cellular mechanism (the 'co-localization' hypothesis) or (ii) reside separately on distinct populations of neurones whose axon collaterals or efferents indirectly subserve such interactions (the 'neurointegrative' hypothesis).

Though behavioural studies were the progenitors of initial formulations of D$_1$: D$_2$ interactions, they have little power to resolve a debate which centres on cellular function(s). The first review thereof (Waddington, 1986) speculated on a neurointegrative basis to cooperative/synergistic D$_1$: D$_2$ interactions apparent in behavioural regulation, with the oppositional roles of these receptors in the regulation of striatal adenylyl cyclase presumed to derive from co-localized receptors; subsequently, others have also argued, on a similar basis, for neurointegrative interactions (Robertson and Robertson, 1987; LaHoste and Marshall, 1990), but there is a great deal of contrary data at other levels of neuronal function. The results of those electrophysiological studies involving iontophoretic drug application have appeared more consistent with co-localization, but their interpretation is not always straightforward; a number of neurochemical studies have given similar indications, but do not allow unqualified interpretation (Waddington and O'Boyle, 1987, 1989; Clark and White, 1987). More recently, using radioligand binding techniques, both Zhang and Segawa (1989) and Seeman et al. (1989) have offered evidence for direct interactions between co-localized D$_1$ and D$_2$ recognition sites via their regulation of guanine nucleotide-binding protein components; by the very nature of these studies, it is not possible to clarify whether such events might subserve cooperative/synergistic or oppositional interactions. The identification of cooperative/synergistic interactions at the levels of Na$^+$/K$^+$-ATPase activity in isolated striatal neurones (Bertorello et al., 1990) and of arachidonic acid release in cells transfected to express both D$_1$ and D$_2$ receptors (Piomelli et al., 1991) would also be consistent with the co-localization hypothesis; additionally, there is recent evidence consistent with oppositional interactions in the nucleus accumbens having some basis in co-localization at the level of adenylyl cyclase-associated protein kinases (Szmigielski and Zalewska-Kaszubska, 1991). However, oppositional interactions evident at the level of striatal ACh release (Bertorelli and Consolo, 1990; Damsma et al., 1991) and cooperative/synergistic interactions at the level of striatal ascorbic acid release (Pierce and Rebec, 1990) both appear more consistent with a neurointegrative mechanism.

Clearly, a fundamental approach to resolving these issues would be to conduct detailed neuroanatomical investigations seeking direct evidence for or against co-localization of 'D$_1$-like' and 'D$_2$-like' receptors; however, previous techniques such as receptor autoradiography have not been of sufficient sensitivity to allow such studies. More recently, the detection of D$_1$ and D$_2$ receptor mRNAs by *in situ* hybridization histochemistry has demonstrated adequate sensitivity for preliminary studies, but the results to date have been far from consistent; thus, Gerfen *et al.* (1990) and Le Moine *et al.* (1991) have each reported that striatal neurones express essentially one or the other receptor, and rarely both, while Weiner *et al.* (1991) and Meador-Woodruff *et al.* (1991) have reported that between one-third and one-half of striatal neurones co-express both receptors. These are early days for such studies, and there remain many methodological problems; considerably more technical refinement will be needed to clarify unambiguously the extent of any substrate for the co-localization hypothesis, and any such neuroanatomical data would not in themselves be able to distinguish readily between substrates for cooperative/synergistic and those for oppositional 'D$_1$-like': D$_2$-like' interactions.

3.5.3 How do changes in D_2 activity influence D_1-mediated function?

Much of the above analysis has centred on the role of tonic/phasic activity through D$_1$ receptors in 'enabling' or 'permitting' and potentiating synergistically the full expression of typical D$_2$-stimulated functions in the intact adult animal. However, there remains the important question of whether such cooperative/ synergistic D$_1$:D$_2$ interactions are complementary; that is, to what extent does tonic/phasic activity through D$_2$ receptors influence the expression of typical D$_1$-stimulated functions?

Just as selective D$_1$ antagonists or DA depletions block typical behavioural responses to selective D$_2$ agonists, studies have indicated that selective D$_2$ antagonists such as metoclopramide and YM 09151 (Waddington, 1989) or piquindone (Murray and Waddington, 1989b) can block grooming behaviour induced by SK & F 38393 and by SK & F 77434 (and by A 68930; see Table 1); this would be consistent with tonic activity through D$_2$ receptors cooperating in the expression of such D$_1$-stimulated behaviour. Other explanations are possible, including non-specific motor depressant or cataleptogenic actions of the D$_2$ antagonists; however, attenuation of typical D$_1$ agonist-induced grooming is evident using only modest doses of these selective D$_2$ antagonists and, as other atypical D$_1$ agonist-induced behaviours are *released* by such pretreatments (Section 3.4.2), such animals are clearly not incapable of motor responses under such circumstances. Some attenuation of SK & F 38393-induced grooming following partial DA depletion with αMPT has been reported, while essentially total depletion of DA with αMPT + reserpine abolished spontaneous levels of grooming which could be reinstated (but not exceeded) by SK & F 38393 (White *et al.*, 1988); on the basis of *some* manifestation of grooming in response to SK & F 38393 following such DA depletions, these authors proposed that D_2 receptor activation was not necessary for the expression of such a response, but there remains the resultant attenuation of this response, as noted also in several previous studies (Waddington, 1989). Similarly, Moody and Spear (1992) have recently reported that in 21-day-old rat pups, αMPT blocks SK & F 38393-induced grooming without affecting responses to quinpirole, while αMPT + reserpine suppressed responses to both the D_1 and the D_2 agonist; they conclude that in such animals there exists a reciprocal co-dependence of the two receptor subtypes, with extensive DA depletion influencing responses to D_1 as well as to D_2 agonists. In one chronic D_1 antagonist treatment paradigm, the data suggested not only that D_1 and D_2 receptors have a cooperative role in the generation of stereotyped behaviour, but also that behavioural evidence of D_1 receptor supersensitivity may be manifested only during concurrent D_2 receptor stimulation (Dall'Olio *et al.*, 1988).

There is evidence (Waddington *et al.*, 1990; Matsumoto *et al.*, 1991) that the action of selective D_2 antagonists in blocking apomorphine-induced stereotypy is accompanied by release of grooming behaviour; the explanation offered was that the D_1 component of this non-selective DA agonist was 'unmasked' through antagonism of its D_2 component, and this might seem at variance with any notion that D_2 receptor activation cooperates in the expression of D_1-mediated grooming. However, the action of D_2 antagonists such as metoclopramide in releasing grooming in response to apomorphine appears to show a biphasic dose–response relationship, being evident at lower but lost at higher doses (Waddington *et al.*, 1990); it may be that modest doses thereof exert sufficient D_2 antagonism to block directly a particular D_2 component of the action of apomorphine, causing abolition of stereotypy and release of grooming, yet do not give sufficient overall reduction in D_2 tone to indirectly attenuate grooming under such conditions. Clearly, the issue of how D_2 manipulations influence typical D_1-dependent behaviour is considerably less straightforward than that of how D_1 manipulations influence D_2-dependent behaviour. The situation is made yet more complex by evidence that there may be differences between classes of selective D_2 antagonists in how they influence responsivity to apomorphine (Vasse and Protais, 1988; Chandler *et al.*, 1990b); also, D_1 agonist-induced grooming appears to be *potentiated* rather than reduced by pretreatment with the atypical substituted benzamide D_2 antagonists sulpiride (Molloy and Waddington, 1987b) and remoxipride (Darney *et al.*, 1991). Nevertheless, the results of a recent intracerebral injection study are provocative in this regard. Intra-accumbens injections of SK & F 38393 (strongly) and of quinpirole (modestly) each induced increases in locomotor activity that showed synergism on co-administration and were suppressed by an antagonist of either receptor subtype, in accordance with local cooperative/synergistic $D_1:D_2$ interactions; furthermore, the locomotor-stimulant action of intra-accumbens

SK & F 38393, like that of quinpirole, was blocked by depletion of DA with αMPT and reserpine (Dreher and Jackson, 1989). It is not clear, on the basis of such data alone, how effects on the D_1 agonist response can have their basis in cooperative/synergistic $D_1:D_2$ interactions while qualitatively similar effects on the D_1 agonist might derive fron non-specific motor-depressant actions of these *same* drugs. Evidence from other levels of physiological function might throw some light on these problems.

At the level of striatal and accumbal electrophysiology, the inhibitory action of iontophoretically applied SK & F 38393 appeared unmodified by acute depletion of DA with αMPT, while that of quinpirole was attenuated (Wachtel *et al.*, 1989); this would imply that while D_1 tone is necessary for the electrophysiological expression of D_2 stimulation, the same may not be true for D_2 tone and D_1 stimulation. However, there are precedents for inconsistencies between such electrophysiological and behavioural phenomena, e.g. the ability of 6-OHDA lesions to 'uncouple' electrophysiological but spare behavioural $D_1:D_2$ agonist synergism (Section 3.3.5). Furthermore, Hu and Wang (1988) have reported that, in the striatum, it is quinpirole that potentiates the neuronal depressant action of SK & F 38393, while Carlson *et al.* (1988) have noted that attenuation of D_2 tone with αMPT can influence the expression of SK & F 38393's effect on the activity of pallidal neurones. Similarly, recent data (Stromberg and Bickford-Wimer, 1991) suggest that the D_1 receptor requires an active D_2 receptor for the full expression of its neuronal function, at least under conditions of 6-OHDA and pertussis toxin lesions. Clearly, the above constitutes a far from substantial and conclusive body of evidence on the issue, and further behavioural and electrophysiological studies will be required to finally resolve these aspects of $D_1:D_2$ interaction.

3.5.4 The enigma of apparent species differences in $D_1:D_2$ interaction

The great bulk of our knowledge and understanding of $D_1:D_2$ interaction derives from studies in rodents, the majority involving rats and a significant minority involving mice; those in rats and mice have generated usually comparable results, though a recent comparative study suggests some differences between these rodent species (Arnt *et al.*, 1992). However, the single study carried out in guinea-pigs (Brent, 1991) indicates a markedly different profile of interactions between D_1 and D_2 agonist and antagonist drugs. More significantly, in non-human primates the evidence indicates more consistently that many presumed forms of $D_1:D_2$ interaction are absent or contrary to those evident in rats and mice (Waddington, 1989; Waddington and O'Boyle, 1989; Loschmann *et al.*, 1991). The nature of these distinct phenomena in non-human primates is fundamental to how we perceive the clinical significance of $D_1:D_2$ interactions, and is therefore the subject of extensive consideration elsewhere (Chapter 10).

3.6 Conclusions

Over recent years, DAergic neuroscience has been profoundly influenced by results from two particular lines of enquiry: (i) that the classical D_1 and D_2 receptor subtypes do not usually act independently but, rather, interact critically in the regulation of multiple aspects of DAergic function; and (ii) that these two receptor subtype designations appear to constitute 'umbrellas' for two families of DA receptor subtypes that are considerably broader than envisaged previously. It will be the task of future studies to integrate these two lines of enquiry; this will be facilitated greatly by the identification of a further generation of selective agents capable of distinguishing between members of these new families of 'D_1-like' and 'D_2-like' receptors, and thus better specifying 'D_1-like':'D_2-like' interactions at various levels of function. From such studies may evolve answers to some of the above problems and current issues regarding those $D_1 : D_2$ interactions through which unconditioned motor behaviour appears to be regulated.

Acknowledgements

The authors' studies are supported by the Wellcome Trust and the Health Research Board.

References

Abbott, B., Starr, B.S. & Starr, M.S. (1991) *Pharmacol. Biochem. Behav.* **38**, 259–263.
Ajima, A., Yamaguchi, T. & Kato, T. (1990) *Brain Res.* **518**, 193–198.
Altar, A.C., Boyar, W.C. & Kim, H.S. (1990) *Eur. J. Pharmacol.* **181**, 17–21.
Anden, N.E. & Grabowska-Anden, M. (1988) *Acta Physiol. Scand.* **134**, 285–290.
Anden, N.E. & Grabowska-Anden, M. (1989) *J. Pharm. Pharmacol.* **41**, 490–492.
Anden, N.E. & Grabowska-Anden, M. (1990) *J. Neurol Transm.* **79**, 209–214.
Andersen, P.H. (1988) *Eur. J. Pharmacol.* **152**, 153–156.
Andersen, P.H., Gingrich, J.A., Bates, M.D., Dearry, A., Falardeau, P., Senogles, S.E. & Caron, M.G. (1990) *Trends Pharmacol. Sci.* **11**, 231–236.
Arnt, J. (1987) In *Dopamine Receptors* (eds Creese, I. & Fraser, C.M.), pp 199–231. New York, Alan R. Liss.
Arnt, J. & Hyttel, J. (1989) *Pharmacol. Toxicol.* **74**, 116–119.
Arnt, J. & Hyttel, J. (1990) *J. Neural Transm.* **80**, 33–50.
Arnt, J., Hyttel, J. & Perregaard, J. (1987) *Eur. J. Pharmacol.* **133**, 137–145.
Arnt, J., Bogeso, K.P., Hyttel, J. & Meier, E. (1988a) *Pharmacol. Toxicol.* **62**, 121–130.
Arnt, J., Hyttel, J. & Meier, E. (1988b) *Eur. J. Pharmacol.* **155**, 37–47.
Arnt, J., Hyttel, J. & Sanchez, C. (1992) *Eur. J. Pharmacol.* **213**, 259–267.
Bertorelli, R. & Consolo, S. (1990) *J. Neurochem.* **54**, 2145–2148.
Bertorello, A.M., Hopfield, J.F., Aperia, A. & Greengard, P. (1990) *Nature* **347**, 386–388.

Bordi, F. & Meller, E. (1989) *Brain Res.* **504**, 276–283.

Braun, A.R. & Chase, T.N. (1988) *Eur. J. Pharmacol.* **147**, 441–451.

Brent, P.J. (1991) *Psychopharmacology* **104**, 201–207.

Breese, G. & Creese, I. (1986) *Neurobiology of Central D$_1$ Dopamine Receptors.* New York, Plenum Press.

Cameron, D.L. & Crocker, A.D. (1988) *Neuropharmacology* **27**, 447–450.

Cameron, D.L., Crosbie, J. & Crocker, A.D. *Prog. Neuro-Psychopharmacol. Biol. Psychiatry* **12**, 595–606.

Carlson, J.H., Bergstrom, D.A., Demo, S.D. & Walters, J.R. (1988) *Eur. J. Pharmacol.* **152**, 289–300.

Carlson, J.H., Bergstrom, D.A., Demo, S.D. & Walters, J.R. (1990) *Synapse* **5**, 83–93.

Carlson, A. (1987) *Annu. Rev. Neurosci.* **10**, 19–40.

Carlsson, M. & Carlsson, A. (1990) *Trends Neurosci.* **13**, 272–276.

Chandler, C.J., Starr, B.S. & Starr, M.S. (1990a) *Pharmacol. Biochem. Behav.* **35**, 285–289.

Chandler, C.J., Wohab, W., Starr, B.S. & Starr, M.S. (1990b) *Neuroscience* **38**, 437–445.

Christensen, A.V., Arnt, J., Hyttel, J., Larsen, J.-J. & Svendsen, O. (1984) *Life Sci.* **34**, 1529–1540.

Civelli, O., Bunzow, J.R., Grandy, D.K., Zhou, Q.Y. & Van Tol, H.H.M. (1991) *Eur. J. Pharmacol.–Mol. Pharmacol. Sect.* **207**, 277–286.

Clark, D. & White, F.J. (1987) *Synapse* **1**, 347–388.

Collins, P., Broekkamp, C.L.E., Jenner, P. & Marsden, C.D. (1991) *Psychopharmacology* **103**, 504–512.

Creese, I., Sibley, D.R., Hamblin, M.W. & Leff, S.E. (1983) *Annu. Rev. Neurosci.* **6**, 43–71.

Dall'Olio, R., Gandolfi, O., Vaccheri, A., Roncada, P. & Montanaro, N. (1988) *Psychopharmacology* **95**, 381–385.

Dall'Olio, R., Roncada, P., Vaccheri, A., Gandolfi, O. & Montanaro, N. (1989) *Psychopharmacology* **98**, 342–346.

Dall'Olio, R., Gandolfi, O., Roncada, P., Vaccheri, A. & Montanaro, N. (1990) *Psychopharmacology* **100**, 560–562.

Daly, S.A. & Waddington, J.L. (1991) *Br. J. Pharmacol.* **104**, 60P.

Daly, S.A. & Waddington, J.L. (1992a) *Neurochem. Int.* **20** (supplement), 135S–139S.

Daly, S.A. & Waddington, J.L. (1992b) *Eur. J. Pharmacol.* **213**, 251–258.

Daly, S.A. & Waddington, J.L. (1992c) *J. Psychopharmacol.* **6**, 50–60.

Daly, S.A. & Waddington, J.L. (1992d) *Br. J. Pharmacol.* **105**, 7P.

Damsma, G., Tham, C.S., Robertson, G.S. & Fibiger, H.C. (1990) *Eur. J. Pharmacol.* **186**, 335–338.

Damsma, G., Robertson, G.S., Tham, C.S. & Fibiger, H.C. (1991) *J. Pharmacol. Exp. Ther.* **259**, 1064–1072.

Darney, K.J., Lewis, M.H., Brewster, W.K., Nichols, D.E. & Mailman, R.B. (1991) *Neuropsychopharmacology* **5**, 187–195.

De Boer, P., Damsma, G., Schram, Q., Stoof, J.C., Zaagsma, J. & Westerink, B.H.C. (1992) *Naunyn-Schmiedeberg's Arch. Pharmacol.* **345**, 144–152.

Delfs, J.M. & Kelley, A.E. (1990) *Neuroscience* **39**, 59–67.

DeNinno, M.P., Schoenleber, R., MacKenzie, R., Britton, D.R., Asin, D.E., Briggs, C., Trugman, J.M., Ackerman, M., Artman, L., Bednarz, L., Bhatt, R., Curzon, P., Gomez, E., Kang, C.H., Stittsworth, J. & Kebabian, J.W. (1991) *Eur. J. Pharmacol.* **199**, 209–219.

Dolezal, V., Jackisch, R., Hertting, G. & Allgaier, C. (1992) *Naunyn-Schmiedeberg's Arch. Pharmacol.* **345**, 16–20.

Double, K.L. & Crocker, A.D. (1990) *Neurosci. Lett.* **113**, 81–85.

Dreher, J.K. & Jackson, D.M. (1989) *Brain Res.* **487**, 267–277.

Drukarch, B. & Stoof, J.C. (1990) *Life Sci.* **47**, 361–376.

Eilam, D., Clements, K.V.A. & Szechtman, H. (1991) *Behav. Brain Res.* **45**, 117–124.

Eilam, D., Talangbayan, H., Canaran, G. & Szechtman, H. (1992) *Psychopharmacology* **106**, 447–454.

Eshel, G., Ross, S.B., Kelder, D., Edis, L.E.M. & Jackson, D.M. (1990) *Pharmacol. Toxicol.* **67**, 123–131.

Ferrari, F., Pelloni, F., Filaferro, M. & Giuliani, D. (1992) *Life Sci.* **50**, 1013–1019.

Fletcher, G.H. & Starr, M.S. (1987) *Neuroscience* **23**, 1001–1010.

Fletcher, G.H. & Starr, M.S. (1989) *Neuroscience* **28**, 171–180.

Friedman, E., Wang, H.-Y. & Butkeriat, P. (1990) *Neuropharmacology* **29**, 537–544.

Gandolfi, O., Dall'Olio, R., Vaccheri, A., Roncada, P. & Montanaro, N. (1988) *Pharmacol. Biochem. Behav.* **30**, 463–469.

Gerfen, C.R. (1992) *Annu. Rev. Neurosci.* **15**, 285–320.

Gerfen, C.R., Engber, T.M., Mahan, L.C., Susel, Z., Chase, T.N., Monsma, F.J. & Sibley, D.R. (1990) *Science* **250**, 1429–1432.

Giorgi, O. & Biggio, G. (1990) *Pharmacol. Biochem. Behav.* **35**, 877–884.

Glenthoj, B., Arnt, J. & Hyttel, J. (1990) *Life Sci.* **47**, 1339–1346.

Goodwin, P., Starr, B.S. & Starr, M.S. (1992) *J. Neural Transm.* **4**, 15–26.

Grabowska-Anden, M. & Anden, N.-E. (1983) *J. Pharm. Pharmacol.* **35**, 543–545.

Grabowska-Anden, M. & Anden, N.-E. (1987) *J. Pharm. Pharmacol.* **29**, 660–661.

Hu, X.T. & Wang, R.Y. (1988) *J. Neurosci.* **8**, 4340–4348.

Hu, X.T. & White, F.J. (1992) *Synapse* **10**, 206–216.

Hu, X.T., Wachtel, S.R., Galloway, M.P. & White, F.J. (1990) *J. Neurosci.* **10**, 2318–2329.

Jackson, D.M., Ross, S.B. & Edwards, S.R. (1989a) *J. Neural Transm.* **75**, 213–220.

Jackson, D.M., Ross, S.B. & Larsson, L.G. (1989b) *Naunyn-Schmiedeberg's Arch. Pharmacol.* **340**, 355–365.

Johansen, P.A., Clark, D. & White, F.J. (1988) *Life Sci.* **43**, 515–524.

Johansen, P.A., Hu, X.-T. & White, F.J. (1991) *J. Neural Transm.* **86**, 97–113.

Johansson, P., Levin, E., Gunne, L. & Ellison, G. (1987) *Eur. J. Pharmacol.* **134**, 83–88.

Karlsson, G., Jaton, A.L. & Vigouret, J.M. (1988) *Neurosci. Lett.* **88**, 69–74.

Kebabian, J.W. & Calne, D.B. (1979) *Nature* **277**, 93–96.

Kelland, M.D., Pitts, D.K., Freeman, A.S. & Chiodo, L.A. (1991) *Naunyn-Schmiedeberg's Arch. Pharmacol.* **343**, 447–457.

Klemm, W.R. & Block, H. (1988) *Pharmacol. Biochem. Behav.* **29**, 223–229.

Konitsiotis, S. & Kafetzopoulos, E. (1990) *Eur. J. Pharmacol.* **179**, 201–205.

Kontani, H., Inque, T. & Sakai, T. (1990) *Japan J. Pharmacol.* **54**, 482–486.

Koshikawa, N., Aoki, S., Hiruta, M., Tomiyama, K., Kobayashi, M., Tsuboi, Y., Iwata, K., Sumino, R. & Stephenson, J.D. (1989) *Eur. J. Pharmacol.* **163**, 227–236.

Koshikawa, N., Mori, E., Maruyama, Y., Yatsushige, N. & Kobayashi, M. (1990a) *Eur. J. Pharmacol.* **178**, 233–237.

Koshikawa, N., Koshikawa, F., Tomiyama, K., de Beltran, K.K., Kamimura, F. & Kobayashi, M. (1990b) *Eur. J. Pharmacol.* **182**, 375–380.

Koshikawa, N., Tomiyama, K., Omiya, K., de Beltran, K.K. & Kobayashi, M. (1990c) *Eur. J. Pharmacol.* **178**, 189–194.

Koshikawa, N., de Beltran, K.K., Tomiyama, K., Kobayashi, M. & Cools, A.R. (1991) *Eur. J. Pharmacol.* **201**, 47–51.

LaHoste, G.J. & Marshall, J.F. (1990) *Behav. Brain Res.* **38**, 233–242.

Lappalainen, J., Hietala, J., Sjoholm, B. & Syvalahti, E. (1990) *Eur. J. Pharmacol.* **179**, 314–321.

Le Moine, C., Normand, E. & Bloch, B. (1991) *Proc. Natl Acad. Sci. USA* **88**, 4205–4209.

Levin, E.D., See, R.E. & South, D. (1989) *Pharmacol. Biochem. Behav.* **34**, 43–48.

Loschmann, P.A., Smith, L.A., Lange, K.W., Jaehnig, P., Jenner, P. & Marsden, C.D. (1991) *Psychopharmacology* **105**, 303–309.

Mahan, L.C., Burch, R.M., Monsma, F.J. & Sibley, D.R. (1990) *Proc. Natl Acad. Sci. USA* **87**, 2196–2200.

Mailman, R.B., Schulz, D.W., Kilts, C.D., Lewis, M.H., Rollema, H. & Wyrick, S. (1986) *Psychopharmacol. Bull.* **22**, 593–598.

Mandel, R.J., Yurek, D.M. & Randall, P.K. (1990) *Brain Res. Bull.* **25**, 285–292.

Martin-Iverson, M.T., Iversen, S.D. & Stahl, S.M. (1988) *Eur. J. Pharmacol.* **149**, 25–31.

Maslowski, R.J. & Napier, T.C. (1991) *Eur. J. Pharmacol.* **200**, 103–112.

Matsumoto, K., Cai, B., Ohta, H., Imamura, L. & Watanabe, H. (1991) *Pharmacol. Biochem. Behav.* **39**, 699–703.

Mattingly, B.A., Rowlett, J.K., Graff, J.T. & Hatton, B.J. (1991) *Psychopharmacology* **105**, 501–507.

McGonigle, P., Boyson, S.J., Reuter, S. & Molinoff, P.B. (1989) *Synapse* **3**, 74–82.

Meador-Woodruff, J.H., Mansour, A., Healy, D.J., Kuehn, R., Zhou, Q.Y., Bunzow, J.R., Akil, H., Civelli, O. & Watson, S.J. (1991) *Neuropsychopharmacology* **5**, 231–242.

Meller, E., Bordi, F. & Bohmaker, K. (1988) *Life Sci.* **42**, 2561–2657.

Meltzer, L.T., Wiley, J.N. & Heffner, T.G. (1989) *Eur. J. Pharmacol.* **170**, 105–107.

Molloy, A.G. & Waddington, J.L. (1984) *Psychopharmacology* **82**, 409–410.

Molloy, A.G. & Waddington, J.L. (1987a) *Psychopharmacology* **92**, 164–168.

Molloy, A.G. & Waddington, J.L. (1987b) *J. Psychopharmacol.* **1**, 177–183.

Moody, C.A. & Spear, L.P. (1992) *Psychopharmacology* **107**, 39–49.

Moore, N.A. & Axton, M.S. (1988) *Psychopharmacology* **94**, 263–266.

Morelli, M., Fenu, S., Pinna, A. & Di Chiara, G. (1991a) *J. Pharmacol. Exp. Ther.* **260**, 402–408.

Morelli, M., Fenu, S., Cozzolino, A. & Di Chiara, G. (1991b) *Neuroscience* **42**, 41–48.

Murray, A.M. & Waddington, J.L. (1989a) *Psychopharmacology* **98**, 245–250.

Murray, A.M. & Waddington, J.L. (1989b) *Eur. J. Pharmacol.* **160**, 377–384.

Neisewander, J.L., Lucki, I. & McGonigle, P. (1991) *J. Pharmacol. Exp. Ther.* **257**, 850–860.

Ogren, S.O. & Fuxe, K. (1988) *Neurosci. Lett.* **85**, 333–338.

Parashos, S.A., Barone, P., Tucci, I. & Chase, T.N. (1987) *Life Sci.* **41**, 2279–2284.

Parashos, S.A., Marin, C. & Chase, T.N. (1989a) *Neurosci. Lett.* **105**, 169–173.

Parashos, S.A., Barone, P., Marin, C.A., Parashos, A.J., Kapitzoglou-Longothetis, V. & Chase, T.N. (1989b) *Psychopharmacology* **98**, 189–192.

Parashos, S.A., Marin, C., Barone, P., Kapitzoglou-Logothetis, V. & Chase, T.N. (1990) *Psychopharmacology* **102**, 411–413.

Pichler, L. & Pifl, C. (1989) *J. Pharm. Pharmacol.* **41**, 690–693.

Pierce, R.C. & Rebec, G.V. (1990) *Eur. J. Pharmacol.* **191**, 295–302.

Piomelli, D., Pilon, C., Giros, B., Sokoloff, P., Martres, M.P. & Schwartz, J.C. (1991) *Nature* **353**, 164–167.

Pizzi, M., Valerio, A., Benarese, M., Missale, C., Carruba, M.O., Memo, M. & Spano, P.F. (1990) *Molec. Neuropharmacol.* **1**, 37–42.

Plaznik, A., Stefanski, R. & Kostowski, W. (1989) *Psychopharmacology* **99**, 558–562.

Robertson, G.S. & Robertson, H.A. (1986) *Brain. Res.* **384**, 387–390.

Robertson, G.S. & Robertson, H.A. (1987) *Trends Pharmacol. Sci.* **8**, 295–299.

Rosengarten, H., Schweitzer, J.W. & Friedhoff, A.J. (1983) *Life Sci.* **33**, 2479–2482.

Rosengarten, H., Schweitzer, J.W. & Friedhoff, A.J. (1986) *Life Sci.* **39**, 29–35.

Rosengarten, H., Schweitzer, J.W. & Friedhoff, A.J. (1989) *Pharmacol. Biochem. Behav.* **34**, 895–897.

Ross, S.B., Jackson, D.M., Wallis, E.M. & Edwards, S.R. (1988) *Naunyn-Schmiedeberg's Arch. Pharmacol.* **337**, 512–518.

Ross, S.B., Jackson, D.M. & Edwards, S.R. (1989) *Pharmacol. Toxicol.* **64**, 72–77.

Rouillard, C. & Bedard, P.J. (1988) *Neuropharmacology* **27**, 1257–1264.

Rouillard, C., Bedard, P., Falardeau, P. & Di Paolo, T. (1988) *Eur. J. Pharmacol.* **157**, 125–133.

Rubinstein, M., Gershanik, O. & Stefano, F.J.E. (1988a) *Naunyn-Schmiedeberg's Arch. Pharmacol.* **337**, 115–117.

Rubinstein, M., Gershanik, O. & Stefano, F.J.E. (1988b) *Eur. J. Pharmacol.* **148**, 419–426.

Rubinstein, M., Schinder, A.F., Gershanik, O. & Stefano, F.J.E. (1989) *Life Sci.* **44**, 337–346.

Schiorring, E. (1979) *Psychopharmacology* **66**, 281–287.

Seeman, P. (1980) *Pharmacol. Rev.* **32**, 229–313.

Seeman, P., Niznik, H.B., Guan, H.-C., Booth, G. & Ulpian, C. (1989) *Proc. Natl. Acad. Sci. USA* **86**, 10156–10160.

Setler, P.E., Sarau, H.M., Zirkle, C.L. & Saunders, H.L. (1978) *Eur. J. Pharmacol.* **50**, 419–430.

Sibley, D.R. & Monsma, F.J. (1992) *Trends Pharmacol. Sci.* **13**, 61–69.

Singh, K. & Jackson, D.M. (1990) *Asia Pacific J. Pharmacol.* **5**, 323–326.

Sonsalla, P.K., Mazino, L. & Heikkila, R.E. (1988) *J. Pharmacol. Exp. Ther.* **247**, 180–185.

Spano, P.F., Govoni, S. & Trabucci, M. (1978) *Adv. Biochem. Psychopharmacol.* **19**, 155–165.

Stahle, L. (1992) *Psychopharmacology* **106**, 1–13.

Starr, M.S. (1988) *Eur. J. Pharmacol.* **151**, 479–482.

Starr, M.S. & Starr, B.S. (1989) *Pharmacol. Biochem. Behav.* **33**, 41–44.

Steulet, A.F., Bernasconi, R., Leonhardt, T., Martin, P., Grunenwald, C., Bischoff, S., Heinrich, M., Bandelier, V. & Maitre, L. (1990) *Eur. J. Pharmacol.* **191**, 19–27.

Stromberg, I. & Bickford-Wimer, P. (1991) *Brain Res.* **564**, 279–285.

Szmigielski, A. & Zalewska-Kaszubska, J. (1991) *Neuropharmacology* **30**, 259–266.

Undie, A.S. & Friedman, E. (1990) *J. Pharmacol. Exp. Ther.* **353**, 987–992.

Vallar, L. & Meldolesi, J. (1989) *Trends Pharmacol. Sci.* **10**, 74–77.

Vasse, M. & Protais, P. (1988) *Eur. J. Pharmacol.* **156**, 1–11.

Vasse, M., Chagraoui, A. & Protais, P. (1988) *Eur. J. Pharmacol.* **148**, 221–229.

Wachtel, S.R., Hu, X.T., Galloway, M.P. & White, F.J. (1989) *Synapse* **4**, 327–346.

Waddington, J.L. (1986) *Biochem. Pharmacol.* **35**, 3661–3667.

Waddington, J.L. (1989) *J. Psychopharmacol.* **3**, 54–63.

Waddington, J.L. & O'Boyle, K.M. (1987) *Rev. Neurosci.* **1**, 157–184.

Waddington, J.L. & O'Boyle, K.M. (1989) *Pharmacol. Ther.* **43**, 1–52.

Waddington, J.L., Molloy, A.G., O'Boyle, K.M. & Mashurano, M. (1986) *Clin. Neuropharmacol.* **9** (supplement 4), 20–22.

Waddington, J.L., Molloy, A.G., O'Boyle, K.M. & Pugh, M.T. (1990) In *Neurobiology of Stereotyped Behaviour* (eds Cooper, S.J. & Dourish, C.T.), pp 64–90. Oxford, Oxford University Press.

Walters, J.R., Bergstrom, D.A., Carlson, J.H., Chase, T.N. & Braun, A.R. (1987) *Science* **236**, 719–722.

Wanibuchi, F. & Usuda, S. (1990) *Psychopharmacology* **102**, 339–342.

Weick, B.G. & Walters, J.R. (1987a) *Brain Res.* **405**, 234–246.

Weick, B.G. & Walters, J.R. (1987b) *Neuropharmacology* **26**, 641–644.

Weiner, D.M., Levey, A.I., Sunahara, R.K., Niznik, H.B., O'Dowd, B.F., Seeman, P. & Brann, M.R. (1991) *Proc. Natl Acad. Sci. USA* **88**, 1859–1863.

White, F.J., Bednarz, L.M., Wachtel, S.R., Hjorth, S. & Brooderson, R.J. (1988) *Pharmacol. Biochem. Behav.* **30**, 189–193.

White, F.J., Hu, X.T. & Brooderson, R.J. (1990) *Eur. J. Pharmacol.* **191**, 497–499.

Yamada, K., Nagashima, M., Kimura, H., Matsumoto, S. & Furukawa, T. (1990) *Psychopharmacology* **100**, 141–144.

Zarrindast, M.R. & Amin, R. (1992) *Psychopharmacology* **106**, 67–70.

Zarrindast, M.R. & Naghashi, H. (1991) *J. Psychopharmacol.* **5**, 160–165.

Zhang, X. & Segawa, T. (1989) *Japan. J. Pharmacol.* **50**, 333–345.

CHAPTER 4

ELECTROPHYSIOLOGICAL CORRELATES OF $D_1 : D_2$ INTERACTIONS

Francis J. White and Xiu-Ti Hu

Neuropsychopharmacology Laboratory, Department of Neuroscience, University of Health Sciences/The Chicago Medical School, 3333 Green Bay Road, North Chicago, IL 60064, USA

Table of Contents

DOPAMINE RECEPTOR INTERACTIONS
ISBN 0–12–729045–1

4.1   Introduction

During the 1980s, drugs selective for the originally defined D_1 and D_2 dopamine (DA) receptors became availaable to researchers interested in testing the concept of this receptor subdivision from a functional perspective. Using a variety of methods, neuroscientists eagerly sought to characterize the DA receptors which might be responsible for the various behavioural, biochemical and electro-physiological effects thought to be mediated by DA. Although numerous biochemical effects were shown to be under the apparent oppositional control of D_1 and D_2 receptors, early behavioural studies yielded perplexing evidence which was not easily assimilated within an oppositional framework of receptor interaction.

As behavioural pharmacologists began to generate findings indicative of cooperative and synergistic interactions between D_1 and D_2 DA receptors, other neuroscientists began the quest for cellular correlates of such interactions. It was at this time, in the mid-1980s, that our laboratory first began to use selective agents for the different DA receptor subtypes to investigate the roles of these receptors in mediating the electrophysiological effects of DA within anatomically defined areas of rat brain. As in the behavioural studies, our early findings regarding the effects of D_1- and D_2-selective agonists within the ventral striatum questioned the extent to which these receptor subtypes worked in functional opposition. As such, they helped lead to the notions of $D_1:D_2$ synergism and the enabling or permissive role of D_1 receptor stimulation for D_2 receptor-mediated functions.

In this chapter, we will review the current literature regarding electrophysio-logical evidence for D_1 and D_2 DA receptor actions and interactions and attempt to integrate such evidence with both behavioural effects and possible mechanisms. It should be noted from the outset that the recent identification of the new D_1-like receptor, D_5 (or D_{1b}), and two new D_2-like DA receptors, D_3 and D_4 (Sokoloff *et al.*, 1990; Sunahara *et al.*, 1991; Van Tol *et al.*, 1991), is likely to add considerable complexity to the concept of DA receptor interaction and may eventually help to resolve many current controversies. However, as with the D_1 and D_2 receptors before them, elucidation of the possible roles of these receptor subtypes must await the development of selective compounds. For the sake of simplicity, we will continue to refer to SK & F 38393 (and related drugs) as selective D_1 agonists and to quinpirole (and other D_2 agonists) as D_2 selective despite the fact that these drugs have high affinities for the D_5 and D_3/D_4 receptors, respectively. We should also note that all of the results obtained from experiments conducted in our laboratory, and many of those from other laboratories, were obtained from anaesthetized rats. Specific preparations used in other studies described herein are noted as necessary.

4.2 Characterization of impulse-regulating somatodendritic autoreceptors

The earliest electrophysiological studies which attempted to characterize DA receptor subtypes were conducted on DA neurones within the rat midbrain. These cells were known to possess autoreceptors along their somatodendritic domains which helped to control firing rates (Aghajanian and Bunney, 1977) by responding to dendritically released DA (Korf et al., 1976; Wang, 1981). White and Wang (1984) first reported that somatodendritic DA autoreceptors were of the D_2 subtype by demonstrating that A10 DA neurones within the ventral tegmental area (VTA) were readily inhibited by iontophoretic administration of D_2-selective agonists, but not by the D_1 agonist SK & F 38393. Antagonism studies also supported the existence of D_2, but not D_1, autoreceptors since the inhibitory effects of DA and DA agonists were blocked or reversed by the D_2 antagonist sulpiride, but not the D_1 antagonist SCH 23390 (White and Wang, 1984). Subsequent studies using systemic injection of these drugs confirmed this observation and extended it to A9 DA cells within the substantia nigra pars compacta (Carlson et al., 1986; Napier et al., 1986; White, 1986). This pharmacological characterization has been supported by a number of subsequent studies, primarily using in vitro slice preparations, which have identified D_2 autoreceptors controlling membrane K^+ conductance (Lacey et al., 1987; Silva and Bunney, 1988), probably via inhibitory guanine nucleotide regulatory (G_i, G_o) proteins (Innis and Aghajanian, 1987). The fact that D_3 receptors are expressed by DA neurones (Sokoloff et al., 1990; Bouthenet et al., 1991) indicates that this subtype may also function as a DA autoreceptor. Thus, the effects of quinpirole, which has a particularly high affinity for D_3 (Sokoloff et al., 1990), may involve both D_2 and D_3 autoreceptors.

Despite the apparent lack of D_1 receptors on DA-containing neurones, D_1 receptor-selective agents have been shown to influence the activity of these cells. Systemically administered SCH 23390 increases the firing of a subpopulation of nigral DA cells (Mereu et al., 1985; Carlson et al., 1986) by activating an inhibitory striatonigral feedback pathway, ultimately leading to an increase in DA cell activity. Extracellular recordings from midbrain DA cells in a slice preparation indicate that SCH 23390 ($10\,\mu M$) excites A9 DA cells without altering the ability of DA to inhibit activity (Suppes and Pinnock, 1987). This suggests that D_1 receptors within the slice, presumably on striatonigral terminals

(Altar and Hauser, 1987; Beckstead, 1988), may also contribute to the excitatory effects of SCH 23390. At higher concentrations, SCH 23390 causes irregular firing and cessation of all activity, which are not reversible by drug washout (Suppes and Pinnock, 1987), suggesting non-receptor-mediated disruption of function. Direct inhibitory effects of the D_1 agonist SK & F 38393 on A9 DA cells have recently been reported in rats depleted of DA by chronic reserpine treatment (Huang and Walters, 1992), although this effect was observed with bolus injections of rather high doses of the agonist (10.0 mg/kg, i.v.). Such doses are considerably higher than those required to produce alterations in either striatal cell activity (0.1–1.0 mg/kg, i.v.) or behaviour (0.5–8.0 mg/kg, s.c. or i.p.) in either normal or DA-depleted rats (Sections 4.3.2, 4.4.1 and 4.7.2).

In addition to the lack of direct effects of D_1 agonists on midbrain DA neurones in normal rats, it is now clear that, unlike postsynaptic D_2 receptors within the striatal complex (Sections 4.3.2 and 4.7.2), D_2 autoreceptors are not modulated by D_1 receptor activity. As mentioned above, D_1 antagonists do not block the effects of D_2 agonists on DA neurones. In addition, neither enhancing D_1 receptor tone with SK & F 38393 nor reducing it by acute DA depletion alters the inhibitory effects of D_2 agonists on DA cells (Carlson et al., 1987; Wachtel et al., 1989). Although recent studies suggest that telencephalic D_1 receptors (presumably within the striatum) may play a role in regulating the rate-dependent nature (White and Wang, 1984) of DA agonist-induced inhibition of A9, but not A10, DA cells (Kelland et al., 1988), the physiological and behavioural relevance of such an effect remains to be established.

4.3 Characterization of dopamine receptors in the ventral striatum (nucleus accumbens)

4.3.1 $D_1:D_2$ synergism

Our laboratory provided the initial electrophysiological evidence for D_1 and D_2 DA receptor effects within the ventral striatum. In these studies (White, 1986; White and Wang, 1986), we tested the effects of iontophoretic administration of D_1 and D_2 agonists on neurones within the rat nucleus accumbens (NAc), which is the primary terminal area for the majority of A10 DA neurones. Because most NAc cells are quiescent or fire at extremely slow rates, glutamate was iontophoretically administered to induce firing of most NAc cells. However, in this and all subsequent studies of the striatal complex described below, both spontaneously active and glutamate-driven neurones were included and in no case was there a significant difference between the two populations with respect to $D_1:D_2$ interactions. Over 80% of NAc cells were inhibited during iontophoretic administration of DA, whereas 40% were inhibited by SK & F 38393 and 75% by the D_2-selective agonist LY 141865 (the racemic form of quinpirole). In addition, receptor selectivity was apparent since sulpiride blocked only the effects of LY 141865 whereas SCH 23390 completely blocked the effects of SK & F 38393 while partially attenuating the effects of LY 141865 (White, 1986; White and Wang, 1986).

In addition to identifying both D_1- and D_2-receptive NAc neurones, we also determined that a subpopulation of neurones was inhibited by both D_1 and D_2 agonists (White, 1986; White and Wang, 1986), a finding that was recently confirmed (Hara *et al.*, 1989). The more important result from our initial studies was that on this set of $D_1:D_2$-responsive NAc cells, co-administration of SK & F 38393 and LY 141865 often produced synergistic (supra-additive) inhibition. These findings suggested that certain NAc neurones possess both D_1 and D_2 receptors which interact in a synergistic, rather than opposing, manner to regulate NAc cell discharge (White and Wang, 1986). Subsequent studies indicated that SK & F 38393 could potentiate the inhibitory effects of quinpirole even on neurones that were not significantly inhibited by the D_1 agonist alone, demonstrating that the percentage of NAc cells responding to the D_1 agonist was more extensive than originally thought (White, 1986, 1987).

4.3.2 The enabling role of D_1 receptors in the ventral striatum

At the time that we first reported the surprising findings of $D_1:D_2$ synergism within the NAc (White and Wang, 1984, 1986), there was only one other published report clearly demonstrating a cooperative $D_1:D_2$ interaction. Gershanik *et al.* (1983) had demonstrated that a combination of D_1- and D_2-selective agonists (SK & F 38393 and LY 141865) was required to reverse reserpine-induced akinesia in mice. Several behavioural findings were soon published to further the notion of synergistic $D_1:D_2$ interactions and to provide hints as to how such synergism might occur (Section 4.7.1). The apparently paradoxical finding that the D_1 antagonist SCH 23390 blocked the behavioural effects of D_2 agonists suggested that D_1 receptor stimulation might be required for the expression of D_2-stimulated behaviour, an effect that was initially described as an 'enabling' or 'permissive' role of the D_1 receptor (Molloy *et al.*, 1986; Waddington, 1986).

In view of the proposed enabling role of D_1 receptors in behavioural effects elicited by D_2 receptor stimulation, we next sought to determine whether this relationship might underly the observed $D_1:D_2$ synergism on NAc cells. To do so, we employed the acute depletion strategy wherein the tyrosine hydroxylase inhibitor α-methyl-*p*-tyrosine (AMPT) was used to reduce striatal levels of DA by 80% (White *et al.*, 1988). In such rats, the normal inhibitory effects of quinpirole on NAc cells were significantly attenuated (White, 1986, 1987; Wachtel *et al.*, 1989). However, they were readily reinstated by co-administration of SK & F 38393 either by iontophoretic administration at low ejection currents which alone produced little inhibition (Figure 1) or by low systemic doses (1.0 mg/kg, i.v.). The reciprocal relationship was not observed (Figure 2) since

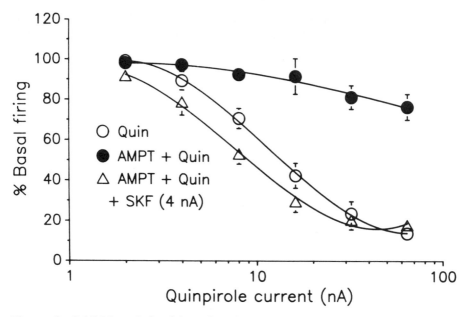

Figure 1 Inhibition of the firing of nucleus accumbens neurones by iontophoretic administration of the D_2 agonist quinpirole (Quin). Current–response curves illustrate attentuation of the inhibitory effect of Quin by pretreatment with α-methyl-*p*-tyrosine (AMPT) and reinstatement of the Quin-induced inhibition on the same neurones with co-iontophoresis of SK & F 38393 (4 nA). Each point represents the mean ± SEM (Quin control, $n = 11$; AMPT, $n = 12$; AMPT + SK & F 38393, $n = 11$). Adapted from Wachtel *et al.* (1989), with permission.

acute DA depletion failed to attenuate the inhibitory effects of SK & F 38393 (White *et al.*, 1987; Wachtel *et al.*, 1989). Our original findings have now been extended to other selective D_1 and D_2 agonists (Johansen *et al.*, 1988, 1991; Wachtel *et al.*, 1989). Thus, activation of D_1 receptors in rats acutely depleted of DA enables D_2 receptor occupation to produce an inhibition of cellular discharge, further suggesting that endogenous DA acts at D_1 receptors to enable D_2-mediated events in the intact rat (White, 1986, 1987).

4.3.3 Intracellular recordings from nucleus accumbens neurones

In contrast to the extracellular recordings obtained from our *in vivo* studies, intracellular recordings from NAc neurones in an *in vitro* slice preparation suggest that D_1 and D_2 receptors can, in fact, exert opposite effects on cellular activity. Selective stimulation of D_1 receptors hyperpolarizes whereas selective stimulation of D_2 receptors depolarizes NAc cells (Uchimura *et al.*, 1986; Uchimura and North, 1990). Both effects appear to be due to alterations in K^+ conductance (Uchimura and North, 1990).

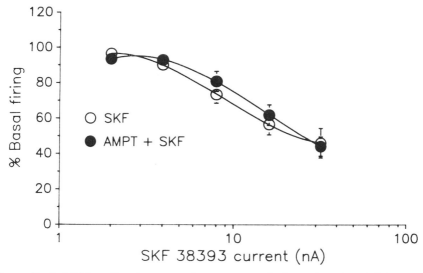

Figure 2 Inhibition of nucleus accumbens neurones by iontophoretic administration of the D$_1$ agonist SK & F 38393. Current–response curves illustrate the failure of AMPT pretreatment to affect the inhibition of NAc neurones by SK & F 38393. Each point represents the mean ± SEM (SK & F 38393 control, $n = 10$; AMPT + SK & F 38393, $n = 11$). Adapted from Wachtel *et al.* (1989), with permission.

The discrepancy between *in vivo* and *in vitro* effects of DA receptor stimulation has yet to be resolved but is likely to involve the presence of afferent activation *in vivo*. Certainly, the presence of functional DAergic and other inputs not present *in vitro* may influence the 'resting' membrane potential of NAc cells, an important factor in the ability of drugs to alter specific conductances. Similar activity- dependent alterations in drug effects can occur *in vivo*. Recent studies from our laboratory indicate that, in addition to inhibiting NAc cells *in vivo*, both D$_1$ and D$_2$ agonists can cause excitatory effects under certain conditions (Section 4.8.2). Thus, the particular effects of D$_1$ and D$_2$ agonists will depend upon both the experimental preparation and the specific manipulations and dependent variables being used to assay drug action.

4.4 Characterization of dopamine receptors in the dorsal striatum (caudate-putamen)

4.4.1 Extracellular recordings

The earliest electrophysiological attempts to characterize DA receptor subtypes within the dorsal striatum were conducted in cats. These studies demonstrated apparent excitation produced by D_2, but not D_1, receptor activation during electrical stimulation of the substantia nigra (Ohno *et al.*, 1985, 1986). This conclusion was based upon the ability of the D_2 receptor agonist domperidome, applied iontophoretically, to reduce the activation of caudate neurones produced by single-pulse stimulation of the nigra. Accordingly, iontophoretic application of D_2 agonists also excited striatal cells (Ohno *et al.*, 1986) whereas D_1 agonists inhibited them (Ohno *et al.*, 1987).

Similar extracellular recordings of rat striatal neurones by a number of investigators have uniformly found that local administration (by either iontophoresis or micropressure ejection) of both D_1- and D_2-selective agonists produces primarily inhibition of activity (Hu and Wang, 1988, 1989; Wachtel *et al.*, 1989; Bickford-Wimer *et al.*, 1990; Hu *et al.*, 1990; White *et al.*, 1990; Hu and White, 1992a), although a potentiation of glutamate-induced activity can be observed with low ejection currents of D_1 and D_2 agonists (Hu and Wang, 1988, 1989; Hu *et al.*, 1990). The reasons for the discrepancy between these various reports and those of Ohno and colleagues (above) may be related to a number of variables, including the different species involved. It is also noteworthy that the Ohno *et al.* reports routinely employed very high ejection currents apparently without current neutralization which can lead to artifactual results. It is also surprising that single-pulse stimulation of the substantia nigra, as employed by Ohno and co-workers, should produce monosynaptic DA-dependent activation, since it is well accepted that such stimulation preferentially activates polysynaptic inputs to the striatum via the cortex and thalamus (Wilson *et al.*, 1982; Ryan *et al.*, 1986). Moreover, long-latency stimulation of striatal neurone action potentials following single-pulse stimulation of the nigra has been shown to be primarily antidromic, rather than orthodromic, in origin (Ryan *et al.*, 1986). Indeed, pulse-train stimulation is required to activate midbrain DA cells which exhibit a relatively high chronaxie (Vives and Mogenson, 1986).

As in the NAc, most neurones in the dorsal striatum are very slow firing or quiescent, such that excitatory amino acids are often used to drive their activity. In contrast to the NAc, where most neurones were more sensitive to D_2 agonists (White and Wang, 1986), the majority of neurones within the medial caudate-putamen (CPu) were inhibited by the D_1 agonist SK & F 38393, whereas fewer cells were inhibited by the D_2 agonist quinpirole (Hu and Wang, 1988). In addition, $D_1:D_2$ synergism was demonstrated following combined intravenous administration of SK & F 38393 (0.1–1.0 mg/kg) and quinpirole (1.0 mg/kg), but not during iontophoretic administration of the two agonists (Hu and Wang, 1988). Later studies (Hu *et al.*, 1990) conducted within the lateral CPu demonstrated a greater percentage of D_2-responsive neurones and a potentiating effect of iontophoretic SK & F 38393 on quinpirole-induced inhibition when low, sub-inhibitory currents were used to apply SK & F 38393 continuously during a quinpirole current–response determination (Figure 3A). The differences between these findings and those of Hu and Wang (1988) suggest possible regional variations in striatal $D_1:D_2$ interactions which may be due to distribution gradients of D_2 receptors throughout the striatal complex (Boyson *et al.*, 1986; Joyce, 1991).

A clear enabling relationship between D_1 and D_2 DA receptors has been shown within the lateral CPu. As in the NAc, acute DA depletion by AMPT treatment nearly abolished the inhibitory effects of quinpirole and another D_2 agonist, RU 24213, on CPu neurones (Figure 3B). This effect was readily reversed by co-iontophoretic administration of SK & F 38393 (Wachtel *et al.*, 1989; Hu *et al.*, 1990). Acute DA depletion failed to alter the inhibitory effects of SK & F 38393 or the mixed D_1/D_2 agonist apomorphine on striatal cells (Wachtel *et al.*, 1989).

4.4.2 Intracellular recordings

The effects of D_1 and D_2 DA receptor agonists on striatal neurones have also been studied with intracellular recordings from *in vitro* slice preparations. Unfortunately, these studies have provided conflicting results. Akaike *et al.* (1987) first reported that low concentrations of DA ($1 \mu M$) produced domperidone-reversible depolarization of striatal cells, whereas higher concentrations ($100 \mu M$) produced SCH 23390-reversible hyperpolarizations, suggesting differential involvement of D_2 and D_1 receptors, respectively. In contrast, Calabresi *et al.* (1987) reported that DA failed to alter the membrane potential of striatal cells but produced a suppression of locally elicited excitatory postsynaptic potentials (EPSPs) via an action on D_1 receptors presumably modulating Na^+ currents. D_2 receptor activation was without effect unless rats were depleted of DA for at least 12 h (Calabresi *et al.*, 1988a, b). More recently, Bertolucci *et al.* (1991) found that either D_1 or D_2 receptor stimulation can suppress EPSPs elicited by local stimulation.

At least two studies have now investigated DA receptor subtypes controlling specific conductances in acutely isolated striatal cells. During cell-attached patch recordings from striatal neurones acutely dissociated from the brains of 31–45-day-old rats, Freedman and Weight (1988) reported that DA and the D_2 agonist quinpirole caused single K^+ channel openings which were blocked by haloperidol and spiperone. Such increased K^+ permeability would be expected to result in an outward current resulting in hyperpolarization, as has been observed with D_2 receptors in other preparations (Lacey *et al.*, 1987; Einhorn *et al.*, 1991). Interestingly, SCH 23390 was also able to prevent the effects of quinpirole on K^+ channels in half of the cells tested (Freedman and Weight, 1988), raising the possibility of an enabling interaction between D_1 and D_2 receptors in this preparation.

A more recent study found that both D_1 and D_2 receptor agonists modulate Na^+ currents in retrogradely labelled striatonigral cells acutely isolated from adult rats (Surmeier *et al.*, 1992). In most neurones, both SK & F 38393 (81%) and the D_2 agonists quinpirole and bromocriptine (55%) reduced evoked whole-cell Na^+ current, an effect which was blocked by appropriate antagonists.

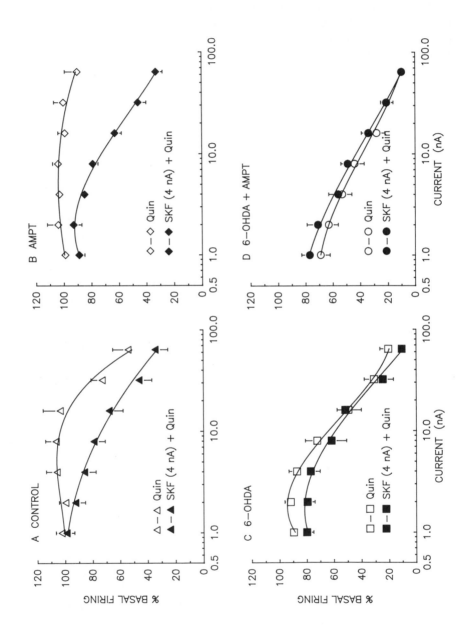

88

In 20% of the whole-cell recordings, D_2 agonists increased the amplitude of the Na^+ current, an effect which was also blocked by sulpiride. In cell-attached patch recordings, bath application of SK & F 38393 decreased currents whereas D_2 agonists consistently enhanced currents. The different effects of D_2 agonists in the two recording preparations suggest the likelihood of two distinct D_2 receptor-mediated actions, perhaps due to the presence of both D_2 and D_3 receptors on these striatonigral neurones (Section 4.8.1). These types of studies have great promise for further elucidation of DA receptor subtype actions and interactions and could help resolve present discrepancies obtained with other recording preparations.

4.5 Effects of D_1 and D_2 agonists on other basal ganglia neurones

4.5.1 Substantia nigra pars reticulata

The substantia nigra pars reticulata is a major output centre of the basal ganglia, receiving a dense innervation from the striatum. DA is known to exert dual effects on neurones within the substantia nigra pars reticulata. In paralysed, artificially respired rats, it increases the firing of about 50% of these neurones and more consistently decreases the inhibitory effects of GABA (Waszczak and Walters, 1983, 1984, 1986). The excitatory effect can be mimicked by 8-bromo-cAMP (Matthews and German, 1986) and by SK & F 38393 (Waszczak, 1990) via interactions with D_1 receptor mechanisms located on the terminals of striatonigral neurones (Altar and Hauser, 1987; Beckstead, 1988).

Figure 3 Comparison of responses of dorsal striatal neurones to co-iontophoretic administration of D_1- and D_2-selective agonists in various treatment groups. (A) In control rats, a low, sub-inhibitory current of SK & F 38393 potentiated the inhibitory effects of quinpirole on the same striatal neurones ($n = 10$). (B) In rats acutely depleted of DA by AMPT, quinpirole-induced inhibition was attenuated without simultaneous stimulation of D_1 receptors ($n = 15$). (C) In rats chronically depleted of DA by 6-OHDA lesions, the requirement of D_1 receptor stimulation for quinpirole-induced inhibition was abolished ($n = 23$), as was the potentiating (synergistic) effect of SK & F 38393 on quinpirole-induced inhibition ($n = 15$). (D) Additional depletion of DA with AMPT in 6-OHDA-lesioned rats not only enhanced the inhibitory effect induced by quinpirole but also failed to produce a synergistic inhibition ($n = 10$), indicating that: (1) the supersensitive response observed in 6-OHDA-pretreated rats was not maximal, thereby masking possible potentiation by SK & F 38393; and (2) the ability of D_2 receptor stimulation to inhibit striatal neurones in 6-OHDA rats was not due to residual DA stimulating supersensitive D_1 receptors (enabling). From Hu *et al.* (1990), with permission.

The ability to modulate GABA-induced inhibition is mimicked by D_2 agonists (Waszczak, 1990).

These findings suggest that dendritically released DA can alter neurotransmission through the reticulata in two distinct ways, depending upon the DA receptor subtype activated. However, at least one study has questioned the extent to which D_1 receptors on striatonigral neurones are stimulated by endogenously released DA (Ryan et al., 1989). A synergistic interaction between D_1 and D_2 agonists in the inhibition of reticulata neurones has also been observed following systemic administration to rats with 6-hydroxydopamine (6-OHDA) lesions of the nigrostriatal pathway (Weick and Walters, 1987), as will be discussed below (Section 4.7.3).

4.5.2 Globus pallidus

The globus pallidus is another major recipient of striatal afferents. The non- selective $D_1 : D_2$ receptor agonist apomorphine, administered intravenously, potently increases the firing of globus pallidus neurones in paralysed rats (Bergstrom et al., 1982). When administered alone, D_2-selective agonists produce modest increases in firing but SK & F 38393 elicits no consistent alterations at reasonable doses (< 10 mg/kg, i.v.) and only modest and inconsistent effects at extremely high doses (20 mg/kg). Combinations of this high SK & F 38393 dose with low doses of D_2 agonists causes a marked excitation similar to that observed with apomorphine, suggesting that concurrent stimulation of D_1 and D_2 receptors is necessary for the full excitatory effect (Carlson et al., 1987; Walters et al., 1987).

Walters and colleagues have also demonstrated $D_1 : D_2$ interactions on pallidal neurones in rats acutely depleted of DA (Carlson et al., 1987; Walters et al., 1987). These fndings closely parallel our own results within the striatal complex. AMPT pretreatment attenuates the partial excitatory effects of intravenous quinpirole, but not the more marked excitatory effects of apomorphine. Subsequent administration of SK & F 38393 to rats which had received quinpirole produces marked increases in pallidal firing equivalent to those produced by apomorphine (Walters et al., 1987). This group has also demonstrated that the excitatory effects of systemic apomorphine on pallidal neurones are attenuated by ipsilateral quinolinic acid lesions of the rostral striatum (Pan et al., 1990; Pan and Walters, 1988), suggesting that the excitatory effects of apomorphine on pallidal neurones result from disinhibition, with the primary effect being suppression of the discharge of GABAergic striatopallidal neurones. This, in turn, suggests that the permissive role of D_1 receptor stimulation for D_2 agonist-induced excitation of globus pallidus neurones may result from the direct enabling actions on striatopallidal GABAergic neurones (Wachtel et al., 1989).

4.5.3 Ventral pallidum

Analogous to the pathway from dorsal striatum to the globus pallidus is a corresponding projection from the ventral striatum (NAc) to the infracommissural extension of the pallidum, i.e. the ventral pallidum/substantia innominata region (Heimer and Wilson, 1975). The response of ventral pallidal neurones to systemic administration of DA agonists is more complex than that reported within the globus pallidus (Napier *et al.*, 1991; Maslowski and Napier, 1991). Systemic administration of SK & F 38393 increases the firing of most ventral pallidal neurones at doses considerably below (0.1–3.2 mg/kg, i.v.) those which are effective within the dorsal pallidum (above). Moreover, D$_2$ agonists produce predominantly inhibitions of ventral pallidal cells, as opposed to the excitations observed within the dorsal pallidum.

Yang and Mogenson (1989) reported that SK & F 38393 enables the ability of quinpirole to increase the firing of rat ventral pallidal neurones, which receive an inhibitory input from NAc GABAergic neurones, when the D$_1$ agonist is infused directly into the NAc prior to the D$_2$ agonist. However, a recent study by Napier (1992) indicates that activation of D$_1$ and D$_2$ receptors within the NAc is not necessary for ventral pallidal responses to systemic DA agonist administration and that D$_1$ receptors within the amygdala may play a role in such responses via an amygdala-ventral pallidal projection.

4.6 Effects of D$_1$ and D$_2$ agonists in other dopaminoceptive regions

4.6.1 Medial prefrontal cortex

The medial prefrontal cortex (mPFC) receives a prominent innervation from VTA DA neurones. Local administration of DA or electrical stimulation of the VTA markedly inhibits the firing of neurones in this area (Bunney and Aghajanian, 1976; Thierry *et al.*, 1986). Pharmacological characterizations of the DA receptors responsible for this inhibition have yielded different results. Sesack and Bunney (1989) first reported that iontophoretic application of either SK & F 38393 or quinpirole, as well as their combined administration, failed to mimick the inhibitory efficacy of DA on mPFC neurones recorded from rats in a low cerveaux isole preparation. Moreover, quinpirole significantly attenuated the inhibitory effect of DA, suggesting that it may exert partial agonist effects. Thus, the D$_2$ receptor in the mPFC was suggested to differ from that within other brain areas. Along a similar line, Yang and Mogenson (1990) reported complex modulatory effects of DA on acetylcholine (ACh)-evoked activity of mPFC neurones in anaesthetized rats. Although DA increased the signal/noise ratio of ACh-evoked responses through a D$_2$-like receptor (sulpiride-sensitive), this effect was not mimicked by quinpirole. At higher ejection currents, DA produced the opposite effect, decreasing the signal/noise ratio of ACh-evoked responses via a D$_1$-like (SCH 23390-sensitive) receptor (Yang and Mogenson, 1990). In contrast to both of these reports, Parfitt *et al.* (1990) found that both

D_1- and D_2-selective agonists, administered locally by pressure ejection, inhibited the great majority of mPFC neurones in anaesthetized rats, but no evidence for synergism was reported. Godbout *et al.* (1991) reported that D_2, but not D_1, agonists mimicked the inhibitory effects of DA on mPFC neurones in anaesthetized rats.

4.6.2 Hippocampus

Smialowski and Bijack (1987) characterized DA receptors responsible for DA's actions within the rat hippocampus. Using extracellular recordings from a slice preparation, these authors first reported that CA1 pyramidal cells could be both excited and inhibited by DA. The excitatory effect was elicited by lower concentrations of DA and was mediated by D_2 receptors whereas the inhibitory effect was less sensitive and mediated by D_1 receptors (Smialowski and Bijack, 1987). Recent intracellular recordings from CA1 pyramidal neurones confirmed that D_1 receptor stimulation produced hyperpolarizations and D_2 receptor stimulation produced depolarizations (Beretta *et al.*, 1990).

4.7   Relationship between electrophysiology and behaviour

When viewing the current status of the literature regarding the electro-physiological actions controlled by D_1 and D_2 DA receptors, it becomes clear that many discrepancies remain to be resolved. In many ways, these discrepancies resemble the long-standing controversy as to whether DA is an excitatory or inhibitory transmitter; for example, see Siggins (1978) and Kitai (1981). It now seems obvious that DA exerts a variety of effects on CNS neurones which are dependent upon a number of factors, including the specific neurone being studied, its prevailing afferent inputs and related membrane voltage state, and the specific subtypes of DA receptor(s) which it possesses. When coupled with an appreciation of the increasing number of identified D_1- and D_2-like receptors and possible transduction mechanisms, it is not surprising that experiments using disparate experimental preparations and procedures have identified so many different effects. For our purpose, one of the critical questions is the extent to which the electrophysiological findings correspond to the effects of D_1 and D_2 agonists observed in behavioural studies. The following discussion will address this question.

4.7.1   The enabling role of D_1 receptors: electrophysiology and behaviour

The types of synergisms which we have observed on striatal neurones (Sections 4.3 and 4.4), and which Walters and colleagues (Section 4.5.2) have observed on pallidal neurones, are closely paralleled by behavioural findings. First, the ability of low, sub-inhibitory currents of D_1 agonists to potentiate the inhibitory effects of D_2 agonists on striatal neurones in normal rats is similar to the ability of D_1 agonists to potentiate locomotor and stereotyped behaviours produced by D_2-selective agonists (Braun and Chase, 1986; Mashurano and Waddington, 1986; Arnt et al., 1987; Walters et al., 1987; Koller and Herbster, 1988; Meller et al., 1988; White et al., 1988). Similar results have been obtained following direct administration of these agonists into the striatal complex. Bilateral administration of either D_1 or D_2 agonists into the ventral striatum can promote locomotion, but the combined administration of such drugs produces a synergistic effect (Bordi and Meller, 1989; Dreher and Jackson, 1989; Plaznik et al., 1989). However, the recent finding that intracranial administration of SK & F 38393 can produce extensive neurotoxicity (Kelly et al., 1990) prescribes caution when interpreting such findings.

The second similarity between our electrophysiological results and behavioural studies is the absolute necessity of D_1 receptor activation for D_2 agonist-induced inhibition of striatal neurones. Behavioural studies using acute DA depletion, produced by vesicular depletion (reserpine) and/or synthesis inhibition (AMPT), have demonstrated that the effects of D_2 agonists are abolished in such rats, but are readily reinstated by D_1 agonists. This has been observed for a variety of D_2 agonist-induced behaviours, including locomotor activity and stereotypy (Braun and Chase, 1986; Jackson and Hashizume, 1986; Longoni et al., 1987b; Walters et al., 1987; White et al., 1988), yawning (Longoni et al., 1987a; Ushijima et al., 1988) and circling in rats with quinolinic acid lesions of the striatum (Barone et al., 1986). As in our electrophysiological experiments (Wachtel et al., 1989), acute DA depletion failed to alter apomorphine-induced stereotyped behaviour because apomorphine supplies the necessary D_1 receptor stimulation (White et al., 1988).

4.7.2   Do D_2 receptors enable the effects of D_1 receptor stimulation?

While there has been near total agreement on the enabling role of D_1 receptor stimulation for many D_2 receptor-mediated functional effects, such has not been the case for a possible role of D_2 receptor stimulation for D_1 receptor-mediated effects. Our electrophysiological studies revealed no alteration in D_1 agonist-induced inhibition of striatal neurones following acute DA depletion (White et al., 1987; Wachtel et al., 1989; Johansen et al., 1991). Similarly, the excitatory effects of systemic SK & F 38393 on rat globus pallidus neurones (Carlson et al., 1988) are still evident in rats acutely depleted of DA. In contrast, the weak inhibitory effects of SK & F 38393 observed on a small subset (14%) of pallidal cells are abolished (Carlson et al., 1988). However, since very weak inhibitory effects of SK & F 38393 were observed only at extremely high doses (20.0 mg/kg, i.v.), far above those required to elicit reliable behavioural effects

(0.5–8.0 mg/kg, s.c.), the physiological relevance of such minor changes in a small subset of pallidal cells is dubious.

Using D_1 agonist-induced grooming behaviour, Waddington and colleagues have recently argued that D_2 receptor stimulation is necessary for D_1 agonist- induced behaviour. This conclusion is based upon the ability of certain selective D_2 antagonists to reduce D_1 agonist-induced grooming (Molloy and Waddington, 1987b; Murray and Waddington, 1989; Waddington, 1989). However, many studies have found that SK & F 38393-induced grooming is not blocked by selective D_2 antagonists such as haloperidol, metoclopramide and sulpiride (Molloy and Waddington, 1984, 1985, 1987a, b; Vasse and Protais, 1988; Chandler et al., 1990). The reason for the differential effects of various D_2 blockers is presently unclear. Our studies indicate that the D_2 antagonist eticlopride reduced, but did not abolish, SK & F 38393-induced grooming, but that the antagonist failed to produce a parallel shift in the SK & F 38393 dose–response curve. This indicates a lack of competitive antagonism as would be expected with physiological or functional blockade (Wachtel et al., 1992). Clearly arguing against a permissive role of D_2 receptors for the expression of D_1-stimulated behaviour is the consistent finding (Molloy and Waddington, 1985; Starr and Starr, 1986; Starr et al., 1987; Vasse and Protais, 1988; Wachtel et al., 1992) that D_2 antagonists, when combined with the non-selective D_1/D_2 agonist apomorphine, unmask D_1 receptor-mediated grooming responses.

Controversy also exists with respect to D_2 receptor influences on D_1 agonist- induced grooming when D_2 activation is reduced by acute DA depletion. Some investigators have reported that acute DA depletion abolished grooming induced by SK & F 38393 (Braun and Chase, 1986; Starr et al., 1987; Ross et al., 1988). However, we reported that pretreatment with either AMPT or the combination of AMPT and reserpine (>99% DA depletion) reduced but did not prevent SK & F 38393-induced grooming in rats (White et al., 1988). In fact, grooming was the only behaviour in which these rats engaged, leading us to conclude that the reduction in grooming was not due to the loss of D_2-mediated enabling of the D_1 response, but rather reflected the severe akinesia produced by such treatments. We believe that the previously reported losses of SK & F 38393-induced grooming following acute depletion may have resulted either from the use of a time-sampling procedure, which may have missed grooming episodes, or from observational periods of insufficient duration. In our studies, wherein rats are watched continuously for 30–45 min, acute DA depletion has been found to delay the onset of SK & F 38393-induced grooming.

A final line of evidence which has been used to support the notion that D_2 receptor stimulation is necessary for SK & F 38393-enhanced grooming is that the behaviour is reduced in aged rats (Molloy and Waddington, 1988), with a reported 26% reduction in D_2 DA receptors, but normal levels of D_1 DA receptors (O'Boyle and Waddington, 1984). However, when the irreversible DA receptor antagonist EEDQ is used to inactivate over 50% of both D_1 and D_2 DA receptors, a similar reduction in SK & F 38393-induced grooming (46%) is observed. When

D_1, but not D_2, receptors are protected from inactivation, no reduction is observed (Wachtel *et al.*, 1992). Thus, in rats with a normal complement of D_1 receptors but with a greater than 50% loss of D_2 receptors, SK & F 38393-elicited grooming is unchanged. This finding questions the extent to which the reduction in grooming reported in aged rats was due to decreases in D_2 receptor density (Molloy and Waddington, 1988). Moreover, many recent investigations have found substantially reduced levels of D_1 DA receptors in aged rats (Giorgio *et al.*, 1987; Hyttel, 1987; Morelli *et al.*, 1990), including those within the lateral striatum (Morelli *et al.*, 1990), the site which appears to be primarily involved in SK & F 38393-induced grooming (Neisewander *et al.*, 1991).

Taken together, these observations lead us to conclude that the attenuation of SK & F 38393-induced grooming behaviour by certain D_2 antagonists, like that produced by acute DA depletion, is the result of an overall decrease in behavioural responsiveness rather than removal of D_2 receptor-mediated enabling of the D_1 response. Certainly, it does not appear that D_2 receptor stimulation by endogenous DA is absolutely required for the production of this D_1 receptor-mediated behaviour in the same manner that D_2 receptor-mediated behaviours require D_1 receptor stimulation by DA. The close parallel between these findings and our electrophysiological evidence is noteworthy given that the cellular relationships were demonstrated within the portion of the lateral striatum (Hu *et al.*, 1990; Wachtel *et al.*, 1989) thought to be involved in SK & F 38393-induced grooming behaviour (Neisewander *et al.*, 1991).

4.7.3 Chronic DA depletion relieves D_2 receptors from necessity of D_1 stimulation

One of the most intriguing aspects of the enabling relationship between D_1 and D_2 receptors is the apparent loss of such interaction following chronic DA depletion. In contrast to their ability to block the unconditioned behaviour effects of D_2 agonists in normal rats, D_1 receptor antagonists fail to block the behavioural effects of both mixed D_1/D_2 agonists and selective D_2 agonists in behavioural models utilizing rats with supersensitive DA receptors (Arnt, 1985a, b; Arnt and Hyttel, 1985; Breese and Mueller, 1985). While both D_1 and D_2 agonists elicit rotation in rats with unilateral 6-OHDA lesions of the nigrostriatal pathway, these effects are blocked only by antagonists selective for those receptors (Arnt and Hyttel, 1984, 1985). Similarly, the hyperactivity produced by D_1 or D_2 agonists in rats with bilateral 6-OHDA lesions (Arnt, 1985b; Breese and Mueller, 1985) or in rats treated repeatedly with reserpine (Arnt, 1985a) is blocked only by the appropriate receptor-selective antagonist. These findings suggest that the necessity of D_1 receptor stimulation for D_2 receptor-mediated functional responses may be relieved after chronic DA depletion.

We have recently investigated these relationships using electrophysiological techniques (Hu *et al.*, 1990). In striking contrast to the effects of acute DA depletion (AMPT), long-term depletion of DA produced by 6-OHDA lesions of the nigrostriatal DA system did not attenuate the inhibitory effects of iontophoretic quinpirole on dorsolateral striatal neurones (Figure 3C). In fact, the inhibitory potency of quinpirole was enhanced (supersensitive) as compared to the intact striatum (Figure 3A versus Figure 3C). The inhibitory effects of quinpirole in the denervated striatum could not be attributed to residual DA stimulating supersensitive D_1 receptors (and thereby enabling D_2 receptor-mediated inhibition) since further DA depletion produced by additional acute administration of AMPT failed to reduce the effects of quinpirole (Figure 3D). Moreover, the lack of necessity for D_1 receptor stimulation for D_2 agonist-induced inhibition in the 6-OHDA rat could not be attributed to the loss of DA terminals and possible cell–cell $D_1:D_2$ interactions since similar findings were observed with repeated reserpine treatment (Hu et al., 1990). In addition to abolishing the enabling relationship between D_1 and D_2 receptors, chronic DA depletion also abolished the ability of the D_1 agonist SK & F 38393 to potentiate quinpirole-induced inhibition (Figure 3C). Thus, these electrophysiological results provide a single-cell correlate of behavioural evidence indicating an uncoupling of $D_1:D_2$ synergisms in rats following chronic DA depletion.

In spite of the apparent uncoupling of D_1 and D_2 receptor function in rats with supersensitive DA receptors, several investigators have reported synergistic rotational responses to D_1 and D_2 DA agonists in rats with unilateral 6-OHDA lesions of the nigrostriatal tract (Koller and Herbster, 1988; Robertson and Robertson, 1986; 1987; Rouillard and Bedard, 1988; Sonsalla et al., 1988). Thus, although there is an apparent lack of 'adjacent' $D_1:D_2$ synergisms within the striatum, D_1 and D_2 receptors can still work in concert to regulate behaviour in DA denervated rats. It is likely that such regulation results from a 'systems-level' or 'distant' interaction involving D_1 and D_2 receptors in distinct, but connected, basal ganglia sites. In fact, Robertson and Robertson (1986) argued that synergistic rotational responses in unilateral 6-OHDA-lesioned rats were due to D_2 receptors within the striatum and D_1 receptors within the substantia nigra pars reticulata. Electrophysiological support for this possibility comes from the work of Weick and Walters (1987), who have demonstrated synergistic inhibitions of reticulata neurones by systemic administration of SK & F 38393 and quinpirole only in 6-OHDA-lesioned rats.

4.7.4 D_1 receptors regulate the development of D_2 receptor supersensitivity following denervation

Because 6-OHDA lesions of the nigrostriatal pathway lead to supersensitive cellular responses mediated by both D_1 and D_2 receptors (Figure 4), it is unclear whether supersensitivity of one or both of these receptors plays a critical role in the uncoupling of $D_1:D_2$ synergisms. To address this question, we conducted additional studies which attempted to prevent 6-OHDA-induced supersensitivity of D_1 or D_2 receptors by initiating a regimen of chronic agonist treatment immediately after producing a lesion. Thus, following postoperative recovery

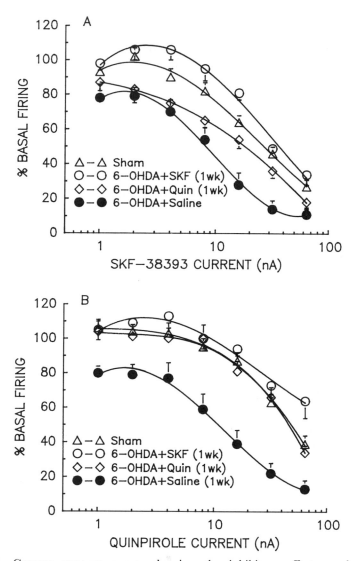

Figure 4 Current–response curves showing the inhibitory effects produced by iontophoretic administration of the selective D_1 receptor agonist SK & F 38393 (A) and the selective D_2 receptor agonist quinpirole (B) on dorsal striatal neurones in sham (ascorbic acid vehicle) and 6-OHDA-lesioned rats. Striatal neurones recorded in saline-treated, DA denervated rats were significantly more sensitive to the inhibitory effects of both SK & F 38393 and quinpirole (12 cells each) as compared to sham-lesioned rats (13 cells each). However, the enhanced inhibitory striatal responses to both SK & F 38393 and quinpirole (10 cells each) were prevented following daily administration of SK & F 38393 (8.0 mg/kg, s.c.). In contrast, daily quinpirole injection (0.5 mg/kg, s.c.) prevented the enhancement of inhibitory responses to quinpirole but failed to affect the supersensitive response to SK & F 38393 (10 cells each) as compared to sham-lesioned rats. Each data point represents the mean percentage inhibition ± SEM. From Hu and White (1992a), with permssion.

(24 h), different groups of rats were treated daily (for 7 days) with either SK & F 38393 (8.0 mg/kg), quinpirole (0.5 mg/kg) or saline and were tested in electrophysiological or behavioural studies 12–24 h after the last injection.

Denervation supersensitivity of neuronal responses within the rat striatum was prevented by this repeated daily treatment with DA receptor agonists (Hu and White, 1992a). Striatal neurones in 6-OHDA-lesioned rats that had received daily repeated administration of the selective D_1 receptor agonist SK & F 38393 failed to exhibit supersensitive inhibitory responses to this agonist administered iontophoretically (Figure 4A). Similar prevention of supersensitive D_2 agonist-induced inhibition was observed following repeated daily treatment with the selective D_2 receptor agonist quinpirole (Figure 4B). When rats were allowed a 4-week withdrawal from the chronic agonist treatment, supersensitivity was evident, indicating that the preventive effect was not permanent. Taken together, these findings suggest that under certain experimental conditions, exogenous DA agonists can supply relatively normal levels of activation of the respective receptors in the near absence of endogenous DA (Hu and White, 1992a).

The unexpected finding of this set of experiments was that daily repeated treatment with a selective D_1 receptor agonist also prevented the ability of DA denervation to induce a functional supersensitivity of striatal D_2 DA receptors (Hu and White, 1992a). Thus striatal neurones from 6-OHDA-lesioned, SK & F 38393-treated rats exhibited normal sensitivity not only to this D_1 agonist but also to quinpirole (Figure 4B). In addition, prevention of D_1 receptor supersensitivity by repeated SK & F 38393 treatment also preserved the normal ability of this D_1 agonist to potentiate D_2 agonist-induced inhibition of striatal neurones when both agonists were administered (Figure 5A). Therefore, it appears that D_1 receptors can regulate the development of D_2 receptor denervation supersensitivity and that D_1 receptor supersensitivity is intricately involved in the uncoupling of adjacent synergistic $D_1 : D_2$ interactions (Hu and White, 1992a). Whether selective D_2 receptor supersensitivity might also cause an uncoupling of $D_1 : D_2$ receptor synergism cannot be determined from our 6-OHDA studies since no such selectivity was afforded by the repeated SK & F 38393 injections in 6-OHDA lesioned rats.

The ability of D_1 receptors to regulate D_2 receptor sensitivity and to uncouple functional $D_1 : D_2$ interactions was not reciprocated since daily repeated administration of quinpirole failed to prevent the development of functional D_1 receptor supersensitivity (Figure 4A) and $D_1 : D_2$ uncoupling (Figure 5B) in 6-OHDA-lesioned rats. In this regard, the present results resemble our previous findings indicating that D_1 receptor stimulation in normal rats is required for certain D_2 agonist-induced electrophysiological and behavioural effects but that similar effects of D_1 agonists do not require D_2 receptor stimulation. Thus, D_1 receptors appear to play an essential regulatory role in the functioning of D_2 receptors (Hu and White, 1992a).

We also observed a behavioural parallel of these electrophysiological results (Hu and White, 1992a). Rats that received unilateral 6-OHDA lesions of the

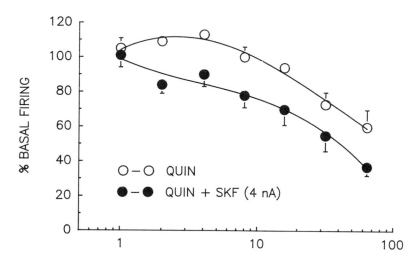

A. 6–OHDA LESION WITH DAILY SKF–38393 TREATMENT

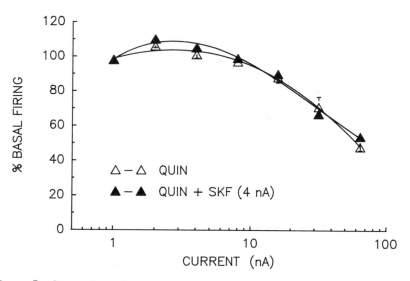

B. 6–OHDA LESION WITH DAILY QUINPIROLE TREATMENT

Figure 5 Comparison of responses of striatal neurones to iontophoretic administration of quinpirole with and without concurrently applied SK & F 38393 in SK & F 38393-treated (8.0 mg/kg, s.c.), or quinpirole-treated (0.5 mg/kg, s.c.) DA denervated rats. (A) A low, sub-inhibitory current of SK & F 38393 (4 nA) significantly potentiated the inhibitory effects of quinpirole on the same striatal neurones in SK & F 38393-pretreated rats. (B) Similar potentiation experiments were unsuccessful in quinpirole-pretreated rats. Adapted from Hu and White (1992a) with permission.

nigrostriatal DA pathway and subsequent daily treatment with SK & F 38393 failed to exhibit contralateral rotation to the non-selective D_1/D_2 DA agonist apomorphine. In contrast, 6-OHDA-lesioned rats that received daily quinpirole injections still exhibited contralateral rotation to apomorphine (Figure 6). The ability of repeated SK & F 38393 treatment to prevent apomorphine-induced rotation was not due solely to prevention of D_1 receptor supersensitivity since rotational responses to apomorphine require stimulation of both D_1 and D_2

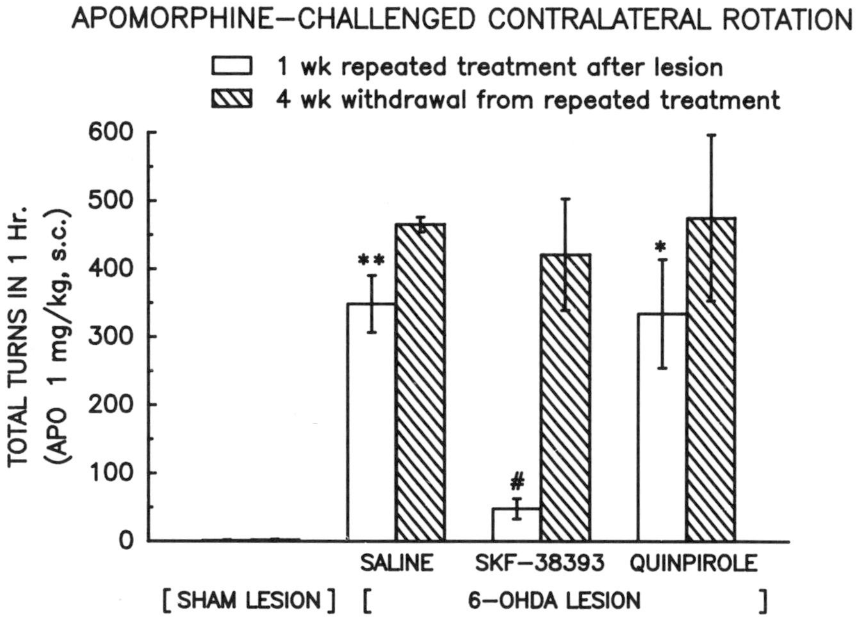

Figure 6 Daily treatment with the selective D_1 agonist SK & F 38393 prevented apomorphine-stimulated contralateral turning in rats with unilateral 6-OHDA lesions of the nigrostriatal pathway. Apomorphine (1 mg/kg, s.c.) induced strong contralateral rotation in daily saline-treated rats ($n = 9$) 9 days after 6-OHDA injection, but failed to produce a similar effect in sham-lesioned controls ($n = 5$, $**p < 0.01$). Daily administration of the selective D_1 agonist SK & F 38393 (8 mg/kg, s.c. for 1 week) almost completely prevented apomorphine-induced rotation ($n = 13$) as compared to saline-treated, DA denervated rats ($^{\#}p < 0.01$). In fact, there was no significant difference in apomorphine-induced turning between sham-lesioned and 6-OHDA-lesioned rats that received daily injections of SK & F 38393. In contrast, daily treatment with the selective D_2 agonist quinpirole (0.5 mg/kg, s.c.) failed to attenuate apomorphine-induced rotation ($n = 11$) as compared to saline-treated, DA denervated rats. The supersensitive behavioural responses to apomorphine lasted at least 5 weeks in daily saline- and quinpirole-treated, 6-OHDA-lesioned rats ($n = 4$ rats). Following a 4-week period of withdrawal from daily agonist injections, the contralateral turning responses to apomorphine were similar in all three groups. From Hu and White (1992a) with permission.

receptors (Arnt, 1985a; Arnt and Hyttel, 1985; Herrera-Marschitz and Ungerstedt, 1985). Moreover, SK & F 38393 treatment in 6-OHDA-lesioned rats also prevented the development of quinpirole-induced rotation (Hu and White, unpublished findings).

Several other laboratories have studied the ability of repeated or continuous treatment with selective D_1 and D_2 receptor agonists to regulate rotational behaviour in rats with unilateral 6-OHDA lesions of the nigrostriatal pathway. Unlike our paradigm, all other studies initiated repeated agonist treatment subsequent to the development of 6-OHDA-induced supersensitivity. These experiments have provided discrepant findings with respect to homologous regulation of D_1 and heterologous regulation of D_2 receptor function. Repeated daily injections of SK & F 38393 diminished contralateral circling induced by this D_1 agonist but increased D_2 agonist-induced turning (Rouillard et al., 1988). Similar daily injections of the new selective D_1 agonist A 68930 prevented rotational responses to this drug (Britton et al., 1991). Continuous administration of SK & F 38393 markedly reduced contralateral rotation induced by the same drug, but not that elicited by D_2 agonists in 6-OHDA-lesioned mice (Winkler et al., 1988). Following repeated injections of l-DOPA, contralateral rotation induced by SK & F 38393 or A 68930 was abolished, whereas rotation elicited by D_2-selective or mixed D_1/D_2 agonists was enhanced (Engber et al., 1989; Britton et al., 1991). When viewed along with our findings (Hu and White, 1992a), these studies suggest that D_1 receptors may regulate the development of D_2 receptor supersensitivity, but once it has occurred, D_2 receptors may be resistant to attempts to normalize their sensitivity.

While our results indicate that D_1 receptor stimulation can affect the sensitivity of D_2 receptors, others have shown that D_1 receptor tone can also influence D_2 receptor density. For example, repeated stimulation of D_1 receptors can suppress 6-OHDA-induced upregulation of D_2 receptors in rats (Rouillard et al., 1988). Similar findings have been reported (Falardeau et al., 1988; Gagnon et al., 1990) in monkeys pretreated with the DA neurotoxin 1-methyl-4-phenyl-1,2,3,6-tetrahydropyridine (MPTP). Repeated injections of SK & F 38393 have also been reported to speed the rate of recovery of D_2 receptors inactivated by alkylation (Cameron and Crocker, 1988). The mechanisms by which D_1 receptors might exert heterologous regulation of D_2 receptor density and functional supersensitivity are important issues for further investigation.

4.7.5   Electrophysiology and behaviour: summary and conclusions

The findings reviewed within this section have demonstrated close parallels between D_1 : D_2 DA receptor interactions at the behavioural and cellular levels. Although the data were never obtained from the same animals, the similarities between D_1 . D_2 interactions regulating unconditioned DA-dependent behaviours and those controlling neuronal discharge within the striatal complex suggest that the behavioural effects may be a reflection of D_1 : D_2 receptor interactions occurring on striatal cells. These findings have not only generated considerable interest in the underlying mechanisms involved in $D_1:D_2$ receptor interactions but also have distinct clinical implications.

Among the most important clinical implications of $D_1:D_2$ synergisms is that for the treatment of Parkinson's disease (reviews: Clark and White, 1987; Waddington and O'Boyle, 1987). With the exception of l-dopa, currently available anti-Parkinsonian drugs (e.g. bromocriptine) are primarily D_2 agonists. With the discovery that D_1 receptor stimulation is required for many effects of D_2 agonists, investigators suggested that mixed D_1/D_2 agonists or combinations of D_1 and D_2 agonists might be more effective in alleviating Parkinsonian symptoms. The more recent finding that D_1 and D_2 receptors are functionally uncoupled in the DA denervated striatum would appear to argue against the need for simultaneous stimulation of D_1 and D_2 receptors in Parkinson's patients. However, our findings suggest that reinstating $D_1:D_2$ synergisms may be an important process in the reversal of abnormal movements caused by DA denervation. Moreover, as mentioned above, synergistic behavioural effects of selective D_1 and D_2 agonists have been reported in the unilateral 6-OHDA rotational model (Koller and Herbster, 1988; Robertson and Robertson, 1986, 1987; Rouillard and Bedard, 1988; Sonsalla et al., 1988).

In view of these findings, it is interesting that DA denervation not only relieved the requirement of D_1 receptor stimulation for D_2 agonist-induced inhibition (enabling), but also abolished the D_1-mediated potentiation of D_2 agonist-induced inhibition (quantitative synergism). Thus the behavioural synergism reported in previous studies of DA denervated rats is not due to synergistic actions at adjacent D_1 and D_2 DA receptors located in the CPu, but may involve distant $D_1:D_2$ interactions (Robertson and Robertson, 1986, 1987). It may be that the loss of adjacent $D_1:D_2$ receptor interactions on striatal neurones unmasks or evokes additional distant (perhaps compensatory) functional interactions between D_1 and D_2 receptors at a system level. Thus, the possible utility of D_1 or combined $D_1:D_2$ stimulation in the treatment of Parkinson's disease cannot be ruled out, as shown in MPTP-lesioned monkeys (Gomez-Mancilla et al., 1992).

4.8 Mechanisms of $D_1:D_2$ interactions

4.8.1 Cellular location of D_1 and D_2 receptors

Perhaps the most hotly debated of current issues concerning $D_1:D_2$ interactions is the extent to which these receptors are located on the same striatal (or other) neurones. Obviously, the answer to this question will have tremendous impact upon the elucidation of mechanisms involved in $D_1:D_2$ receptor interactions. The discovery that D_2 receptor stimulation can inhibit D_1 receptor-stimulated cAMP formation within the striatum (e.g. Onali et al., 1985) was the initial impetus leading to models in which the two receptors were considered to be on the same striatal cells. Studies of DA-regulated adenylyl cyclase activity in cultured striatal cells suggest the validity of such a model (Chneiweiss et al., 1988). However, recent anatomical studies have questioned this assumption.

Despite differing in the specific effects reported to be mediated by D_1 and D_2 receptors, early electrophysiological studies agreed that many striatal cells appeared to be responsive to both D_1 and D_2-selective agonists (Uchimura et al., 1986; White and Wang, 1986; Akaike et al., 1987; Ohno et al., 1987; White, 1987). However, results from iontophoretic studies cannot be definitively attributed to drug actions on the neurone being recorded because surrounding neuronal elements, particularly nerve terminals, are also reached by drugs ejected from micropipettes. Nevertheless, the consistence with which D_1 and D_2 agonists act and interact to influence striatal cells (nearly 80% of striatal cells respond in a similar manner) during iontophoretic drug administration is highly suggestive evidence for co-localization of the two receptors on individual neurones. Intracellular recordings from striatal cells in slice preparations are more definitive with respect to receptor localization and almost every study reported to date has found that the majority of striatal cells respond to both D_1- and D_2-selective agonists and antagonists (Uchimura et al., 1986; Akaike et al., 1987; Calabresi et al., 1988a, b; Uchimura and North, 1990; Bertolucci et al., 1991).

A quite different story has begun to emerge from recent investigations using in situ hybridization histochemical localization of mRNA encoding the D_1 and D_2 receptors. Some investigators have reported considerable segregation of striatal output neurones with respect to receptor expression. Thus, the D_1 receptor is reportedly expressed primarily by striatonigral (primarily GABAergic) neurones which also contain substance P and dynorphin mRNA, whereas the D_2 receptor is primarily expressed by striatopallidal (also primarily GABAergic) neurones containing enkephalin mRNA (Gerfen et al., 1990; Le Moine et al., 1990, 1991). Studies using selective lesioning procedures and receptor autoradiography have supported this concept of receptor segregation (e.g. Beckstead, 1988; Harrison et al., 1990). However, immunohistochemical identification of striatal output neurones containing the dopamine and adenylyl cyclase-related phosphoprotein DARPP-32, another marker for D_1 receptor-containing neurones, have demonstrated that essentially all striatal medium spiny projection neurones contain DARPP-32 (Anderson and Reiner, 1991). This latter finding suggests either that another D_1-like receptor may be linked to DARPP-32 and expressed by a subpopulation of striatal cells or that this protein is not specifically associated with DA receptors. Another possibility is that mRNA studies may be underestimating the proportion of D_1 and D_2 receptor-expressing striatal neurones due to sensitivity limitations of the techniques. Indeed, when retrograde tracing techniques were used in combination with immuno-fluorescence of various D_2 receptor amino acid sequences, a minimum of 60% of striatonigral neurones were found to be D_2 receptor positive (Ariano et al., 1992).

Although Gerfen *et al.* (1990) found only a small subset of striatal cells (15–20%) containing both D_1 and D_2 receptor mRNA, more recent reports suggest a higher percentage (as much as 50%) of co-localization (Meador-Woodruff *et al.*, 1991; Weiner *et al.*, 1991). Additional studies using fluorescently labelled ligands have also reported substantial overlap of D_1 and D_2 receptor protein within the striatum (Ariano *et al.*, 1991), with estimates of 50% of striatal neurones possessing both subtypes. One potentially important difference between these reports and that of Gerfen *et al.* (1990) is that the latter used primarily 6-OHDA-lesioned rats. Given that 6-OHDA lesions cause a functional uncoupling of D_1 and D_2 receptors (Section 4.7.3) and a loss of specific association of D_1 receptors with cAMP-immunoreactive neurones (Ariano, 1988), it seems possible that DA denervation may alter the expression of striatal receptors. Clearly, such findings dictate caution in generalizing from the denervated to the normal striatum.

Differences between anatomical and electrophysiological estimates of $D_1:D_2$ co-localization might also involve the existence of multiple D_1-like and D_2-like receptors. All functional studies are limited by the lack of selectivity of currently available compounds within these receptor classes. Such studies actually report the response of cells or animals to these 'selective' drugs whereas molecular anatomical studies are using more specific probes for the various receptor mRNAs. Because it is possible that cells may express differing combinations of D_1-class and D_2-class receptors, such as D_1 and D_3 or D_4 and D_5, differences in functional and anatomical studies are not surprising. Such cells would be identified by electrophysiological studies as being both D_1 and D_2 responsive, but not by *in situ* hybridization immunohistochemical approaches as co-expressing the D_1 and D_2 receptors.

While this reasoning may help to account for existing discrepancies, at least one recent study has attempted to reconcile these electrophysiological and molecular anatomical findings more directly. Surmeier *et al.* (1992) recently combined the two approaches to study the functional and anatomical properties of striatal neurones. Striatonigral projection neurones were labelled by prior injections of retrogradely transported rhodamine-impregnated fluorescent microbeads into the substantia nigra. The striatum was then dissected and striatonigral cells were isolated in dissociated culture. Whole-cell and cell-attached patch recordings clearly indicated that almost all striatonigral neurones respond to both D_1 and D_2 agonists (Section 4.4.2). Following the physiological recordings, an antisense RNA (aRNA) technique was used to amplify and detect the mRNA from single striatonigral cells. All neurones which were subjected to this analysis were found to express mRNA not only for D_1 and D_2 receptors, but for D_3 receptors as well (Surmeier *et al.*, 1992). These provocative findings raise the possibility that previous studies of mRNA expression may have underestimated the percentage of $D_1:D_2$ co-expressing neurones. Certainly, $D_1:D_3$ cells would not have been identified by other investigators since D_3 mRNA probes were not used in the previous reports.

Clearly, this elegant and powerful approach will be influential in further addressing the important question of receptor co-localization.

4.8.2 Molecular mechanisms of $D_1:D_2$ synergisms

Although there has been considerable speculation as to the mechanisms involved in $D_1:D_2$ receptor synergisms, few published reports have directly addressed this issue. Berterello et al. (1990) reported that DA inhibits the Na^+/K^+-ATPase activity of acutely dissociated, cultured striatal cells via a synergistic effect on D_1 and D_2 receptors. Activation of both receptor subtypes was necessary to achieve inhibition of Na^+/K^+-ATPase activity in cells taken from rats acutely depleted of endogenous DA. This effect clearly indicates $D_1:D_2$ interaction at the level of single striatal cells. It was proposed that the inhibition of the electrogenic Na^+/K^+-ATPase would lead to a rise in intracellular Na^+ and a transient membrane depolarization. Such an effect may be related to earlier electrophysiological findings that DA, at low ejection currents, can enhance the ability of glutamate to excite striatal cells (Chiodo and Berger, 1986).

We have reported that in addition to inhibiting the firing of striatal neurones when administered at moderate to high ejection currents, both D_1 and D_2 agonists can potentiate the excitatory effects of glutamate when they are administered at low ejection currents (Hu and Wang, 1988; Hu et al., 1990). Recently, we have found that this effect of either a selective D_1 or D_2 agonist, but not of DA, is significantly reduced by acute DA depletion (Hu and White, 1992b), suggesting yet another form of $D_1:D_2$ synergism on striatal cells. Thus, it appears possible that inhibition of the Na^+/K^+ pump by DA stimulation of D_1 and D_2 receptors (Berterello et al., 1990) may be involved in regulation of neuronal excitability in vivo and that, in this case, stimulation of both receptors is always necessary for the effect to occur. Thus, this mechanism would not appear to account for the enabling of D_2 receptor function by D_1 receptors since this relationship is not always reciprocated.

A second mechanism which has been postulated to account for $D_1:D_2$ synergisms involves enhancement of arachidonic acid release. Piomelli et al. (1991) reported that in Chinese hamster ovary (CHO) cells transfected with the D_2 complementary DNA, quinpirole potently potentiated arachidonic acid release produced by increasing intracellular Ca^{2+}. This effect was not observed in CHO cells expressing D_1 receptors. However, a synergistic effect was observed when D_1 and D_2 receptors were co-expressed in CHO cells. The authors suggested that this mechanism might account for the synergistic regulation of Na^+/K^+-ATPase activity since arachidonic acid and its metabolites are potent inhibitors of this enzyme. However, the effect of D_2 agonists on arachidonic acid release occurred in the absence of D_1 receptor stimulation unlike the regulation of Na^+/K^+-ATPase. In this respect, the synergistic regulation of arachidonic acid release also differs from previous in vivo electrophysiological and behavioural studies. Nevertheless, this report indicates yet another possible form of $D_1:D_2$

synergism. It will be of interest to determine whether such interaction occurs within intact mammalian brain.

4.8.3 Non-cyclase-linked D_1 receptors and $D_1 : D_2$ synergisms

In addition to the well-characterized D_1 receptor linked to adenylyl cyclase, there is considerable evidence that D_1 receptors exist which are not coupled to this transduction mechanism. A non-cyclase-linked D_1 receptor was first postulated to exist within the rat amygdala based upon evidence indicating a significant density of $[^3H]SCH$ 23390 binding within the central amygdaloid nucleus, but a lack of apparent DA-stimulated adenylyl cyclase activity in this region (Mailman *et al.*, 1986; Kilts *et al.*, 1988). The existence of a non-cyclase-linked striatal D_1 receptor was first postulated by Andersen and Braestrup (1986), who suggested a two-state model of the D_1 receptor. Further suggestions came from studies indicating differing sensitivities of D_1 receptors to guanine nucleotide regulation (De Keyser *et al.*, 1988, 1989). More definitive evidence was provided by the demonstration that mRNA derived from rat striatum and expressed in *Xenopus* oocytes results in a functional D_1 receptor which regulates Ca^{2+}-dependent Cl^- currents by coupling to inositol phosphate formation and mobilization of intracellular Ca^{2+} (Mahan *et al.*, 1990). Enhanced inositol phosphate formation following D_1 agonist administration has also been reported within the rat striatum (Undie and Friedman, 1990).

Several recent behavioural studies have demonstrated dissociations between the activity of D_1 agonists in adenylyl cyclase assays and certain responses. Arnt and colleagues have reported such dissociations with respect to the ability of various D_1 agonists to convert quinpirole-induced stereotyped sniffing to oral forms of stereotyped behaviour (Arnt *et al.*, 1987, 1988), to potentiate quinpirole-induced circling in rats with hemitransections (Arnt and Perregaard, 1987; Arnt *et al.*, 1988) and to substitute for the discriminative stimulus effects of SK & F 38393 (Arnt, 1988). Murray and Waddington (1989) reported a similar finding with respect to induction of D_1 receptor-mediated grooming behaviour. In addition, inactivation of D_1 and D_2 receptors by the irreversible aklylating agent EEDQ abolished apomorphine-induced stereotyped behaviour while leaving striatal adenylyl cyclase activity unchanged (Cameron and Crocker, 1988).

We have also provided two lines of evidence which have questioned the extent to which the effects of D_1 agonists on striatal neurones involve activation of adenylyl cyclase (Johansen *et al.*, 1991). First, despite widely different relative efficacies in stimulating adenylyl cyclase, the D_1 agonists SK & F 38393 (46–69% as compared to 100 μM DA), SK & F 75670 (18–33%) and SK & F 81297 (88%) exhibited nearly identical current–response curves for the inhibition of NAc neurones. Following acute DA depletion, all three D_1 agonists enabled quinpirole-induced inhibition of NAc neurones, but SK & F 38393 proved to be significantly more active than the more potent full agonist SK & F 81297. Finally, although iontophoretic administration of the stable cAMP analogue 8-bromo-cAMP readily inhibited NAc cells, this agent failed to enable the inhibitory effects of quinpirole in AMPT-pretreated rats (Figure 7). Therefore, although increases in intracellular cAMP levels may be related to inhibition of NAc neuronal firing, it is not necessarily the case that the effects of D_1 agonists (inhibition, enabling) are mediated by this mechanism.

These various findings have provided considerable, albeit only suggestive, evidence that the D_1 receptor involved in important behavioural and electrophysiological effects of D_1-selective agonists might be, at least in part, distinct from the 'classical' D_1 receptor. Although such a non-cyclase-linked receptor has not yet been identified with molecular biological approaches, it is likely to be discovered in due course. Such a receptor has important implications for our current classification scheme of DA receptor subtypes, and for our understanding of the mechanisms underlying $D_1:D_2$ interactions.

4.8.4   Multiple forms of $D_1:D_2$ interactions

As demonstrated and discussed by Waddington and colleagues (Murray and Waddington, 1989; Waddington, 1989), behavioural data are suggestive of both $D_1:D_2$ opposition and $D_1:D_2$ synergism, each of which has its own underlying mechanistic support. It now appears that multiple forms of $D_1:D_2$ synergism may also exist. It is presently unclear whether the necessity of D_1 stimulation for D_2 agonist-induced inhibition of striatal cells, observed in rats acutely depleted of DA (enabling), is mediated by the same mechanisms which result in D_1 agonist potentiation of D_2-mediated inhibitions in intact rats. Because such a possibility should be appraised, we have been careful to describe them separately, as qualitative and quantitative synergisms (Hu et al., 1990), and to test for the presence of each effect during all experimental manipulations of the DA system. The finding that both forms of adjacent $D_1:D_2$ synergisms are abolished in DA denervated rats indicates that behavioural evidence for $D_1:D_2$ synergism observed in such animals must result from some form of 'distant' interaction between D_1 and D_2 receptors on distinct neuronal elements within the basal ganglia. The substantia nigra pars reticulata may represent a convergence site of such distant interactions (Weick and Walters, 1987; Robertson and Robertson, 1987). Finally, new evidence indicates synergistic interactions between D_1 and D_2 receptors in controlling Na^+/K^+-ATPase activity, modulation of glutamate-induced excitation of striatal neurones and stimulation of arachidonic acid release. All of these synergisms exhibit characteristics distinct from those of qualitative and quantitative synergisms previously described.

Despite these findings suggesting different forms of $D_1:D_2$ synergism, it appears that many researchers have not yet considered this possibility. It is not uncommon to read papers describing $D_1:D_2$ synergism as though it were a unitary phenomenon. It will be essential for future investigations to concentrate on the precise nature of the interaction(s) under investigation and the extent to which

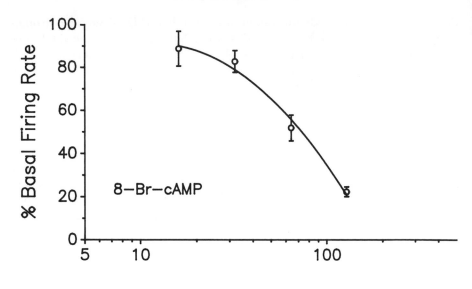

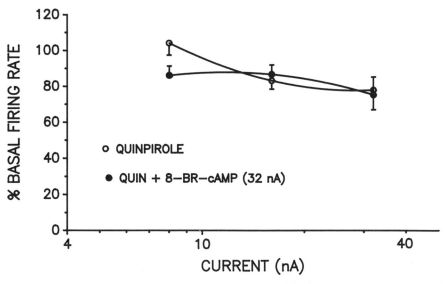

Figure 7 (A) Inhibitory effect of iontophoretically applied 8-bromo-cAMP on the firing of nucleus accumbens neurones in AMPT-pretreated rats. Each point represents the mean ± SEM ($n = 10$). Note that the inhibitory effect of 8-Br-cAMP was statistically significant at all but the lowest current as determined by ANOVA followed by Dunnett's test ($p < 0.05$). (B) Failure of 8-Br-cAMP to enable the inhibitory effect of quinpirole on nucleus accumbens neurones in AMPT-treated rats. Each point represents the mean ± SEM ($n = 9$). From Johansen *et al.* (1991), with permission.

the characteristics of the D_1 : D_2 synergism (s) resemble those described by other investigators. Only with such recognition will it be possible to elucidate the mechanisms underlying each of the apparently disparate forms of DA receptor interaction.

4.9 Summary and conclusions

The D_1 and D_2 receptors were originally defined according to the association and lack of association with the adenylyl cyclase/cAMP transduction mechanism. This classification has been modified to incorporate the inhibitory effect of some D_2 receptors on adenylyl cyclase activity. The concept of two DA receptors was extremely useful from a heuristic perspective. Based upon this classification scheme, the latter half of the 1980s witnessed a successful 'search for a function' of the D_1 receptor. This search yielded abundant information regarding several functional roles of both D_1 and D_2 receptors and the varied forms of D_1 : D_2 interactions (Clark and White, 1987; Waddington and O'Boyle, 1987).

With respect to the neurophysiological actions mediated by D_1 and D_2 receptors, many different effects have now been identified and several distinct membrane conductances have been demonstrated as being under the control of the two receptors. There is now an extensive literature indicating behaviourally relevant alterations in the discharge of specific sets of D_1- and D_2-responsive neurones. The related literature regarding possible mechanisms responsible for the different forms of D_1 : D_2 interactions is currently evolving. The discovery of several distinct D_1-class and D_2-class receptors promises to provide new insights into mechanisms and forms of DA receptor interactions. As these new receptor subtypes begin their 'search for a function', we can expect a burgeoning literature and increasing calls for modification of the current scheme of DA receptor subtypes. In fact, recent reviews have called for reappraisals of DA receptor nomenclature, based primarily on the multiple forms of DA receptors identified with molecular biological approaches (Andersen et al., 1990; Sibley and Monsma, 1992). As these discussions proceed, it will be essential that additional consideration is afforded to pharmacological properties and functional aspects of the receptor subtypes.

It seems quite likely that the number of identified DA receptors will continue to increase. Even as we complete this chapter, we must wonder how many more subtypes will be known before this volume is actually published. From our perspective, one thing is clear. Further elucidation of the functional roles of these various receptors must await the development of pharmacological probes with some degree of selectivity for the various DA receptor subtypes. Until such time, we are restricted to speculations, however well founded, on the physiological and behavioural relevance of the many D_1 and D_2-class receptors. It seems quite likely that with appropriate drug development, the mechanisms underlying the many identified DA receptor interactions will be unravelled and many discrepancies described herein will be resolved. Undoubtedly, the 1990s loom as another exciting decade in the field of DA receptor research.

Acknowledgements

This research from our laboratory which is presented and described herein was supported by US Public Health Service grants DA 04093 from the National Institute on Drug Abuse and MH 40832 from the National Institute of Mental Health and by the American Parkinsons Disease Association. We thank Drs Marjorie Ariano, James Surmeier and Michael Levine for helpful discussions and access to their unpublished data.

References

Aghajanian, G.K. & Bunney, B.S. (1977) *Naunyn Schmiedeberg's Arch. Pharmacol.* **247**, 1–7.
Akaike, A., Ohno, Y., Sasa, M. & Takaori, S. (1987) *Brain Res.* **418**, 262–272.
Altar, C.A. & Hauser, K. (1987) *Brain Res.* **410**, 1–11.
Andersen, K.D. & Reiner, A. (1991) *Brain Res.* **568**, 235–243.
Andersen, P.H. & Braestrup, C. (1986) *J. Neurochem.* **47**, 1822–1831.
Anderson, P.H., Gingrich, J.A., Bates, M.D., Dearry, A., Falardeau, P., Senogles, S.E. & Caron, M.G. (1990) *Trends Pharmacol. Sci.* **11**, 231–235.
Ariano, M.A., Stronski, C.J., Smyk-Randall, E.M. & Sibley, D.R. (1988) *Brain Res.* **443**, 204–214.
Ariano, M.A. (1992) *Neurosci. Lett.* **144**, 215–220.
Ariano, M.A., Kang, H.C., Haugland, R.P. & Sibley, D.R. (1991) *Brain Res.* **547**, 208–222.
Arnt, J. (1985a) *Eur. J. Pharmacol.* **113**, 79–88.
Arnt, J. (1985b) *Life Sci.* **37**, 717–723.
Arnt, J. (1988) *Life Sci.* **42**, 567–574.
Arnt, J. & Hyttel, J. (1984) *Eur. J. Pharmacol.* **102**, 349–354.
Arnt, J. & Hyttel, J. (1985) *Psychopharmacology* **85**, 346–352.
Arnt, J. & Perregaard, J. (1987) *Eur. J. Pharmacol.* **143**, 45–53.
Arnt, J., Hyttel, J. & Perregaard, J. (1987) *Eur. J. Pharmacol.* **133**, 137–145.
Arnt, J., Hyttel, J. & Meier, E. (1988) *Eur. J. Pharmacol.* **155**, 37–44.
Barone, P., Davis, T.A., Braun, A.R. & Chase, T.N. (1986) *Eur. J. Pharmacol.* **123**, 109–114.
Beckstead, R.M. (1988) *Neuroscience* **27**, 851–863.
Beretta, N., Berton, F., Bianchi, R., Capogna, M., Francesconi, W. & Brunelli, M. (1990) *Exp. Brain Res.* **83**, 124–130.
Bergstrom, D.A., Bromley, S.D. & Walters, J.R. (1982) *Brain Res.* **238**, 266–271.
Bertolucci, M., Cepeda, C., Buchwald, N.A. & Levin, M.S. (1991) *Soc. Neurosci. Abstr.* **17**, 852.
Bertorello, A.M., Hopfield, J.F., Aperia, A. & Greengard, P. (1990) *Nature* **347**, 386–388.
Bickford-Wimer, P., Kim, M., Boyajian, C., Cooper, D.M.F. & Freedman, R. (1990) *Brain Res.* **533**, 263–267.
Bordi, F. & Meller, E. (1989) *Brain Res.* **504**, 276–283.

Bouthenet, M.-L., Souil, E., Martres, M.-P., Sokoloff, P., Giros, B. & Schwartz, J.-C. (1991) *Brain Res.* **564**, 203–219.
Boyson, S.J., McGonigle, P. & Molinoff, P.B. (1986) *J. Neurosci.* **6**, 3177–3188.
Braun, A. & Chase, T.N. (1986) *Eur. J. Pharmacol.* **131**, 301–306.
Breese, G.R. & Mueller, R.A. (1985) *Eur. J. Pharmacol.* **113**, 109–114.
Britton, D.R., Kebabian, J.W. & Curzon, P. (1991) *Eur. J. Pharmacol.* **200**, 89–93.
Bunney, B.S. & Aghajanian, G.K. (1976) *Life Sci.* **19**, 1783–1792
Calabresi, P., Mercuri, N., Stanzione, P., Stefani, A. & Bernardi, G. (1987) *Neuroscience* **20**, 757–771.
Calabresi, P., Benedetti, M., Mercuri, N.B. & Bernardi, G. (1988a) *Neuropharmacology* **27**, 579–588.
Calabresi, P., Benedetti, M., Mercuri, N.B. & Bernardi, G. (1988b) *Neuroscience* **27**, 145–157.
Cameron, D.L. & Crocker, A.D. (1988) *Neurosci. Lett.* **90**, 165–171.
Carlson, J.H., Bergstrom, D.A. & Walters, J.R. (1986) *Eur. J. Pharmacol.* **23**, 237–251.
Carlson, J.H., Bergstrom, D.A. & Walters, J.R. (1987) *Brain Res.* **400**, 205–218.
Carlson, J.H., Bergstrom, D.A., Demo, S.D. & Walters, J.R. (1988) *Eur. J. Pharmacol.* **152**, 289–300.
Chandler, C.J., Starr, B.S. & Starr, M.S. (1990) *Pharmacol. Biochem. Behav.* **35**, 285–289
Chiodo, L.A. & Berger, T.W. (1986) *Brain Res.* **375**, 198–203
Chneiweiss, H., Glowinski, J. & Premont, J. (1988) *J. Neurosci.* **8**, 3376–3382.
Clark, D. & White, F.J. (1987) *Synapse* **1**, 347–388.
De Keyser, J., Dierckx, R., Vanderhyden, P., Ebinger, G. & Vauquelin, G. (1988) *Brain Res.* **443**, 77–84.
De Keyser, J., Walraevens, H., Ebinger, G. & Vauquelin, G. (1989) *J. Neurochem.* **53**, 1096–1102.
Dreher, J.K. & Jackson, D.M. (1989) *Brain Res.* **487**, 267–277.
Einhorn, L., Gregerson, K.A. & Oxford, G.S. (1991) *J. Neurosci.* **11**, 3727–3737.
Engber, T.M., Susel, Z., Juncos, J.L. & Chase, T.N. (1989) *Eur. J. Pharmacol.* **168**, 291–298.
Falardeau, P., Bouchard, S., Bedard, P., Boucher, R. & Di Paolo, T. (1988) *Eur. J. Pharmacol.* **150**, 59–66.
Freedman, J.E. & Weight, F.F. (1988) *Proc. Natl Acad. Sci. USA* **85**, 3618–3622.
Gagnon, C., Bedard, P.J. & Di Paolo, T. (1990) *Eur. J. Pharmacol.* **178**, 15–120.
Gerfen, C.R., Engber, T.M., Mahan, L.C., Susel, Z., Chase, T.N., Monsma, F.J. Jr & Sibley, D.R. (1990) *Science* **250**, 1429–1432.
Gershanik, O., Heikkila, R.E. & Duvoisin, R.C. (1983) *Neurology* **33**, 1489–1492.
Giorgio, O., De Montis, G., Porceddu, M.L., Mele, S., Calderini, G., Toffano, G. & Biggio, G. (1987) *Dev. Brain Res.* **35**, 283–291.
Godbout, R., Mantz, J., Pirot, S., Glowinski, J. & Thierry, A.-M. (1991) *J. Pharmacol. Exp. Ther.* **258**, 728–738.
Gomez-Mancilla, B., Boucher, R. & Bédard, P.J. (1992) *Movement Disord.* **7**, 43–47.
Hara, M., Sasa, M. & Takaori, S. (1989) *Neuropharmacology* **28**, 1203–1209.
Harrison, M.B., Wiley, R.G. & Wooten, G.F. (1990) *Brain Res.* **528**, 317–322.
Heimer, L. & Wilson, R.D. (1975) In *Golgi Centennial Symposium Proceedings* (ed. Santini, M.), pp 177–193. New York, Raven Press.
Herrera-Marschitz, M. & Ungerstedt, U. (1985) *Eur. J. Pharmacol.* **109**, 349–354.
Hu, X.-T. & Wang, R.Y. (1988) *J. Neurosci.* **8**, 4340–4348.
Hu, X.-T. & Wang, R.Y. (1989) *Brain Res.* **486**, 325–333.
Hu, X.-T. & White, F.J. (1992a) *Synapse* **10**, 206–216.
Hu, X.-T. & White, F.J. (1992b) *Soc. Neurosci. Abstracts* **18**, 279.
Hu, X.-T., Wachtel, S.R., Galloway, M.P. & White, F.J. (1990) *J. Neurosci.* **10**, 2318–2329.

Huang, K.-X. & Walters, J.R. (1992) *J. Pharmacol. Exp. Ther.* **260**, 409–416.
Hyttel, J. (1987) *Pharmacol. Toxicol.* **61**, 126–129.
Innis, R.B. & Aghajanian, G.K. (1987) *Brain Res.* **411**, 139–143.
Jackson, D.M. & Hashizume, H. (1986) *Psychopharmacology* **90**, 147–149.
Johansen, P.A., Clark, D. & White, F.J. (1988) *Life Sci.* **43**, 515–524.
Johnsen, P.A., Hu, X.-T. & White, F.J. (1991) *J. Neural Transm.* **86**, 97–113.
Joyce, J.N. (1991) *Exp. Neurol.* **113**, 277–290.
Kelland, M.D., Freeman, A.S. & Chiodo, L.A. *Synapse* **2**, 416–423.
Kelly, A.E., Delfs, J.M. & Chu, B. (1990) *Brain Res.* **532**, 342–346.
Kilts, C.D., Anderson, C.M., Ely, T.D. & Mailman, R.B. (1988) In *The Mesocortical Dopamine System* (eds Kalivas, P.W. & Nemeroff, C.B.), pp 173–187. New York, Ann. NY Acc. Sci.
Kitai, S.T. (1981) In *Handbook of Physiology—The Nervous System* (eds Brookhalt, J.M., Mountcastle, V.B. & Brooks, V.B.), vol. II, pp 997–1015. American Physiology Society.
Koller, W.C. & Herbster, G. (1988) *Clin. Neuropharmacol.* **11**, 221–231.
Korf, J., Zielman, M. & Westerink, B.H.C. (1976) *Nature* **260**, 257–258.
Lacey, M.G., Mercuri, N.B. & North, R.A. *J. Physiol. (Lond.)* **392**, 397–416.
Le Moine, C., Normand, E., Guitteny, A.F., Fouque, B., Teoule, R. & Bloch, B. (1990) *Proc. Natl Acad. Sci. USA* **87**, 230–234.
Le Moine, C., Normand, E. & Bloch, B. (1991) *Proc. Natl Acad. Sci. USA* **88**, 4205–4209.
Longoni, R., Spina, L. & Di Chiara, G. (1987a) *Eur. J. Pharmacol.* **134**, 163–173.
Longoni, R., Spina, L. & Di Chiara, G. (1987b) *Life Sci.* **41**, 2135–2145.
Mahan, L.C., Burch, R.M., Monsma, F.J. Jr & Sibley, D.R. (1990) *Proc. Natl Acad. Sci. USA* **87**, 2169–2200.
Mailman, R.B., Schulz, D.W., Kilts, C.D., Lewis, M.H., Rollema, H. & Wyrick, S. (1986) In *Neurobiology of Central D₁-dopamine Receptors* (eds Breese, G.R. & Creese, I.), pp 53–72. New York, Plenum Press.
Mashurano, M. & Waddington, J.L. (1986) *Neuropharmacology* **25**, 947–949.
Maslowski, R.J. & Napier, C.T. (1991) *Eur. J. Pharmacol.* **200**, 103–112.
Matthews, R.T. & German, D.C. (1986) *Eur. J. Pharmacol.* **120**, 87–93.
Meador-Woodruff, J.H., Mansour, A., Bunzow, J.R., Van Tol, H.H.M., Watson, S.J. Jr & Civelli, O. (1991) *Proc. Natl Acad. Sci. USA* **86**, 7625–7628.
Meller, E., Bordi, F. & Bohmaker, K. (1988) *Life Sci.* **42**, 2561–2567.
Mereu, G., Fanni, B., Collu, M., Diena, A. & Glasser, A. (1985) *Life Sci.* **36**, 459–464.
Molloy, A.G. & Waddington, J.L. (1984) *Psychopharmacology* **82**, 409–410.
Molloy, A.G. & Waddington, J.L. (1985) *Eur. J. Pharmacol.* **116**, 183–186.
Molloy, A.G. & Waddington, J.L. (1987a) *Psychopharmacology* **92**, 164–168.
Molloy, A.G. & Waddington, J.L. (1987b) *J. Psychopharmacol.* **1**, 177–183.
Molloy, A.G. & Waddington, J.L. (1988) *Br. J. Pharmacol.* **95**, 335–342.
Molloy, A.G., O'Boyle, K.M., Pugh, M.T. & Waddington, J.L. (1986) *Pharmacol. Biochem. Behav.* **25**, 249–253.
Morelli, M., Mennini, T., Cagnotto, A., Toffano, G. & Di Chiara, G. (1990) *Neuroscience* **36**, 403–410.
Murray, A.M. & Waddington, J.L. (1989) *Eur. J. Pharmacol.* **160**, 377–382.
Napier, T.C. (1992) *Synapse* **10**, 110–119.
Napier, T.C., Givens, B.S., Schulz, D.W., Bunney, B.S., Breese, G.R. & Mailman, R.B. (1986) *J. Pharmacol. Exp. Ther.* **236**, 838–845.
Napier, T.C., Simson, P.E. & Givens, B.S. (1991) *J. Pharmacol. Exp. Ther.* **258**, 249–262.
Neisewander, J.L., Ong, A. & McGonigle, P. (1991) *Soc. Neurosci. Abst.* **17**, 677.
O'Boyle, K.M. & Waddington, J.L. (1984) *Eur. J. Pharmacol.* **106**, 219–220.
Ohno, Y., Sasa, M. & Takaori, S. (1985) *Life Sci.* **37**, 1515–1521.
Ohno, Y., Sasa, M. & Takaori, S. (1986) *Life Sci.* **38**, 1867–1873.
Ohno, Y., Sasa, M. & Takaori, S. (1987) *Life Sci.* **40**, 1937–1945.

Onali, P., Olianas, M.C. & Gessa, G.L. (1985) *Mol Pharmacol.* **28**, 138–145.
Pan, H.S. & Walters, J.R. (1988) *Synapse* **2**, 650–656.
Pan, H.S., Engber, T.M., Chase, T.N. & Walters, J.R. (1990) *Life Sci.* **46**, 73–80.
Parfitt, K.D., Gratton, A. & Bickford-Wimer, P.C. (1990) *J. Pharmacol. Exp. Ther.* **254**, 539–545.
Piomelli, D., Pilon, C., Giros, B., Sokoloff, P., Martres, M.-P. & Schwartz, J.-C. (1991) *Nature* **353**, 164–167.
Plaznik, A., Stefanski, R. & Kostowski, W. (1989) *Psychopharmacology* **99**, 558–562.
Robertson, G.S. & Robertson, H.A. (1986) *Brain Res.* **384**, 387–390.
Robertson, G.S. & Robertson, H.A. (1987) *Trends Pharmacol. Sci.* **8**, 295–299.
Ross, S.B., Jackson, D.M. & Edwards, S.R. (1988) *Pharmacol. Toxicol.* **64**, 72–77.
Rouillard, C. & Bedard, P.J. (1988) *Neuropharmacology,* **27**, 1257–1264.
Rouillard, C., Bedard, P., Falardeau, P. & Di Paolo, T. (1988) *Eur. J. Pharmacol.* **157**, 125–133.
Ryan, L.J., Young, S.J. & Groves, P.M. (1986) *Exp. Brain Res.* **63**, 449–460.
Ryan, L.J., Diana, M., Young, S.J. & Groves, P.M. (1989) *Exp. Brain Res.* **77**, 161–165.
Sesack, S.R. & Bunney, B.S. (1989) *J. Pharmacol. Exp. Ther.* **248**, 1323–1333.
Sibley, D.R. & Monsma, F.J. Jr (1992) *TIPS* **150**, 61–69.
Siggins, G.R. (1978) In *Psychopharmacology—A Generation of Progress* (eds Lipton, M.A., DiMascio, A. & Killam, K.F.), pp 143–157. New York, Raven Press.
Silva, N.L. & Bunney, B.S. (1988) *Eur. J. Pharmacol.* **149**, 307–315.
Smialowski, A. & Bijack, M. (1987) *Neuroscience* **23**, 95–101.
Sokoloff, P., Giros, B., Martres, M.-P., Bouthenet, M.-L. & Schwartz, J.-C. (1990) *Nature* **347**, 146–151.
Sonsalla, P.K., Manzino, L. & Heikklia, R.E. (1988) *J. Pharmacol. Exp. Ther.* **247**, 180–195.
Starr, B.S. & Starr, M.S. (1986) *Neuropharmacology* **25**, 455–463.
Starr, B.S., Starr, M.S. & Kilpatrick, I.C. (1987) *Neuroscience* **22**, 179–188.
Sunahara, R.K., Guan, H.-C., O'Dowd, B.F., Seeman, P., Laurier, L.G., Ng, G., George, S.R., Torchia, J., Van Tol, H.H.M. & Niznik, H.B. (1991) *Nature* **350**, 614–619.
Suppes, T. & Pinnock, R.D. (1987) *Neuropharmacology* **26**, 331–337.
Surmeier, D.J., Eberwine, J., Wilson, C.J., Cao, Y., Stefani, A. & Kitai, S.T. (1992) *Proc. Natl. Acad. Sci. USA* **89**, 10178–10182.
Thierry, A.M., Le Douarin, C., Penit, J., Ferron, A. & Glowinski, J. (1986) *Brain Res. Bull.* **16**, 155–160.
Uchimura, N. & North, R.A. (1990) *Br. J. Pharmacol.* **99**, 736–740.
Uchimura, N., Higashi, H. & Nishi, S. (1986) *Brain Res.* **375**, 368–372.
Undie, A.S. & Friedman, E. (1990) *J. Pharmacol. Exp. Ther.* **253**, 987–992.
Ushijima, I., Mizuki, Y. & Yamada, M. (1988) *Psychopharmacology* **95**, 29–33.
Van Tol, H.H.M., Bunzow, J.R., Guan, H.C., Sunahara, R.K., Seeman, P., Niznik, H.B. & Civelli, O. (1991) *Nature* **350**, 610–614.
Vasse, M. & Protais, P. (1988) *Eur. J. Pharmacol.* **156**, 1–11.
Vives, F. & Mogenson, G.J. (1986) *Neuroscience* **17**, 349–359.
Wachtel, S.R., Hu, X.-T., Galloway, M.P. & White, F.J. (1989) *Synapse* **4**, 327–346.
Wachtel, S.R., Brooderson, R.J. & White, F.J. (1992) *Psychopharmacology* **109**, 41–48.
Waddington, J.L. (1986) *Biochem. Pharmacol.* **35**, 3661–3667.
Waddington, J.L. (1989) *J. Psychoparmacol.* **3**, 54–63.
Waddington, J.L. & O'Boyle, K.M. (1987) *Rev. Neurosci.* **1**, 157–184.
Walters, J.R., Bergstrom, D.A., Carlson, J.H., Chase, T.H. & Braun, A.R. (1987) *Science* **236**, 719–722.
Wang, R.Y. (1981) *Brain Res. Rev.* **3**, 141–151.
Waszczak, B.L. (1990) *Brain Res.* **513**, 125–135.
Waszczak, B.L. & Walters, J.R. (1983) *Science,* **220**, 218–221.

Waszczak, B.L. & Walters, J.R. (1984) *Eur. J. Pharmacol.* **105**, 369–373.
Waszczak, B.L. & Walters, J.R. (1986) *J. Neurosci.* **6**, 120–126.
Weick, B.G. & Walters, J.R. (1987) *Brain Res.* **405**, 234–246.
Weiner, D.M., Levey, A.I., Sunahara, R.K., Niznik, H.B., O'Dowd, B.F., Seeman, P. & Bram, M.R. (1991) *Proc. Natl. Acad. Sci. USA* **88**, 1859–1863.
White, F.J. (1986) *Clin. Neuropharmacol.* **9**, 29–31.
White, F.J. (1987) *Eur. J. Pharmacol.* **135**, 101–105.
White, F.J. & Wang, R.Y. (1984) *J. Pharmacol. Exp. Ther.* **231**, 275–280.
White, F.J. & Wang, R.Y. (1986) *J. Neurosci.* **6**, 274–280.
White, F.J., Wachtel, S.R., Johansen, P.A. & Einhorn, L.C. (1987) In *Neurophysiology of Dopamine Systems—Current Status and Clinical Perspectives* (eds Chiodo, L.C. & Freeman, A.S.), pp 317–365. Detroit, Lakeshore Publishing Co.
White, F.J., Bednarz, L.M., Wachtel, S.R., Hjorth, S. & Brooderson, R.J. (1988) *Pharmacol. Biochem. Behav.* **30**, 189–193.
White, F.J., Hu, X.-T. & Brooderson, R.J. (1990) *Eur. J. Pharmacol.* **191**, 497–499.
Wilson, C.J., Chang, H.T. & Kitai, S.T. (1982) *Exp. Brain Res.* **45**, 157–167.
Winkler, J.D., Callison, K., Cass, S.A. & Weiss, B. (1988) *Neuropharmacology* **27**, 439–442.
Yang, C.R. & Mogenson, G.J. (1990) *Brain Res.* **524**, 271–281.

————————— CHAPTER 5 —————————

ROLE OF D_1 AND D_2 RECEPTORS IN LEARNING

Richard J. Beninger

Department of Psychology, Queen's University, Kingston, K7L 3N6, Canada

Table of Contents

DOPAMINE RECEPTOR INTERACTIONS
ISBN 0-12-729045-1

The neurotransmitter dopamine (DA) appears to play a role in the control of locomotor activity and reward-related incentive learning. Rewarding stimuli include, for example, food for a food-deprived animal, sexual stimuli, safety from aversive stimuli, and water for a water-deprived animal. Reward is the presentation of a rewarding stimulus and may affect behaviour by increasing the ability of stimuli immediately preceding reward to elicit approach and other responses in the future. Stimuli that acquire this ability are termed conditioned incentive motivational stimuli or, more simply, conditioned incentive stimuli, and the process is referred to as incentive motivational learning or, more simply, incentive learning (Bindra, 1974; Bolles, 1972). There is now extensive evidence implicating DA in reward-related incentive learning (Beninger, 1983; Le Moal and Simon, 1991; Liebman and Cooper, 1989; Wise and Rompré, 1989).

The neuronal mechanisms underlying incentive learning have not been identified. However, in recent years there has been extensive research effort directed towards understanding the mechanisms of plasticity in the nervous system (e.g. Alkon, 1987; Byrne and Berry, 1989; Martinez and Kesner, 1991). A common finding is that the intracellular second messengers, activated through synaptic inputs to the cell, play a role in altering future responsiveness of the cell (e.g. Schwartz and Greenberg, 1987). It is possible that DA-mediated changes in responsiveness to stimuli signalling reward involve second messengers activated by stimulation of DA receptors. This possibility is supported by the finding that some DA receptors are linked in an excitatory manner to intracellular enzyme systems that influence second messengers.

One of the earliest and most influential classifications of DA receptors was made by Kebabian and Calne (1979). D_1 receptors were defined as those linked in an excitatory manner to the enzyme adenylate cyclase. Stimulation of adenylate cyclase leads to the formation of cAMP, a second messenger. D_2 receptors were defined as those not linked to adenylate cyclase. Subsequent studies found that stimulation of some receptors may lead to the inhibition of cAMP formation (Stoof and Kebabian, 1981); these receptors also were classified as D_2. Recently, the use of molecular biological techniques has led to the identification of a number of distinct DA receptor proteins, designated D_1 to D_5 (Bunzow et al., 1988; Dearry et al., 1990; Monsma et al., 1990; Sokoloff et al., 1990; Sunahara et al., 1990, 1991; Van Tol et al., 1991; Zhou et al., 1990). Although these receptors differ with respect to absolute protein sequence and some aspects of neuroanatomical distribution, their pharmacological profiles suggest that they fall into two categories. Waddington (1992) has suggested that they be classified as D_1-like (D_1 and D_5) and D_2-like (D_2, D_3, D_4). As few pharmacological agents are available that are specific for subclasses of D_1-like or D_2-like receptors, the remainder of this chapter will refer to DA receptor subtypes as 'D_1' or 'D_2'.

There is now an extensive selection of pharmacological agents that have relatively specific dopamimetic or antagonistic action at D_1 and D_2 receptors (Waddington and O'Boyle, 1989). These agents have permitted an evaluation of the possible differential roles of DA receptor subtypes in incentive learning (reviews: Beninger, 1991, 1992; Beninger et al., 1989; Miller et al., 1990). Incentive learning can be assessed with the use of a wide range of behavioural paradigms and many of these have been used in tests of the role of DA receptor subtypes. Section 5.1 will be organized around specific paradigms and the effects of agonists or antagonists with relative selectivity for D$_1$ or D$_2$ receptors will be compared. Section 5.2 will propose a possible mechanism for DA-mediated reward-related incentive learning. Results of the reviewed studies will then be considered in Section 5.3 in the light of this proposed mechanism.

5.1 Role of D$_1$ and D$_2$ receptors in incentive learning

Many paradigms use rewarding stimuli to alter the behaviour of animals. By definition, these paradigms involve incentive learning. Paradigms include: lever pressing for food, water, electrical stimulation of the brain and drug self-administration; the acquisition of lever pressing for a conditioned reward, a previously neutral stimulus that has acquired rewarding properties by having been associated with a rewarding stimulus such as food; place conditioning; the establishment of certain environments as conditioned stimuli for stimulant drug effects; and avoidance learning paradigms, where reward is provided by the presentation of safety-related stimuli. Some studies evaluate the effects of post-training treatments with agents that affect DA neurotransmission on subsequent performance of tasks possibly involving incentive learning. The effects of pharmacological agents relatively specific for D$_1$ or D$_2$ receptors on performance in paradigms using reward to alter behaviour, and therefore involving incentive learning, will be reviewed in this section. Note that many paradigms have been used to evaluate the effects of agents such as pimozide or haloperidol, DA antagonists relatively specific for D$_2$ receptors; only paradigms where data are also available for the effects of antagonists relatively specific for D$_1$ receptors will be reviewed here.

5.1.1 Lever pressing for food

Some of the earliest studies implicating DA in reward-related learning evaluated the effects of systemic pimozide, a DA antagonist relatively specific for D$_2$ receptors (e.g. Seeman, 1981), on responding according to a schedule of continuous food reward. Results revealed that drugged animals showed an intra- and/or intersession pattern of decline in responding similar to that seen in animals undergoing extinction, i.e. no longer receiving food reward following lever press responses (Faustmann and Fowler, 1982; Mason et al., 1980; Tombaugh et al., 1979, 1982; Wise et al., 1978a, b). Similarly, Nakajima and Baker (1989) reported gradually decreased intrasession responding for food with the D$_2$ antagonist raclopride. Pimozide also produced intersession declines in responding for sucrose (Gramling *et al.*, 1987). These results suggest that DA acting at D_2 receptors plays a role in incentive learning. Recently, Hammond *et al.* (1991) used a sophisticated version of this procedure in conjunction with pharmacological compounds affecting either DA or, by other mechanisms, motor capacity, to confirm that the effects of pimozide are to block the rewarding effects of food.

Others have found that responding rewarded with food presented according to a number of different schedules of intermittent reward similarly underwent intra- and/or intersession declines when animals were treated with D_2 antagonists, including pimozide, haloperidol, metoclopramide and raclopride. These effects were observed in animals trained on fixed interval (Greenshaw *et al.*, 1981; Tombaugh *et al.*, 1980), variable interval (Beninger *et al.*, 1987; Gray and Wise, 1980; Nakajima and Baker, 1989; Phillips and Fibiger, 1979; Tombaugh *et al.*, 1980; Willner *et al.*, 1988) and fixed ratio schedules (Salamone, 1986; Sanger, 1986; Tombaugh *et al.*, 1980). Faustman and Fowler (1981) reported that responding for food on a fixed ratio schedule did not show a session-to-session decline following haloperidol but their dose (0.5 mg/kg) was higher than that (0.1 mg/kg) used by Salamone (1986) or those (0.03, 0.1, 0.3 mg/kg) used by Sanger (1986). Perhaps, with the high dose, responding may have decreased rapidly to a low level in the first drug session leading to little further decrease in subsequent drug sessions. One study trained pigeons to respond to a variable ratio schedule of food reward. Using chlorpromazine, a drug that blocks D_2 receptors, Dearing and Branch (1981) reported intrasession declines in pecking responses. It would appear from the results of these studies that antagonists acting at D_2 receptors block the usual effects of reward on behaviour.

Fewer studies have evaluated the effects of antagonists relatively specific for D_1 receptors. Beninger *et al.* (1987) reported that the D_1 antagonist SCH 23390 produced both inter- and intrasession declines in responding rewarded with food according to a variable interval schedule. In contrast, Sanger (1987) found no significant intrasession decline in SCH 23390-treated rats responding for food according to a fixed ratio schedule. It is possible that the latter finding reflects the prior experience of the rats. Sanger (1987) reported that his rats treated with SCH 23390 had received previous injections of several other drugs while participating in an earlier study. As reviewed above, repeated injections with DA antagonists in the context of behavioural testing lead to a progressively greater drug effect. It is possible that the earlier drug history of these animals may have influenced the results of the SCH 23390 test. This might be expected to be the case only if the drug history had been with DA antagonists in the context of lever pressing for food. Unfortunately, this type of information is not available in the paper.

One other study reported the effects of SCH 23390 on lever pressing for food. Nakajima (1986) trained groups of rats on schedules of continuous reward or variable interval schedules. He reported neither intra- nor intersession data, making the assessment of patterns of responding produced by SCH 23390 impossible. However, he found that responding on the schedule of continuous reward was more resistant to the effects of SCH 23390 than responding on the variable interval schedules; for example, a dose of 40 μg/kg almost completely abolished variable interval responding while reducing continuously rewarded responding by less than 50%. This makes it difficult to attribute the effects of SCH 23390 to purely motoric consequences of the drug. There is a need for further studies of the effects of D_1 antagonists on lever pressing according to classical schedules of food presentation. Studies to date seem to suggest that treatments with either a D_1 or D_2 receptor antagonist block the usual effects of reward on behaviour.

This conclusion is supported by another small set of studies using Herrnstein's (1970) matching law to separate the effects of drugs on reward versus performance in operant responding tasks. Herrnstein used an equation to describe the relationship between the rate of responding on interval schedules and the frequency of reward. By fitting the equation to response rate data it is possible to derive two constants, one reflecting the theoretical maximum response rate (k) and the other reflecting the reward frequency needed to maintain a half-maximal rate (R_e). Verification studies showed that these two constants were indeed affected in the predicted manner by experimenter-induced changes. For example, reductions in reward magnitude affected R_e whereas changes in response parameters such as force requirements for a lever press affected k (Heyman et al., 1986). Thus, if DA receptor antagonists produce their effects on responding for food reward primarily by affecting ability to perform the response, k should be altered; if the effects of DA antagonists are to reduce the amount of reward, R_e should be altered.

Results of experiments using the matching law analysis to assess the effects of D_1 and D_2 antagonists on reward versus performance generally have revealed changes in both parameters. This was found with the D_2 antagonists pimozide and sulpiride and with the D_1 antagonist SCH 23390 (Heyman, 1983; Heymann et al., 1986; Porter and Villanueva, 1989; Willner et al., 1990). Morley et al. (1984) found that pimozide affected k but failed to find an effect on R_e, suggesting that the effects were attributable to performance decrements. However, Willner et al. (1990), by varying the number of variable interval components in the multiple schedule used to derive values of k and R_e, were able to show that results were more reliable with a larger number of components. They suggested that Morley et al. (1984) may have used too few components in their multiple schedule, leading to unreliable results. Willner et al. (1990) further suggested that the unequal session lengths for the two schedules may have complicated interpretation of the results of Morley et al. (1984). This latter point was supported by reports from Willner et al. (1989, 1990) of significant time-dependent effects of both D_1 and D_2 antagonists on R_e with relatively constant effects on k. The gradual effect of DA antagonists on responding points up the importance of session length in any analysis of their effects. These observations, suggesting that the effects of DA antagonist on reward may be gradual (producing an extinction-like pattern), are in excellent agreement with studies reviewed above. The observation of an effect of D_1 and D_2 antagonists on motor performance in the matching law analysis is consistent with an extensive literature demonstrating that antagonists selective for either receptor subtype decrease locomotor activity (reviews: Beninger *et al.*, 1991; Clark and White, 1987; Daly and Waddington, 1992; Joyce, 1983; Kebabian *et al.*, 1986; O'Boyle *et al.*, 1986; Waddington, 1989; Waddington and O'Boyle, 1987, 1989). Finally, the observation of an effect of D_1 and D_2 antagonists on R_e, the parameter reflecting amount of reward in the matching law analysis, supports the hypothesis that both receptor subtypes play an important role in mediating the effects of reward on behaviour.

Some studies have evaluated the effects of DA agonists acting preferentially at the D_1 or D_2 receptor on operant responding for food. The D_1 agonist SK & F 38393 and the D_2 agonists N-0437 or quinpirole reduced responding on variable interval (Hoffman and Beninger, 1989b) or fixed ratio schedules (Rusk and Cooper, 1988, 1989b). Hoffman and Beninger (1989b) found that quinpirole but not SK & F 38393 produced a gradual decrease in intrasession response rates; Rusk and Cooper (1988, 1989b) found no intrasession effects with either SK & F 38393 or N-0437. These results make it difficult to attribute the effects of D_1 and D_2 agonists to an action on reward in this paradigm. Furthermore, both D_1 and D_2 agonists have been found to decrease food consumption (Clifton *et al.*, 1989; Cooper *et al.*, 1990; Rusk and Cooper, 1989a, b; Timmerman *et al.*, 1989), raising the possibility that the effects of D_1 and D_2 agonists on operant responding for food may be secondary to their anorectic effect.

In conclusion, studies evaluating the role of DA receptor subtypes in lever pressing for food reveal that antagonists acting at either the D_1 or D_2 receptor produce extinction-like declines in responding. Studies using the matching law to assess drug effects similarly reveal a role for both DA receptor subtypes in reward. It is difficult to interpret the results of studies of the effects of DA receptor subtype-specific agonists on lever pressing for food since these agents produce anorexia. In general, results with antagonists implicate both D_1 and D_2 receptors in food reward-related incentive learning.

5.1.2 Lever pressing for water

Water-deprived animals have been trained to lever press for water reward and the effects of D_1 and D_2 antagonists evaluated. The D_2 antagonists pimozide, haloperidol, metoclopramide and sulpiride produced inter- and/or intrasession declines in responding for water presented according to a schedule of continuous reward (Gerber *et al.*, 1981; Ljungberg, 1987, 1990). Intrasession responding for water on a fixed ratio schedule was affected similarly by haloperidol (Ljungberg, 1987). Only one study has reported the effects of a D_1 antagonist on patterns of operant responding for water. Ljungberg (1990) found that continuously rewarded lever pressing for water decreased on the first day of treatment with SCH 23390 but recovered over the next 3 days. In two studies, it was reported that SCH 23390 dose-dependently decreased water-rewarded lever pressing but patterns of responding were not presented (Ljungberg, 1989; Nakajima, 1986). As patterns of lever press responding for water have been evaluated with only one dose of SCH 23390 in only one study, there is a clear need for further studies in this area.

In conclusion, there is good evidence that treatments with antagonists specific for the D_2 receptor produce patterns of responding consistent with a block of the usual effects of water reward on behaviour. At present there is no evidence that treatments with a D_1 antagonist block the effects of water reward; results from the one relevant study suggest that the effects of SCH 23390 get weaker with repeated administration and testing, an effect opposite to that expected when a block of reward occurs.

5.1.3 Lever pressing for electrical stimulation of the brain (ESB)

The results of numerous studies support the conclusion that DA neurones play an important role in mediating the rewarding effects of ESB (reviews: Le Moal and Simon, 1991; Milner, 1991; Phillips and Fibiger, 1989; Stellar and Rice, 1989; Wise, 1982, 1991; Wise and Rompré, 1989). Some studies have reported the pattern of responding after treatment with pharmacological agents relatively specific for D_2 receptors making it possible to assess the contribution of this receptor subtype to reward-related incentive learning. Thus, it has been found that responding continuously rewarded with ESB delivered to various target regions (e.g. lateral hypothalamus, ventral tegmental area, medial forebrain bundle in posterior hypothalamus) shows an extinction-like intrasession decline following treatment with a number of D_2 antagonists, including haloperidol, pimozide, metoclopramide, raclopride, sulpiride and sultopride (Fenton and Liebman, 1982; Fouriezos and Wise, 1976; Fouriezos et al., 1978; Franklin and McCoy, 1979; Gallistel et al., 1982; Hori et al., 1983; Nakajima and Baker, 1989). Although not reporting response patterns, Gallistel and Davis (1983) demonstrated that the effects of pimozide on responding for ESB were task specific, making it difficult to attribute the results to a drug-induced motor deficit. Zarevics and Setler (1979) used a sophisticated two-lever titration technique to show similarly that pimozide decreased the usual amount of ESB reward.

Animals are capable of responding for ESB presented on schedules of intermittent reward (Beninger et al., 1977, 1978) but few studies have investigated the effects of DA antagonists in this paradigm. Phillips and Fibiger (1979) and Greenshaw et al. (1981) trained rats to respond for ESB on a variable interval or fixed interval schedule, respectively. In both studies, treatment with a D_2 antagonist led to a gradual extinction-like decrease in responding. To my knowledge, no studies have reported the effects of systemically delivered D_1 antagonists on patterns of lever pressing for ESB delivered according to schedules of continuous or intermittent reward. However, the effects of SCH 23390 and haloperidol on ESB-produced continuous reward using spout contact as the required operant have been reported. Nakajima and McKenzie (1986) found that these compounds produced gradual extinction-like decreases in intrasession responding. The results from studies using schedules of continuous or intermittent reward seem to show a role for D_1 and D_2 receptors in mediating the effects of reward on behaviour.

Another paradigm that has been used extensively is the reward summation function. Variations in the number or frequency of pulses per train of ESB produce systematic changes in rates of lever press responding or running down an alley for ESB. Once frequency is increased to a threshold value, response rates show a rapid rise with each additional increase in frequency until an asymptote is reached (Gallistel, 1986; Stellar *et al.*, 1988). Validation studies have shown that manipulations that increase performance demands on the animals reduce the asymptote of the reward summation function without affecting the locus of rise (defined as the frequency needed to produce half-maximal levels of responding) whereas manipulations that reduce reward (e.g. a decrease in current level) shift the locus of rise to the right without affecting the asymptote (Gallistel, 1986; but see Fouriezos *et al.*, 1990). Some studies have evaluated the effects of DA antagonists on lever pressing for ESB using the reward summation function. Both D_1 and D_2 antagonists have been reported to shift the locus of rise to the right (Gallistel, 1986; Nakajima and O'Regan, 1991; Rompré and Bauco, 1990). Similar effects of D_1 and D_2 antagonists have been reported when running was the ESB-rewarded response (Franklin, 1978; Nakajima and McKenzie, 1986; Stellar *et al.*, 1983).

One study has evaluated the effects of D_1- and D_2-specific *agonists* using the reward summation function. Previous studies have shown that the indirect-acting DA agent amphetamine shifts the locus of rise to the left (Gallistel and Karras, 1984). Nakajima and O'Regan (1991) similarly found that the D_2 agonists quinpirole and CV 205-502 shifted the locus of rise to the left. In contrast, the D_1 agonist SK & F 38393 was without significant effect at low doses and led to a cessation of responding at high doses. Results of these studies, contrary to the many studies using antagonists, might suggest that D_1 and D_2 receptors may be differentially involved in mediating the effects of reward on behaviour.

Some investigators have used central microinjection techniques in conjunction with tests of ESB reward to evaluate the possible contribution of DA in specific terminal regions. One approach has been to place electrodes into the ventral tegmental region, an area containing DA cell bodies, and cannulae into the nucleus accumbens, an important target structure for the DA cells of the ventral tegmental region. DA antagonists could then be injected into the nucleus accumbens and their effect on ESB reward evaluated. Using this approach, the D_1 antagonist SCH 23390 and the D_2 antagonist spiperone were shown to reduce ESB reward (Kurumiya and Nakajima, 1988; Mogenson *et al.*, 1979). N.L. Freedman and I have recently replicated this finding with SCH 23390 (Figure 1). Pure motor effects of the injections were ruled out by injecting some rats with the antagonists into the nucleus accumbens contralateral to the electrode; these injections had little influence on responding for ESB. Using a similar approach, Ferrer *et al.* (1983) placed both electrode and cannula into the DA terminal region of the medial frontal cortex. They found that the D_2 antagonist pimozide, when injected ipsilateral to the electrode, blocked ESB reward while contralateral injections had little effect. These studies further implicate both D_1 and D_2 receptors in mediating the effects of reward on behaviour.

In conclusion, experimenters studying animals responding for ESB reward have used many ingenious approaches to evaluate the possible contribution of D_1 and D_2 receptors. There is broad agreement in the results with antagonists relatively specific for D_1 or D_2 receptors; both block the usual effects of ESB reward on behaviour. There are few studies evaluating the effects of agonists. In the one study reported by Nakajima and O'Regan (1991), a differential effect of a D_1 versus D_2 agonist was found in the reward summation function. This result raises the intriguing possibility that studies using agonists in other paradigms may begin to reveal differential roles for D_1 and D_2 receptors in reward-related incentive learning.

5.1.4 Stimulant self-administration

Animals have been surgically prepared with chronic intravenous cannulae allowing them to self-inject stimulant drugs when placed into an operant test cubicle. They were attached by tubing to a syringe that was filled with the stimulant drug and mounted on an infusion pump. Animals could activate the pump by pressing a lever. With the use of this procedure rats and monkeys have been found to self-administer a number of dopaminergic agents, including apomorphine, amphetamine and cocaine (reviews: Koob and Goeders, 1989; Le Moal and Simon, 1991; Wise and Rompré, 1989). Results from studies using the self-administration procedure provide strong support for the hypothesis that DA is involved in reward-related incentive learning.

There is one aspect of this procedure that makes it especially attractive to experimenters trying to sort out the possible motoric versus reward-reducing effects of DA antagonist. That is that rates of stimulant self-administration *increase* with reductions in the concentration of injected drug. If a low dose of a DA antagonist produced an increase in rate, it would not be possible to attribute the effect of the DA antagonist to a motor impairment. Rather, it would be concluded that the rewarding effects of the stimulant were reduced. Precisely this effect has been seen when rats or dogs were self-administering cocaine or amphetamine and then treated with low doses of either the D_1 antagonist SCH 23390 or the D_2 antagonists spiperone, haloperidol, pimozide, sulpiride or metoclopramide (Corrigall and Coen, 1991; de Wit and Wise, 1977; Koob *et al.*, 1987; Risner and Jones, 1976; Roberts and Vickers, 1984, 1987; Yokel and Wise, 1975, 1976). These results suggest that stimulation of both D_1 and D_2 receptors may be necessary for reward to occur.

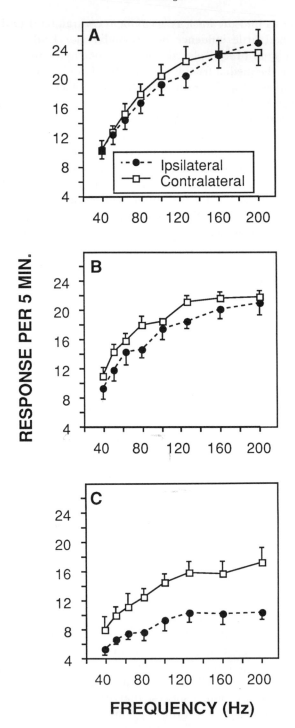

Two studies with monkeys self-administering cocaine have failed to find results in full agreement with those reported above. Woolverton and Virus (1989) found that both SCH 23390 and pimozide caused a decrease in self-administration and Woolverton (1986) reported that pimozide led to an increase whereas SCH 23390 produced a decrease. The discrepancy in the results with pimozide from these two studies may be related to details of the procedure, as suggested by Corrigall and Coen (1991). Thus, Woolverton and Virus (1989) used a time-out following cocaine infusions, possibly limiting the ability of monkeys to increase the dose by pressing the lever more. Woolverton (1986) did not use a time-out and observed increases in self-administration rates with low doses of pimozide, an effect frequently observed by others, as reviewed above.

This explanation also would account for the self-administration rate-decreasing effects of SCH 23390 reported in the study of Woolverton and Virus (1989) but not the apparent differential effects of SCH 23390 and pimozide in the study of Woolverton (1986). However, inspection of Woolverton's (1986) figure 1 reveals that in four of four monkeys receiving SCH 23390, there was a small increase in responding following a low dose of SCH 23390; in two cases, the magnitude of this increase was as great as or greater than that produced by pimozide. This observation and the findings of several investigators who have now reported that low doses of SCH 23390, like D_2 antagonists, have rate-increasing effects in animals responding to self-administered cocaine (Corrigall and Coen, 1991; Koob et al., 1987), suggest that the negative results of Woolverton (1986) should be viewed with caution. It is noteworthy that a recent paper from the laboratory of Woolverton reports that SCH 23390 differentially affected cocaine- and food-maintained behaviour. This observation ruled out a purely motoric interpretation of the effects of SCH 23390. It was concluded that D_1 antagonists may decrease the rewarding properties of cocaine (Kleven and Woolverton, 1990).

A related paper reported effects of DA antagonists on self-administration in a complex paradigm. Bergman et al. (1990) trained monkeys to respond for cocaine self-administration on a second order schedule. According to this

---

Figure 1 Mean (±SEM) responses per 5 min, rewarded with electrical stimulation of the brain (ESB) delivered to the ventral tegmental area, at frequencies ranging from 40 to 200 Hz, for groups ($n = 6$) implanted with cannulae in the ipsilateral (filled symbols) or contralateral (open symbols) nucleus accumbens. Each frequency was available for 5 min in ascending order during 40-min test sessions. There were three treatments: (A) no injections preceded the test session; (B) both groups were injected with drug vehicle (2.0 μl) into the nucleus accumbens prior to the test session; (C) both groups were injected with the D_1 antagonist SCH 23390 (5.0 μg in 2.0 μl) into the nucleus accumbens immediately prior to the session. Analysis of variance revealed a significant group by treatment interaction; the interaction was due to the significantly greater effect of SCH 23390 in the nucleus accumbens on the side ipsilateral to the electrode (N.L. Freedman and R.J. Beninger, unpublished).

schedule, responding was rewarded with a conditioned stimulus previously associated with cocaine injection on a fixed ratio 10 or 30, depending on the monkey, until 10 min had elapsed. Completion of the first ratio after 10 min was rewarded with the conditioned stimulus and an intravenous injection of cocaine. After establishing dose–response curves for cocaine, the effects of SCH 23390 and the D_2 antagonist eliclopride were tested. Both drugs shifted the cocaine dose–response curves to the right, suggesting a blunting of the effffects of cocaine reward. It was concluded that antagonism at either D_1 or D_2 receptors reduced the usual effects of reward on behaviour.

In some studies rats have been trained to self-administer extremely low doses of cocaine directly into DA-innervated regions of the brain. It was found that injections into the medial prefrontal cortex would support this behaviour (Goeders and Smith, 1983, 1986; Goeders et al., 1986). Furthermore, the rewarding effects of these injections seemed to be mediated by D_2 receptors. Thus, the addition of the D_2 antagonist sulpiride, but not the D_1 antagonist SCH 23390, to the cocaine solution significantly reduced self-administration (Goeders and Smith 1983, 1986; Goeders et al., 1986). Although few studies have been carried out, from these results it would appear that cocaine reward in the medial prefrontal cortex is mediated by D_2, not D_1, receptors.

Another approach has been to evaluate the ability of D_1 and D_2 receptor-specific agonists to support self-administration. In two studies it has been reported that the D_2 agonist bromocriptine, but not the D_1 agonist SK & F 38393, were self-administered by rats (Wise et al., 1990; Woolverton et al., 1984). SK & F 38393 was tested only in the Woolverton et al. (1984) study and further studies are needed to confirm these findings. One possible explanation is that systemic SK & F 38393 has an aversive effect in some brain region other than the nucleus accumbens (Section 5.1.1), leading to its failure to support self-administration. On the basis of the data available, it would appear that agonists acting at the D_2 but not the D_1 receptor are rewarding.

In conclusion, the self-administration paradigm provides a powerful tool for assessing the role of DA receptor subtypes in reward-related incentive learning. Results with antagonists were generally in good agreement with those from studies of lever pressing for food, water or ESB. Both D_1 and D_2 antagonists blunted the usual effects of stimulant reward on behaviour. In the case of agonists, few studies have been carried out. Based on the two studies available, it appears that D_2 but not D_1 agonists are capable of supporting self-administration behaviour.

5.1.5 Lever pressing for conditioned reward

When a neutral stimulus (e.g. tone or light) is repeatedly paired with a rewarding stimulus such as food, that stimulus, now termed a conditioned reward, can be shown to have acquired the properties of reward. Thus, animals will learn an operant response such as lever pressing when the only reward for that response is the presentation of the conditioned reward. Of course, with each presentation of the conditioned reward in the absence of primary reward, the rewarding properties of the conditioned reward will weaken. Thus, the acquired resonse will quickly undergo an extinction-like decline with repeated testing (Mackintosh, 1974, pp. 233–237).

This paradigm has been used to assess the effects of DA agonists on responding for reward. One advantage over the use of lever pressing for food, for example, is that possible anorexic properties of DA agonists may be less of a problem when the rewarding stimulus is not food but a conditioned stimulus based on food. The procedure frequently used involves first pairing a neutral stimulus with food during several sessions. Then animals are given access to a chamber with two levers, presses on one of which produce the stimulus previously paired with food. If the level producing that stimulus is pressed more, the food-associated stimulus can be said to be a conditioned reward. Numerous experiments have demonstrated this effect; additionally, treatments with a number of agents that augment DA neurotransmission have been found to produce a relatively specific enhancement of responding on the lever producing conditioned reward. This effect has been seen with amphetamine, pipradrol and several similarly acting drugs (Beninger et al., 1980a, 1981; Hill, 1970; Mazurski and Beninger, 1986; Robbins, 1975, 1976, 1978; Robbins and Koob, 1978; Robbins et al., 1983). Several recent studies have shown this effect with direct injections of amphetamine or DA into the nucleus accumbens (Cador et al., 1991; Kelley and Delfs, 1991a, b; Taylor and Robbins, 1984, 1986). The relatively selective effect on responding on the lever producing conditioned reward suggests that DA may participate in mediating the effects of conditioned rewarding stimuli on behaviour.

An interesting dissociation has been noted between the effects of amphetamine, a DA agent with the action of enhancing the release and blocking the uptake of DA, and apomorphine, a dopamimetic acting at both D$_1$ and D$_2$ receptors (Cooper et al., 1982). As reviewed above, amphetamine enhances responding for conditioned reward. Apomorphine, on the other hand, produces an indiscriminate increase in responding on both levers so that a conditioned reward effect is not seen (Mazurski and Beninger, 1986; Robbins et al., 1983). This differential effect might be related to the different mechanisms of action of the two drugs (e.g. Stellar and Rice, 1989). However, it is noteworthy that DA itself, which, like apomorphine, would directly stimulate DA receptors, produced a specific enhancement of responding for conditioned reward when it was applied directly to the nucleus accumbens (Cador et al., 1991). The reconciliation of these findings awaits further study.

In a series of studies, the effects of the D$_1$ agonist SK & F 38393 and the D$_2$ agonists quinpirole and bromocriptine on responding of rats for conditioned reward were assessed (Beninger and Ranaldi, 1992). Results revealed that the D$_2$ agonists, like amphetamine, enhanced responding for conditioned reward. SK & F 38393, on the other hand, appeared to impair responding for conditioned reward. The finding that systemically administered direct-acting D$_2$ agonists produced amphetamine-like effects was surprising since systemic apomorphine, also direct acting, led to a loss of specific responding for conditioned reward. This finding and the observation that SK & F 38393 appeared to lead to a loss of responding for conditioned reward might suggest that apomorphine produced an impairment of the conditioned reward effect through its action at D_1 receptors. This possibility will be discussed in further detail in Section 5.3.

5.1.6 Place conditioning

One of the simplest paradigms for assessing reward-related incentive learning is place conditioning. The test apparatus often consists of a rectangular box with two distinct sides attached by a tunnel that can be closed with guillotine doors. After several sessions of pairing one side with a rewarding stimulus such as food or a stimulant drug, animals are given access to both sides by removing the guillotine doors. Incentive learning is said to have taken place if animals are observed to spend significantly more time on the side previously associated with the rewarding stimulus. There is now a large body of data showing that DA plays an important role in reward-related incentive learning assessed with the use of place conditioning procedures (reviews: Carr et al., 1989; Hoffman, 1989).

Conditioned place preferences based on systemic injections of amphetamine have been found to be blocked by both D_1 and D_2 antagonists, including SCH 23390, and haloperidol, pimozide, sulpiride and metoclopramide (Hiroi and White, 1991; Hoffman and Beninger, 1989a; Mackey and van der Kooy, 1985; Mithani et al., 1986; Spyraki et al., 1982b). The rewarding effects, in a place conditioning paradigm, of some non-dopaminergic compounds also have been shown to be affected by receptor subtype-specific DA antagonists. The μ-opioid agonist morphine produced a place preference that was blocked by SCH 23390 but not sulpiride, spiperone or haloperidol (Mackey and van der Kooy, 1985; Shippenberg and Herz, 1987, 1988). Rewarding effects of the 5-hydroxy-tryptamine (5-HT_{1A}) receptor agonist 8-hydroxy-2-(di-n-propylamine)tetralin were similarly blocked by SCH 23390 but not sulpiride (Shippenberg, 1991). On the other hand, the rewarding effects of the benzodiazepine diazepam were blocked by the D_2 antagonist haloperidol; a D_1 antagonist was not studied (Spyraki and Fibiger, 1988). These results suggest that D_1 and D_2 receptors may play a role in mediating reward produced by amphetamine and strongly implicate each receptor subtype in mediating the rewarding effects of some non-dopaminergic agents.

Some studies have reported that animals show an aversion to an environment associated with the pharmacological effects of the D_1 antagonists SCH 23390 and A-69024 (Shippenberg and Herz, 1988; Shippenberg et al., 1991) although this effect of SCH 23390 was not seen in another study (Hoffman and Beninger, 1989a). The D_2 antagonists sulpiride, haloperidol, pimozide and spiperone have been reported to be neutral in place conditioning tests (Bozarth and Wise, 1981; Martin-Iverson et al., 1985; Shippenberg and Herz, 1988; Shippenberg et al.,

1991; Spyraki and Fibiger, 1988; Spyraki et al., 1982a, b) but one study found a place preference with the D_2 antagonist metoclopramide (Hoffman and Beninger, 1989a). Shippenberg et al. (1991) used intracranial microinjection techniques to show that injections of SCH 23390 into the nucleus accumbens but not the caudate-putamen, ventral tegmental area or medial prefrontal cortex produced a place aversion. Overall, it appears that D_1 and D_2 antagonists may differ with respect to their ability to produce place aversions, D_1 antagonists being effective and D_2 antagonists generally having little effect. The localization of these effects to the nucleus accumbens is in good agreement with related studies with agonists (see below).

The ability of agonists with relative specificity for D_1 or D_2 receptors to produce place conditioning has also been evaluated. It has been found that the D_2 agonists bromocriptine and quinpirole produced a place preference (Hoffman and Beninger, 1988, 1989a; Hoffman et al., 1988; Morency and Beninger, 1986; White et al., 1991). The D_1 agonist SK & F 38393, on the other hand, was found to produce an aversion (Hoffman and Beninger, 1988, 1989a; White et al., 1991). These results seemed to indicate a differential role for D_1 and D_2 receptors in place conditioning; however, recent studies using central injection techniques have challenged this conclusion.

Carr and White (1983, 1986) were the first to show that amphetamine place conditioning could be produced by microinjections into the nucleus accumbens but not a number of other DA-innervated structures, including the dorsolateral, anteromedial or lateroventral caudate, medial prefrontal cortex, amygdala and region of the area postrema. Recently, researchers in White's laboratory have shown that place conditioning can be produced by either the D_1 agonist SK & F 38393 or the D_2 agonist quinpirole injected directly into the nucleus accumbens (White et al., 1991). The discrepant results with systemic versus intra-accumbens SK & F 38393 might suggest that the aversive effects of this drug are related to an action in the periphery or an action in some other part of the central nervous system. The first of these alternatives was tested by Hoffman and Beninger (1988), who evaluated the effects of systemic SK & F 82526 (fenoldopam), a D_1 agonist that does not readily cross the blood–brain barrier, in a place conditioning experiment. Results revealed no effect. This suggests that the aversive effects of peripherally administered SK & F 38393 may result from its action in some region of the central nervous system other than the nucleus accumbens. It would appear that direct stimulation of either D_1 or D_2 receptors in the nucleus accumbens leads to reward-related learning in place conditioning studies.

Finally, in one study the effects of DA receptor subtype-specific antagonists on receptor subtype-specific agonist-produced place conditioning have been evaluated. Hoffman and Beninger (1989a) found that at least one dose of either SCH 23390 or metoclopramide was effective in antagonizing the place preference or aversion produced by systemic quinpirole or SK & F 38393, respectively.

In the previous study, antagonists and agonists were given during conditioning sessions. In a recent paper, Hiroi and White (1991) compared the effects of DA antagonists giving during conditioning to their effect when given during the test phase on the establishment and expression, respectively, of place preference conditioning produced by intra-accumbens amphetamine. Results revealed that systemic injections of the D_1 antagonist SCH 23390 and the D_2 antagonists sulpiride and metoclopramide dose-dependently blocked both the establishment and expression of place preference conditioning. For the D_2 antagonists, effective doses for blocking the expression were higher than those needed to block establishment. Although the differential effects were weaker, the D_1 antagonist seemed to produce a similar profile; at one dose ($120 \mu g/kg$) SCH 23390 blocked establishment but not expression of conditioning. Hiroi and White (1991) also showed that intra-accumbens injections of DA receptor subtype-specific antagonists were effective in blocking the expression of place preference conditioning. These results show that both D_1 and D_2 antagonists are effective in blocking place conditioning and replicate previous studies showing that the expression of incentive conditioning is more resistant to the effects of DA antagonists than its establishment (Beninger and Hahn, 1983; Horvitz and Ettenberg, 1991).

In summary, place conditioning produced by amphetamine was blocked by either D_1 or D_2 antagonists. Both D_1 and D_2 agonists produced place preferences but the D_1 agonist had to be given directly into the nucleus accumbens to produce this effect. Place conditioning produced by agonists at either DA receptor type appears to be blocked by antagonists at either receptor type.

5.1.7 Conditioned activity

When animals receive treatments with stimulant drugs repeatedly in a particular environment, stimuli in that environment apparently acquire the ability to elicit responses like those produced by the drug itself (e.g. increased locomotor activity). This can be seen in two ways: (1) as an enhanced response to the drug upon repeated administrations in the test environment (i.e. sensitization); or (2) when animals are returned to the drug-associated environment in a drug-free state, as a drug-like response (conditioned activity). Control animals with a similar drug history but never having received the drug in the test environment do not show these effects. Thus, the observed response in the animals previously receiving the drug–environment pairings is a genuine conditioned effect rather than an unconditioned effect related to previous treatments with the drug. This section will be concerned with sensitization and conditioned activity, phenomena that can be understood as further examples of incentive learning (Stewart, 1992; Stewart and Vezina, 1988).

The establishment of sensitization with the DA agents amphetamine or methamphetamine has been reported to be blocked by co-administration with the D_1 antagonist SCH 23390 or the D_2 antagonist YM 09151-2 (Hammamura et al., 1991; Ujike et al., 1989). In contrast, others have found that the establishment of conditioned activity or sensitization following repeated injections of amphetamine was blocked by co-administration of SCH 23390 but not the D$_2$ antagonists metoclopramide, pimozide and Ro 22-2586 (Drew and Glick, 1990; Mazurski and Beninger, 1991; Vezina and Stewart, 1989). In agreement with these findings with D$_1$ antagonists, one study showed that the direct microinjection of SCH 23390 into the ventral tegmental area blocked the establishment of sensitization to the stimulant effects of amphetamine (Stewart and Vezina, 1989). The experiments that reported that D$_2$ antagonists failed to block the establishment of conditioned activity or sensitization found that D$_2$ antagonists were effective in decreasing the unconditioned effects of amphetamine. From this it would appear that a manifestation of the unconditional stimulant effect of amphetamine is not necessary for it to produce conditioned effects.

One recent study has reported that neither a D$_1$ nor a D$_2$ antagonist was effective in blocking the establishment of conditioned activity based on amphetamine (Martin-Iverson and McManus, 1990). The findings with SCH 23390 are inconsistent with those from a number of other studies. Perhaps the 20 μg/kg dose of racemic SCH 23390 used by Martin-Iverson and McManus (1990) was lower than that used in other studies. Thus, with one exception, the papers reporting that SCH 23390 blocked the establishment of conditioned activity or sensitization used doses of the racemate ranging from 40 to 500 μg/kg. The one exception is the paper by Drew and Glick (1990). They found effects with SCH 23390 doses of 1.0 and 10 μg/kg but used many fewer conditioning sessions than Martin-Iverson and McManus (1990). If drug dose interacts with amount of conditioning, this would provide a possible explanation for these inconsistent data. In general, results seem to suggest that intact D$_1$ receptors but possibly not D$_2$ receptors are necessary for the establishment of conditioned activity or sensitization to amphetamine.

It has been found that either the D$_1$ agonist SK & F 38393 or the D$_2$ agonists quinpirole or (+)-4-propyl-9-hydroxynapthoxazine (PHNO) can produce conditioned activity (Martin-Iverson and McManus, 1990; Mazurski and Beninger, 1991). The effect of SK & F 38393 was blocked by SCH 23390 but not metoclopramide; the effects of quinpirole were blocked by metoclopramide but, surprisingly, not by SCH 23390 (Mazurski and Beninger, 1991). The effects of PHNO were blocked by neither SCH 23390 nor haloperidol (Martin-Iverson and McManus, 1990). The failure of SCH 23390 to block the effects of PHNO may be related to the dose as discussed above; alternatively, D$_1$ antagonists may not block D$_2$ agonist-produced conditioned activity, as reported by Mazurski and Beninger (1991). The failure of haloperidol to block conditioning based on PHNO was surprising, as these two compounds should compete for the same receptors. Perhaps the dose of haloperidol was also too low. In the study of Martin-Iverson and McManus (1990), animals treated with haloperidol and PHNO during conditioning were more active than vehicle-treated controls, providing some support for this speculation. It is difficult to draw conclusions from the current small number of studies in this area.

Some researchers have found that conditioned activity based on stimulant drugs like amphetamine is more resistant to the effects of DA antagonist than the unconditioned activity produced by the drug itself. Thus, it has been found that SCH 23390 or haloperidol blocked the unconditioned effects of apomorphine but not the conditioned effects (Carey, 1990). Others have reported that the D_2 antagonists pimozide or haloperidol produced this effect in animals conditioned with apomorphine or amphetamine (Beninger and Hahn, 1983; Welsh-Kunze et al., 1988). These results might suggest that during conditioning DA receptors mediate a plastic change in the brain that is non-dopaminergic.

In summary, both D_1 and D_2 agonists produce conditioned activity. In most cases, co-treatment with D_1 but not D_2 antagonists during conditioning sessions seems to block the establishment of conditioned activity or sensitization responses.

5.1.8   Conditioned avoidance responding

Animals quickly learn to avoid noxious stimuli. Acquisition of this ability may involve different types of learning. Thus, animals may learn the association between stimuli signalling the noxious event and the noxious event itself and they may learn the location of safety. Safety is rewarding and safety-related stimuli may acquire the ability to elicit approach and other responses that lead to successful avoidance. It appears that DA plays an important role in this latter incentive learning component of avoidance responding but not the learning of associations among stimuli (Beninger, 1983, 1989a, b, 1991).

Just as was the case in evaluating the effects of DA antagonists on responding for food, water or ESB, the pattern of avoidance responding seen in animals treated with DA antagonists provides insight into effects that may not be simply motor. Thus, trained animals have been observed to show significant intra- and/or intersession declines in avoidance responding following treatment with D_2 antagonists, including pimozide, haloperidol, metoclopramide and spiperone (Anisman et al., 1982; Beninger et al., 1980b, c, 1983; Blackburn and Phillips, 1989, 1990; Carey, 1987; Carey and Kenney, 1987a, b; Fibiger et al., 1975; Hillegaart et al., 1987; Ranje and Ungerstedt, 1977; Sanger, 1986, 1987). Similar effects have been seen in animals trained to lever press to avoid shock and then treated with haloperidol, metoclopramide, sulpiride or sultopride (Hori et al., 1983). This extinction-like pattern of responding is consistent with a block of the usual effects of reward on behaviour.

There is ample evidence that D_1 antagonists also block avoidance responding. Thus, a dose-dependent decrease in avoidance responding of rats or monkeys has been seen following treatments with the D_1 antagonists SCH 23390, SCH 39166 and SCH 12697 (Breese et al., 1990; Chipkin et al., 1988; Iorio et al., 1983, 1991; McQuade et al., 1991). The authors of these studies emphasized that the D_1 antagonists produced effects on avoidance responding at doses that neither affected escape responses nor produced catalepsy, making it difficult to attribute avoidance deficits to an action of the drugs on motor capacity. Unfortunately, in none of these studies were changes over time reported. In one study, Sanger (1987) evaluated the effects of SCH 23390 and haloperidol on avoidance responding of trained rats and separated the first ten-trial session into two five-trial blocks. He found that the D$_2$ antagonist produced a significant decrease in responding from the first block to the second; SCH 23390, on the other hand, although producing an overall decrease in avoidance responding and a small intrasession decline at one dose, did not produce a significant intrasession decline. Sanger (1987) also evaluated the effects of SCH 23390 and haloperidol over 4 days of avoidance testing and found that the D$_2$ antagonist but not the D$_1$ antagonist produced an intersession decline. These results led Sanger (1987) to conclude that antagonists relatively selective for the two receptor subtypes acted in a dissimilar manner.

From these studies it is clear that D$_2$ antagonists produce extinction-like decreases in avoidance responding consistent with an effect of the drug on reward-related incentive learning. It is equally clear that D$_1$ antagonists produce decreases in avoidance responding but there is currently no strong evidence to tie this effect to an action of the drugs on incentive learning. More studies with D$_1$ antagonists in avoidance paradigms are eagerly awaited.

5.1.9 Post-training treatments

There is one final paradigm in which DA receptor subtype-specific agonists have been evaluated that will be covered in this section. The post-training treatment literature is extensive and only a few recent studies will be the focus of this section. It may not be immediately clear how these studies relate to those reviewed above. However, an attempt to link these studies to those reviewed above and to show how their results can be understood in relation to possible molecular mechanisms involved in DA-mediated reward-related incentive learning will be made in the final section of this chapter.

The presentation of rewarding stimuli a short time *after* a brief period of training in some tasks repeatedly has been found to lead to improved recall of that task when retesting was carried out a day or more later. This has been found whether the task involved classical or operant conditioning and whether it involved appetitive or aversive stimuli (review: Huston et al., 1977). For example, post-training memory-improving effects have been seen with a number of rewarding stimuli, including ESB (Coulombe and White, 1980, 1982; Huston and Mueller, 1978) and glucose (Messier and White, 1984). Further studies implicated DA in these effects. Thus, memory improvement was found with ESB when electrodes were placed into the substantia nigra (Staubli and Huston, 1978) or into the nigrostriatal dopaminergic pathway (Major and White, 1978). Further studies showed that post-training injections of the DA-releasing agent amphetamine could produce memory enhancement and that the effect was abolished by lesions of the nigrostriatal pathway (Carr and White, 1984; White, 1988). It appeared that the post-training stimulation of DA neurones led to enhanced memory.

Subsequent studies assessed the role of DA receptor subtypes. White and Major (1978) found that the D_2 antagonist pimozide blocked the memory-improving effects of ESB. Packard and White (1989) reported that post-training systemic treatments with the D_2 agonist quinpirole but not the D_1 agonist SK & F 38393 improved memory on two different radial maze tasks. White and Viaud (1991) reported similar differential effects of the two agonists injected directly into the caudate nucleus. However, in a recent study, Packard and White (1991) found memory-improving effects of both D_1 and D_2 agonists injected into either the caudate or the hippocampus. This latter study used higher doses of SK & F 38393 than those used in the earlier studies, possibly accounting for the significant effects in the recent study. These studies seem to be leading to the conclusion that post-training stimulation of either D_1 or D_2 receptors may lead to memory enhancement.

One final study may be relevant to this section. Weldon *et al.* (1991) trained rat pups in an odour conditioning task by pairing odours with a rewarding tactile stimulus. They observed that post-pairing injections with the D_1 antagonist ($\pm$) SK & F 83566 but not the D_2 antagonist spiperone impaired conditioning assessed 1 day later. This interesting finding strongly implicates D_1 receptors as playing a role in the formation of memories.

Post-training treatment experiments have progressed over the last 20 years from implicating rewarding stimuli in memory improvement to beginning to identify a role for DA in this effect and the possible contribution of DA receptor subtypes. Studies to date have not ruled out either subtype. There is at least some evidence in favour of both D_1 and D_2 receptors being involved in the process of establishing memories.

5.1.10 Summary

D_1 antagonists have been found to block the usual effects of reward in animals lever pressing for food, ESB and stimulant self-administration. They block place conditioning and conditioned activity produced by stimulant drugs. Their effects in conditioned avoidance paradigms have not been studied extensively; the one available study does not provide evidence that a block of D_1 receptors leads to an extinction-like effect. On the other hand, the one study of post-training treatments with a D_1 antagonist implicates D_1 receptors in memory.

D_2 antagonists block the usual effects of reward in animals lever pressing for food, ESB and stimulant self-administration. They block place conditioning and conditioned activity produced by stimulant drugs. They produce an extinction-like decrease in avoidance responding and block the memory improving effects of post-training reward.

D_1 agonists have little effect or block responding for ESB in the reward summation paradigm and may impair responding for conditioned reward. In the one available study, they failed to support self-administration. They have been reported to support place conditioning and conditioned activity. When given immediately following a brief training trial, they improve memory assessed a day or more later.

D_2 agonists, like amphetamine, shift the reward summation function to the left and enhance responding for conditioned reward. They support self-administration, place conditioning and conditioned activity. They have been found to produce memory-improving effects when given after the training of a number of tasks.

5.2 Possible mechanism for dopamine-mediated incentive learning

Throughout the twentieth century, learning theorists have proposed various schemes for understanding the influence that reinforcing or rewarding stimuli have on behaviour (Mackintosh, 1974). There has never been a generally agreed upon scheme, perhaps partly because previous theories were not constrained by knowledge of the anatomical organization and neurochemical systems of the brain. Research over the past 20 years providing strong evidence that the neurotransmitter dopamine forms a critical link in the neurocircuitry mediating the effects of reward on behaviour, in the context of extensive refinements in knowledge about the anatomical organization and neurochemistry of the brain, provide new possibilities for understanding mechanisms underlying the effects of reward on behaviour. One such mechanism will be proposed in this section. In Section 5.3, the results reviewed in Section 5.1 will be considered in the context of this mechanism.

5.2.1 Reward and dopamine

As reviewed above, many data support the conclusion that DA is involved in reward-related incentive learning. It might be possible, therefore, to measure elevated levels of DA or its metabolites in various DA terminal regions of the brain in association with the presentation of rewarding stimuli. This approach has been taken by a number of researchers and results provide strong evidence that DA is released in association with the presentation of unconditioned or conditioned rewarding stimuli (reviews: Phillips *et al.*, 1989, 1991). In subsequent sections, this reward-related DA release will be referred to as the DA signal.

The earliest results were provided by neurochemical studies using postmortem tissue. Levels of DA metabolites and/or content of DA were measured in a number of brain regions of rats that had eaten food just prior to being killed. Results revealed increased levels of DA metabolites and/or decreased content of

DA, both indicative of increased DA neurotransmission, in the nucleus accumbens, caudate-putamen and/or amygdala (Blackburn *et al.*, 1986; Church *et al.*, 1986; Heffner *et al.*, 1980; Holmes *et al.*, 1989). Similar results were seen in animals lever pressing on various schedules for food, water or ESB reward just prior to being killed (Church *et al.*, 1986; Heffner and Seiden, 1980; Heffner *et al.*, 1981; Phillips *et al.*, 1987). Some studies reported that neurochemical indices of DA release in the nucleus accumbens or caudate-putamen were increased in rats exposed to conditioned stimuli signalling food, i.e. conditioned rewarding stimuli, without presentation of food itself, just prior to death (Blackburn *et al.*, 1989; Holmes *et al.*, 1989). A similar effect was seen in rats exposed to a conditioned stimulus for the DA agonists amphetamine or apomorphine prior to being killed (Schiff, 1982). These data strongly suggest that unconditioned and conditioned rewarding stimuli can lead to DA release, i.e. can produce a DA signal, in some regions of the brain.

A number of electrophysiological studies have recorded from DA cells in the ventral tegmental area of monkeys or rats during the performance of behavioural tasks rewarded with food. Results have generally shown that these cells often increase their firing rate in response to stimuli signalling reward (Fabre *et al.*, 1983; Miller *et al.*, 1981; Nishino *et al.*, 1987). For further discussion of these studies see Grace (1991).

Recently developed *in vivo* electrochemical and microdialysis techniques have made it possible to monitor intracerebral levels of DA and DA metabolites in active animals. Results have shown an elevation of DA and/or DA metabolites in the caudate-putamen or nucleus accumbens for food- or water-deprived rats eating or drinking (Keller *et al.*, 1983; Phillips *et al.*, 1991). Phillips *et al.* (1991) also found that DA levels increased during a conditioned stimulus signalling food, prior to food consumption. Others showed that caudate or accumbens levels of DA or DA metabolites increased in rats lever pressing for food or ESB (Joseph and Hodges, 1990; Joseph *et al.*, 1989; Nakahara *et al.*, 1989; Phillips *et al.*, 1989). A number of recent studies have evaluated brain DA in association with male sexual behaviour. Results have revealed increases in nucleus accumbens DA during a period of exposure to stimuli associated with a sexually receptive female or during sexual reward (Louilot *et al.*, 1986, 1991; Mas *et al.*, 1990; Pfaus *et al.*, 1990; Pleim *et al.*, 1990). Results from studies using *ex vivo* and *in vivo* techniques provide strong evidence that DA neurones are activated in association with the presentation of unconditioned or conditioned rewarding stimuli, producing a reward-related DA signal.

5.2.2 Dopamine in the brain

The anatomical organization of the brain's dopaminergic systems has been worked out in great detail (e.g. Lindvall, 1979). Although DA is to be found in many areas, projections from ventral mesencephalic nuclei to basal forebrain structures collectively termed the striatum have received much attention with respect to reward-related learning. Another DA-innervated area that has been found to play a role in reward is the medial prefrontal cortex (e.g. Ferrer *et al.*, 1983; Goeders and Smith, 1983, 1986; Goeders *et al.*, 1986). This area will not be considered further in the following; this is not intended to suggest that DA in the medial prefrontal cortex is any less important in reward-related learning. The focus for this section will be DA in the striatum.

The striatum consists of the caudate-putamen, nucleus accumbens and olfactory tubercle. These areas receive massive neo- and allocortical input and project to dorsal and ventral pallidum, respectively. They are also major targets of the dopaminergic cells of the substantia nigra and the ventral tegmental area (Heimer and Wilson, 1975; Heimer *et al.*, 1982; Nauta and Domesick, 1984). As DA has been found to play an important role in reward-related incentive learning and many studies have implicated dopaminergic projections to the striatum, it may be there that DA produces changes in connectivity that constitute the substrate of incentive learning.

In recent years, many details of the synaptic, neurochemical and ultrastructural organization of the striatum have become known (e.g. Bolam, 1984; Graybiel, 1990; Smith and Bolam, 1990). For present purposes, the focus will be on a subset of afferents of the most common neurones of the striatum, the medium spiny cells. These striatal efferent cells receive glutamatergic inputs from the cortex and dopaminergic inputs from the ventral mesencephalon (Figure 2). The dopaminergic inputs are noteworthy in that they come from a relatively small number of cells that have been found to arborize extensively; it has been estimated that a single DA neurone may form as many as 500 000 to 1 000 000 synaptic connections in the striatum (Andén *et al.*, 1966; Doucet *et al.*, 1986). The ultrastructural studies of Bolam and his co-workers have revealed that glutamatergic terminals are found on dendritic spines of the medium spiny cells; furthermore, dopaminergic terminals have been found on the same spines (Smith and Bolam, 1990). This arrangement may provide a locus where DA can modify the effectiveness of cortical afferents to the striatum.

5.2.3 Dopamine and glutamate

In recent years, *in vitro* electrophysiological studies have shown that DA may modify the effectiveness of glutamate synapses. Using fish retinal cells, Knapp and Dowling (1987) found that DA enhanced ionic conductances gated by L-glutamate or the glutamate receptor subtype agonist kainic acid. Furthermore, they found that this effect was produced by application of a membrane-permeable form of cAMP. It is known that DA receptors in the fish retina can stimulate the formation of cAMP, making them, by definition, of the D$_1$ subtype. Thus, DA, acting via D$_1$ receptors, stimulated second messenger formation that led to modification of a glutamate synapse. The authors concluded that their data '.., provide the first direct evidence for dopaminergic regulation of excitatory amino-acid neurotransmission in the vertebrate nervous system.' Two subsequent

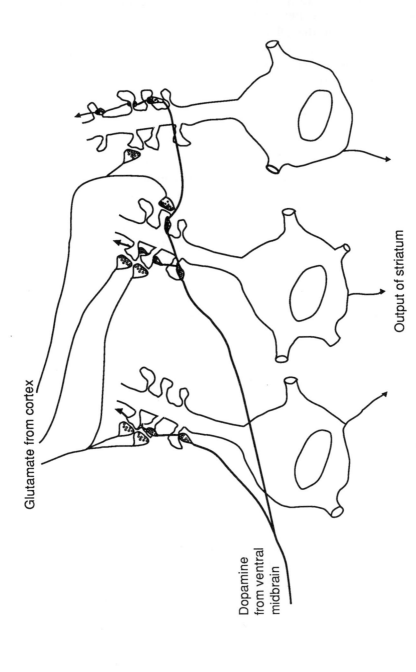

Figure 2 Three striatal medium spiny neurones and some of their afferents. These include glutamatergic inputs from the cortex making axospinous contact with dendritic spines that also receive dopaminergic synapses from the ventral midbrain. There are additional inputs that are not shown (see Smith and Bolam, 1990).

Glutamate from cortex

Dopamine from ventral midbrain

Output of striatum

papers elaborated on this basic finding. In one, it was shown that intracellular application of a cAMP-dependent protein kinase similarly modified the response of the cell to kainate. This suggested that DA may modify kainate-type glutamate receptor-gated channels by a phosphorylation event (Linman et al., 1989). In the other, the authors sought to identify the mechanism by which DA enhanced channels activated by kainate. Results revealed that DA led to a change in the kinetics of the ion channel to favour the open state (Knapp et al., 1990).

Two recent studies used cultured hippocampal cells to show a similar DA-produced modification of a glutamate synapse. In one, the response to kainate was shown to be enhanced by stimulation of cAMP-dependent protein kinase or by intracellular injection of the catalytic subunit of protein kinase. An inhibitor of protein phosphatase also enhanced the response to kainate (Wang et al., 1991). In the other, forskolin, an activator of adenylyl cyclase, modified responses to kainate. Cyclic AMP-dependent protein kinase similarly modified kainate responses and the mechanism was identified as an increased opening frequency and open time of kainate channels, similar to the effect reported above for retinal cells (Greengard et al., 1991). The authors concluded that glutamatergic neurotransmission could be modulated by a variety of receptors that are coupled to adenylyl cyclase and the activation of protein kinases. An obvious candidate is the D$_1$ receptor.

5.2.4   A possible mechanism

Making the leap from structure to function is always difficult. In the present enterprise, making this leap will require oversimplifications and generalizations; however, these will provide a general framework allowing for a focus on the striatum and the possible molecular mechanisms that may take place there in association with reward-related incentive learning.

Sensory stimuli are processed by the central nervous system from receptor organs often through several sensory nuclei, sometimes with parallel pathways concerned with different aspects of the sensory input, ultimately to the cortex where there may be many additional levels of processing as there is in the case of vision and audition (e.g. Imig and Morel, 1983; Maunsell and Newsome, 1987). As mentioned in Section 5.2.2 above, one of the major projection areas of the cortex is the striatum. Therefore, it is suggested that much of the input to the striatum from the cortex be viewed as sensory in nature, bringing to the striatum representations of events in the environment that are encountered by an animal. It is further suggested that striatal output be viewed as motor, influencing locomotion in part through a series of brainstem nuclei (Garcia-Rill, 1986). There is a long tradition in anatomy of viewing the striatum as part of the extrapyramidal motor system and many pathologies of the striatum produce neurological disorders with a motor component (e.g. Garcia-Rill, 1986). These considerations would make it possible to view the striatum as a sensory–motor interface in the brain.

Dopaminergic neurones project heavily to the striatum. They are well positioned to modulate the influence that striatal inputs have on striatal outputs. From the present point of view, DA may modify the influence that sensory events have on motor behaviour of an animal. Numerous investigators have drawn similar conclusions concerning the modulating influence of DA in the striatum (e.g. Divac et al., 1987; Lidsky et al., 1985; Mogenson, 1984; West et al., 1987). Figure 3 is a schematic representation of the connections of glutamatergic corticostriatal projections with the dendritic spines of striatal medium spiny cells and the common dopaminergic connection with each spine, as was illustrated in Figure 2. When reward-related incentive learning occurs, a reward-related DA signal may lead to a modification of these glutamatergic synapses.

As an animal encounters various different stimuli in its environment, different sets of cortical cells would be expected to be activated. Since the cortex projects heavily to the striatum, an associated set of corticostriatal gluatamatergic synapses would be expected to be active. When reward occurs producing the DA signal, DA would be expected to be released widely in the striatum because of the extensive arborization of DA axons there. This event could modify the strength of the *most recently active* corticostriatal glutamatergic synapses forming the structural basis of incentive learning. One requirement for this scheme is that there be a means for selection of the most recently active synapses, which are the only ones to be modified.

Previous authors have suggested that activity in corticostriatal synapses may produce a state of readiness during which these synapses may be modifiable (Miller, 1981; Miller et al., 1990; Wickens, 1990). Wickens (1990) proposed that the state of readiness might be mediated by the concentration of calcium ($[Ca^{2+}]$) in the spines of striatal medium spiny neurones. In an earlier paper, Wickens (1988) argued that spine $[Ca^{2+}]$ may be brought to the critical level for permitting synaptic modification by a conjunction of activity at the glutamate input to the spine and dendritic depolarization, fulfilling the elements of the rule for synaptic modification proposed by Hebb (1949). Wickens (1990) proposed that spine $[Ca^{2+}]$ might decrease to a level ineffective for synaptic modification within a short time following synaptic activation (e.g. 1.0 s).

Reward-related incentive learning might take place as follows. When reward occurs producing a DA signal in the striatum, glutamatergic axospinous synapses activated by the most recently encountered environmental stimuli would be in a state of readiness. The action of DA at D_1 receptors would lead to the stimulation of cAMP formation which, in turn, would activate cAMP-dependent protein kinase. This would lead to the phosphorylation of proteins that may participate in modifying the effectiveness of the glutamate synapse. Wickens (1990) suggested that one candidate for phosphorylation by the action of cAMP-dependent protein kinases is the DA- and cAMP-regulated phosphoprotein DARPP-32 (Hemmings et al., 1987). This protein, when in the phosphorylated state, inhibits protein phosphatase I. Wickens (1990) suggested that when protein phosphatase I is inhibited, calcium- and calmodulin-dependent protein kinase II may be able to

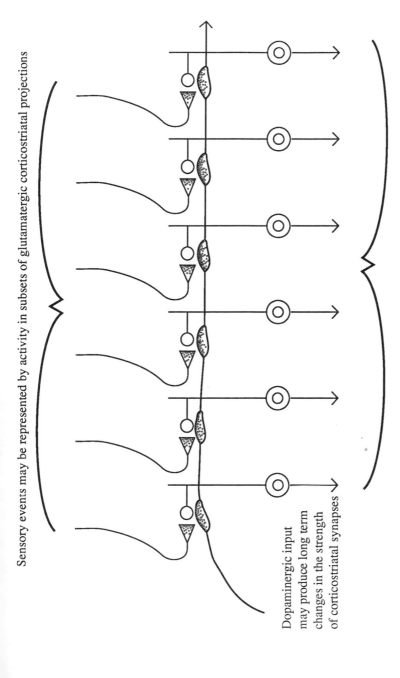

Sensory events may be represented by activity in subsets of glutamatergic corticostriatal projections

Dopaminergic input may produce long term changes in the strength of corticostriatal synapses

Responses may be controlled by striatal output

Figure 3 Highly schematized drawing of a possible locus of putative DA-mediated changes in the strength of corticostriatal glutamatergic synapses onto striatal output cells that may influence approach and other behaviours of an animal.

bring about long-term effects that lead to the enhanced efficacy of the glutamate synapse. By this mechanism, DA could lead to changes in glutamate synaptic effectiveness, like those that have now been shown to take place (Section 5.2.3), but only when the synapse is in a state of readiness defined as an increase in intracellular $[Ca^{2+}]$ (Figure 4).

An interesting aspect of the model proposed by Wickens (1990) is that each time a glutamate synapse is active and participates in activating the postsynaptic cell, an increase in $[Ca^{2+}]$ in the dendritic spine would occur. This increase

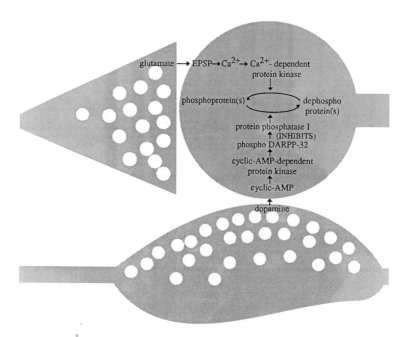

Figure 4 Possible mechanism for reward-related incentive learning. The release of dopamine in association with reward (the dopamine signal) may lead to the production of cAMP that activates a cAMP-dependent protein kinase, leading to the phosphorylation of proteins. One candidate for phosphorylation is DARPP-32; the phosphorylated form of this protein inhibits protein phosphatase I. If there had been a glutamatergic input to this dendritic spine just prior to the dopaminergic input, the increase in $[Ca^{2+}]$ resulting from the excitatory postsynaptic potential (EPSP) may have activated a calcium-dependent protein kinase that may be able to bring about long-term changes in efficacy of the glutamatergic synapse. In the absence of a dopaminergic signal, the consequences of activation of the calcium-dependent protein kinase may have been reversed by protein phosphatase I. If there was a dopaminergic input, the inhibition of protein phosphatase I by DARPP-32 may permit a long-term change (mediated by phosphoproteins) to take place. In this way, activation of D_1 receptors may lead to long-term changes in glutamatergic synapses. For further details see Hemmings *et al.* (1987) and Wickens (1990).

would lead to the activation of calcium- and calmodulin-dependent protein kinase that could potentially produce a long-term change in glutamate synaptic effectiveness. However, in the absence of reward and a DA signal leading to stimulation of D$_1$ receptors, protein phosphatase I may reverse the effects of the kinase. When there is reward and a DA signal, the stimulation of cAMP formation, activation of cAMP-dependent protein kinase and phosphorylation of DARPP-32 may lead to inhibition of protein phosphatase I, removing the normal inhibition of the effects of calcium- and calmodulin-dependent protein kinase. This may permit the changes that lead to increased effectiveness of the glutamate synapse. The postulated interactions are shown in Figure 4. Although some aspects of this model remain speculative, there is strong evidence to support many of its details, as reviewed above.

How permanent might the changes in glutamate synaptic effectiveness be? If this is the structural basis of reward-related learning, it should be relatively permanent without use but gradually should weaken if the modified glutamate synapses are used in the absence of reward, showing a normal extinction effect. Studies of the regulatory effects of cAMP-dependent protein kinase on the kainic acid glutamate receptor subtype provide some relevant data. Thus, Wang *et al.* (1991) found that the enhanced effectiveness of kainate receptors produced by cAMP-dependent protein kinase (PKA) was gradually lost when an inhibitor of the kinase was given (Section 5.2.3). They concluded that '... kainate receptors may be directly phosphorylated and dephosphorylated by PKA and phosphatases, respectively'. They also acknowledged that these effects could be mediated by an intermediate regulatory protein. This would provide a basis for understanding the gradual loss of incentive learning when reward is no longer given.

5.3 Consideration of the results of psychopharmacological studies of the role of D$_1$ and D$_2$ receptors in incentive learning from the point of view of the mechanism

The mechanism proposed in Section 5.2 makes stimulation of D$_1$ receptors crucial for DA-mediated reward-related incentive learning to take place. It would follow that treatments with D$_1$ antagonists in reward paradigms would lead to a block of the usual effects of reward on behaviour. D$_1$ agonists might be expected to affect incentive learning but the direction of their effect may depend on the paradigm under consideration and the relative importance of the timing of the DA signal. D$_2$ antagonists, by influencing the release of DA, may also affect the DA signal and therefore incentive learning. D$_2$ agonists may stimulate locomotor activity, leading to an enhancement of activity in DA neurones and increased stimulation of D$_1$ receptors, thereby influencing incentive learning in an indirect manner. These points will be considered in greater detail below. For related discussions, see Beninger (1991, 1992), Beninger *et al.*(1989) and Miller *et al.* (1990).

5.3.1 D_1 antagonists

The proposed mechanism for DA-mediated reward-related incentive learning requires the stimulation of D_1 receptors. Therefore, any paradigm involving reward should be affected by D_1 antagonists. They might be expected to block the establishment of incentive learning. In general, results support this prediction. Thus, D_1 antagonists impaired the establishment of incentive learning in place conditioning or conditioned activity tasks using amphetamine as the unconditioned rewarding stimulus (Drew and Glick, 1990; Hiroi and White, 1991; Hoffman and Beninger, 1989a; Mazurski and Beninger, 1991; Stewart and Vezina, 1989; Vezina and Stewart, 1989).

D_1 antagonists also might be expected to produce a gradual loss of incentive learning in animals trained prior to drug tests. Here, too, many data support this conclusion. D_1 antagonists have been found to produce declines, consistent with a block of the usual effects of reward, in animals responding for food (Beninger *et al.*, 1987; Nakajima, 1986; Willner *et al.*, 1990), ESB (Kurumiya and Nakajima, 1988; Nakajima and McKenzie, 1986; Nakajima and O'Regan, 1991; Rompré and Bauco, 1990) and stimulant self-administration (Bergman *et al.*, 1990; Corrigall and Coen, 1991; Kleven and Woolverton, 1990; Koob *et al.*, 1987).

Results to date provide strong evidence that D_1 receptor antagonists block the usual effects of reward on behaviour. These data are in good agreement with the mechanism described in Section 5.2 proposing that it is the action of DA at D_1 receptors that leads to reward-related incentive learning.

5.3.2 D_1 agonists

Some incentive learning paradigms require that animals learn to respond to a specific stimulus in the test environment (e.g. a lever). Others only evaluate the time that animals spend in a particular place (place conditioning) or their level of activity in a particular place (conditioned activity). Incentive learning involves the acquisition by certain stimuli of an enhanced ability to elicit approach and other responses. It was proposed that those glutamate synapses activated by stimuli encountered just prior to the reward-related DA signal may undergo the DA-mediated change in effectiveness. From this it follows that treatment with D_1 agonists might mask the reward-related DA signal in paradigms where incentive learning of particular cues in the test environment is required to perform the task. On the other hand, where there is no need to select a particular cue in the test environment to control responding, D_1 agonists might be effective at producing incentive learning. These possibilities are discussed in further detail below.

Paradigms where a particular environmental stimulus must come to control responding include lever-pressing tasks. Animals responding for food show a decrease in lever pressing following treatment with a D_1 agonist but this may reflect drug-produced anorexia (Hoffman and Beninger, 1989b; Rusk and Cooper, 1989b). Anorexia may not be a problem when animals are responding for ESB, stimulant self-administration or conditioned reward. In two of these paradigms, a D_1 agonist has been found to lead to an impairment in the ability of the lever and lever-related stimuli to control responding (Beninger and Ranaldi, 1992; Nakajima and O'Regan, 1991). The D_1 agonist produced effects similar to those seen following treatment with the direct-acting DA agonist apomorphine. A consideration of the effects of apomorphine and amphetamine may provide some insight into the effects of D_1 agonists.

A number of authors have suggested that the differential effects of amphetamine and apomorphine on responding for ESB or conditioned reward may be related to their different mechanisms of action (Beninger and Ranaldi, 1992; Herberg et al., 1976; Mazurski and Beninger, 1986; Robbins et al., 1983; Stellar et al., 1988). Amphetamine enhances responding for ESB or conditioned reward whereas apomorphine leads to a loss of control of responding by the reward-related stimuli. Amphetamine enhances neurogenic release of DA and blocks uptake whereas apomorphine mimics the action of DA at DA receptors (Cooper et al., 1982). It has been proposed that amphetamine may enhance the DA signal, leading to increased responding for reward, whereas apomorphine may mask the DA signal associated with reward, leading to the observed loss of control of responding by reward-related stimuli. The mechanism proposed in Section 5.2 might lead to a complementary explanation but with different emphases.

When animals press a lever and receive reward, there is a putative DA signal. Presumably the subset of glutamatergic synapses in a state of readiness are those activated by environmental stimuli associated with the lever. The release of DA might lead to a modification in the strength of those synapses; therefore, lever-related stimuli might become incentive stimuli controlling responding in the test environment. Treatment with amphetamine, at least at moderate doses, might preserve the temporal relationship between the lever-related stimuli and the DA signal, but the DA signal might be larger, possibly leading to greater incentive learning and more vigorous lever pressing. Treatment with apomorphine, on the other hand, might lead to an indiscriminate stimulation of DA receptors, uncoupling the usual relationship between the lever-related stimuli and the reward-produced DA signal. Control of responding by the lever-related stimuli in this latter case may be lost. As the crucial DA receptor for incentive learning has been proposed to be the D_1 subtype, agonists acting at the D_1 receptor might be expected to produce apomorphine-like effects. This is exactly what has been found (Figure 5). The possible importance of the D_1 receptor in the reward-masking action of apomorphine is suggested further by the observation that D_2 agonists produce amphetamine-like effects in animals

Stimuli from the test environment

Other stimuli

floor | lever | wall | corner

Motor output

lever pressing for ESB or conditioned reward. Apparently, with D_2 agonists the putative reward signal is not lost.

D_1 agonists have been found to produce a place preference (White et al., 1991) and conditioned activity (Mazurski and Beninger, 1991), both examples of incentive learning. This may be understood in the present context when task demands are taken into consideration. Thus, in both of these tasks, a particular environment is paired with injections of a D_1 agonist. The D_1 agonist would be expected to stimulate D_1 receptors tonically. This should lead to an increase in the effectiveness of gluatamatergic synapses brought into a state of readiness while the drug is active. The stimuli encountered while the animals are drugged are those associated with the test environments. Thus, those stimuli would acquire increased ability to elicit approach and other responses. This conditioning would be manifested as more time spent approaching the drug-paired side in the place conditioning task and increased activity in the conditioned activity task (Figure 5).

In summary, D_1 agonists impair responding for ESB or conditioned reward but produce place conditioning and conditioned activity. These results can be understood when the different nature of the tasks is taken into consideration. Lever pressing tasks require that *specific* stimuli in the test environment control responding. Place and activity conditioning tasks require simply that animals approach *any* stimuli in the test environment. In both cases, treatment with a D_1 agonist may lead to many stimuli in the test environment acquiring the ability to control responding. In the former case, this learning impairs control of responding by lever-related stimuli. In the latter, it produces the effect.

Figure 5 Schematized diagram of synaptic interactions in the striatum that may provide a basis for understanding the reported effects of D_1 agonists in different incentive learning tasks. According to the mechanism described in Section 5.2.4 and Figure 4, glutamatergic terminals (see Figure 3) brought into a state of readiness while D_1 receptors are being stimulated in a relatively tonic manner by a D_1 agonist might be expected to be strengthened (*). Various stimuli from the test environment (e.g. floor, lever, wall, corner) might undergo this modification while stimuli from elsewhere (other stimuli), not being encountered in association with stimulation of D_1 receptors, might not. This learning can be seen to have different consequences depending on the task. If an animal was lever pressing for conditioned reward, for example, the ability of the lever to control responding might be lost due to the increase in the ability of other stimuli in the test environment to control responding. This could explain the detrimental effects of apomorphine or SK & F 38393 on selective responding for conditioned reward. If an animal was simply placed into an environment while drugged and then later tested for approach to that environment (place conditioning) or level of activity in that environment (conditioned activity), both effects should be seen. This would indicate that stimuli from the test environment had acquired an enhanced ability to elicit approach and other responses. As no specific response is required in these tasks, D_1 agonists are effective in producing conditioning.

5.3.3 D_2 antagonists

If D_1 receptors are critical for reward-related incentive learning to take place, why are D_2 antagonists so effective at blocking the effects of reward on behaviour? There are two aspects of the effects of D_2 antagonists that may be relevant to answering this question. D_2 antagonists are well known to produce decreases in motor activity (e.g. Beninger, 1983; Beninger et al., 1991). As motor activity has been shown to lead to activation of DA neurones (Freed and Yamamoto, 1985; Heyes et al., 1988; Speciale et al., 1986; Szostak et al., 1986, 1988, 1989; Yamamoto and Freed, 1984; Yamamoto et al., 1982), it is possible that treatment with D_2 antagonists leads to a reduction in the drive on DA neurones. This may have the effect of reducing the strength of the reward signal and, therefore, reducing the stimulation of D_1 receptors in association with reward. The second aspect of D_2 antagonist effects that may influence stimulation of D_1 receptors in association with the reward-related DA signal is that D_2 antagonists have been shown to produce an increase in DA release, probably as a result of blocking presynaptic receptors (Blaha and Lane, 1984; Di Chiara and Imperato, 1985, 1988; Imperato and Di Chiara, 1985; Louilot et al., 1985; Nielson and Moore, 1982; O'Neill and Fillenz, 1985). These elevated levels of synaptic DA may mask the DA signal associated with reward in a similar manner to D_1 agonists, as discussed in the previous section.

By decreasing the drive on DA neurones, thereby weakening the DA signal associated with reward, and/or by increasing the level of DA release, thereby masking to some degree the DA signal associated with reward, D_2 antagonists may critically reduce the ability of rewarding stimuli to control responding. Both of these effects would influence the ability of DA released during the reward-related DA signal to produce a temporally discrete stimulation of D_1 receptors. Thus, D_2 antagonists, although acting primarily at the D_2 receptor, may have an important effect on events at the D_1 receptor that are critical for incentive learning.

Either the putative weakening of the reward signal or the masking of the reward signal at the D_1 receptor would be expected to produce the observed reward-blocking effects of D_2 antagonists in a number of paradigms. Thus, D_2 antagonists reduce the effects of reward in animals lever pressing for food, water, ESB and stimulant self-administration (Section 5.1). The action of D_2 antagonists on avoidance responding can similarly be understood as resulting from either of the above effects on the reward signal.

In considering the effects of D_2 antagonists in place conditioning and conditioned activity paradigms, both of the above-mentioned actions of D_2 antagonists cannot account for the observations. Recall that tonic stimulation of D_1 receptors with a D_1 agonist resulted in place preference conditioning and conditioned activity (Section 5.3.2). If the action of D_2 antagonists was to lead to enhanced concentrations of synaptic DA (as shown by the data, see above) and tonic stimulation of D_1 receptors, D_2 antagonists might be expected to produce place preferences and conditioned activity. In general, they do not. This might suggest that the reward-attenuating effects of D$_2$ antagonists are more importantly related to their reducing the drive on DA neurones and thereby weakening the DA signal than to their increasing striatal synaptic DA concentrations and putatively masking the reward signal. It is interesting to note, however, that there are reports of a D$_2$ antagonist producing place preference conditioning (Hoffman and Beninger, 1989a) and conditioned activity (Mazurski and Beninger, 1991). I am currently evaluating the possibility that the place conditioning effect is related to the stimulation of D$_1$ receptors by increased synaptic DA concentrations following blockade of D$_2$ receptors.

In summary, the ability of D$_2$ antagonists to mitigate the usual effects of reward on behaviour does not require rejection of the D$_1$-based mechanism of reward-related incentive learning proposed in Section 5.2. D$_2$ antagonists have been shown to have effects on the level of activation of DA neurones and on the concentrations of synaptic DA in the striatum. Either of these actions could influence the DA signal associated with reward and its action at D$_1$ receptors.

5.3.4   D$_2$ agonists

D$_2$ agonists have been reported to have amphetamine-like reward-enhancing effects on responding for ESB and conditioned reward and are self-administered (Section 5.1). As described in Section 5.3.3, increases in activity appear to lead to increases in the level of drive on DA neurones. As D$_2$ agonists have potent stimulant effects, they may increase the drive on DA neurones and thereby increase the magnitude of the reward signal. It is noteworthy that D$_2$ agonists, although directly and tonically stimulating D$_2$ receptors, produce effects like the DA release enhancer amphetamine, and do not produce effects like the direct-acting DA (D$_1$ and D$_2$) agonist apomorphine. These observations would suggest that tonic stimulation of D$_2$ receptors does not mask the reward signal; rather, D$_2$ agonists seem to increase motor output and enhance the ability of rewarding stimuli to control responding.

D$_2$ agonists also produce place preferences and conditioned activity. These effects can similarly be understood as resulting from an enhancement of drive on DA neurones leading to increased stimulation of D$_1$ receptors and incentive learning, as proposed in Section 5.2.

There is a clear prediction from these considerations. D$_1$ antagonists should block the reward-enhancing effects of D$_2$ agonists. Very few studies have addressed this question. Ranaldi and Beninger (unpublished) have investigated the effects of the D$_1$ antagonist SCH 23390 on the stimulation of responding for conditioned reward produced by the D$_2$ agonist bromocriptine. We found that SCH 23390 reduced the magnitude of this effect. Hoffman and Beninger (1989a) found that some doses of SCH 23390 were effective at blocking place preference conditioning based on the D$_2$ agonist quinpirole. Mazurski and Beninger (1991), on the other hand, found that SCH 23390 failed to block the establishment of conditioned activity based on quinpirole. There is an urgent need for more studies of this type.

There is at least some direct evidence that the apparent rewarding effects of D_2 agonists are mediated through the D_1 receptor. Although there is a need for further studies, results to date can be seen as consistent with the mechanisms proposed in Section 5.2.

5.3.5 Post-training treatments

Experiments involving the injection of DA receptor-subtype-specific agonists immediately following training are more difficult to understand from the point of view of the proposed mechanism. Only speculation is possible. It would appear that once the mechanism of reward-related learning has been initiated, post-training stimulation of either D_1 or D_2 receptors enhances the strength of learning. In only one study, a D_1 antagonist was injected immediately after pairing an odour with reward and it was found to impair memory for the incentive conditioning task (Weldon *et al.*, 1991). Interestingly, a D_2 antagonist was without effect. Further studies using this paradigm may provide valuable insights into the mechanism involved in incentive learning. An experiment that would be of great interest would be to evaluate the effects of D_1 antagonists on the memory-enhancing effects of D_1 and D_2 agonists. The present mechanism would lead to the prediction that the effects of agonists at either receptor subtype would be blocked.

5.4 Conclusions

In recent years there has been a rapid increase in the number of published papers evaluating the role of D_1 and D_2 receptors in learning. Results of these studies, in conjunction with findings from anatomical and neurochemical experiments, have led to the development of a possible mechanism for how DA may change the ability of reward-related stimuli to elicit approach and other responses. The results of most experiments can be understood from the point of view of this mechanism. However, there is a continuing need for further studies of the interactions of agonists and antagonists specific for DA receptor subtypes in paradigms evaluating incentive learning. The time is also right to begin a more thorough investigation of possible DA–glutamate interactions in studies of reward-related incentive learning.

Acknowledgements

This chapter is dedicated to L.O. Hanson. Thanks go to Robert Ranaldi for helpful comments on an earlier draft of this manuscript. The author wishes to acknowledge support from the Natural Sciences and Engineering Research Council of Canada.

References

Alkon, D.L. (1987) *Memory Traces in the Brain*. Cambridge, Cambridge University Press.
Andén, N.-E., Fuxe, K., Hamberger, B. & Hökfelt, T. (1966) *Acta Physiol. Scand.* **67**, 306–312.
Anisman, H., Irwin, J., Zacharko, R.M. & Tombaugh, T.N. (1982) *Behav. Neural Biol.* **36**, 280–290.
Beninger, R.J. (1983) *Brain Res. Rev.* **6**, 173–196.
Beninger, R.J. (1989a) In *Neuromethods, 13: Psychopharmacology* (eds Bolton, A.A., Baker, G.B. & Greenshaw, A.L.), pp 623–685. Clifton, NJ, Humana Press.
Beninger, R.J. (1989b) In *Aversion, Avoidance and Anxiety: Perspectives on Aversively Motivated Behavior* (eds Archer, T. & Nilsson, L.-G.), pp 265–284. New Jersey, Lawrence Erlbaum Associates.
Beninger, R.J. (1991) In *The Mesolimbic Dopamine System: From Motivation to Action* (eds Willmer P. & Scheel-Krüger, J.), pp 273–299. New York, John Wiley.
Beninger, R.J. (1992) *J. Psychopharmacol.* **6**, 34–42.
Beninger, R.J., Bellisle, F. & Milner, P.M. (1977) *Science* **196**, 547–549.
Beninger, R.J., Laferrière, A. & Milner, P.M. (1978) *Can J. Psychol.* **32**, 106–115.
Beninger, R.J., Hanson, D.R. & Phillips, A.G. (1980a) *Psychopharmacology* **69**, 235–242.
Beninger, R.J., Mason, S.T., Phillips, A.G. & Fibiger, H.C. (1980b) *Psychopharmacology* **69**, 11–18.
Beninger, R.J., Mason, S.T., Phillips, A.G. & Fibiger, H.C. (1980c) *J. Pharmacol. Exp. Ther.* **213**, 623–627.
Beninger, R.J., Hanson, D.R. & Phillips, A.G. (1981) *Br. J. Pharmacol.* **74**, 149–154.
Beninger, R.J. & Hahn, B.L. (1983) *Science* **220**, 1304–1306.
Beninger, R.J., Phillips, A.G. & Fibiger, H.C. (1983) *Pharmacol. Biochem. Behav.* **18**, 619–624.
Beninger, R.J., Cheng, M., Hahn, B.L., Hoffman, D.C., Mazurski, E.J., Morency, M.A., Ramm, P. & Stewart, R.J. (1987) *Psychopharmacology* **92**, 343–349.
Beninger, R.J., Hoffman, D.L. & Mazurski, E.J. (1989) *Neurosci. Biobehav. Rev.* **13**, 113–122.
Beninger, R.J., Mazurski, E.J. & Hoffman, D.C. (1991) *Pol. J. Pharmacol. Pharmac.* **43**, 507–528.
Beninger, R.J. & Ranaldi, R. (1992) *Behav. Pharmacol.* **3**, 155–163.
Bergman, J., Kamien, J.B. & Spealman, R.D. (1990) *Behav. Pharmacol.* **1**, 355–363.
Bindra, D. (1974) *Psychol. Rev.* **81**, 199–213.
Blackburn, J.R. & Phillips, A.G. (1989) *Psychopharmacology* **98**, 453–459.
Blackburn, J.R. & Phillips, A.G. (1990) *Psychopharmacology* **18**, 35–42.
Blackburn, J.R., Phillips, A.G., Jakubovic, A. & Fibiger, H.C. (1986) *Pharmacol. Biochem. Behav.* **25**, 1095–1100.
Blackburn, J.R., Phillips, A.G., Jakubovic, A. & Fibiger, H.C. (1989) *Behav. Neurosci.* **103**, 15–23.
Blaha, C.D. & Lane, R.F. (1984) *Eur. J. Pharmacol.* **98**, 113–117.
Bolam, J.P. (1984) In *Ciba Foundation Symposium 107: Functions of the Basal Ganglia* (eds Evered, D. & O'Connor, M.), pp 30–42. London, Pitman.
Bolles, R.C. (1972) *Psychol. Rev.* **79**, 394–409.
Bozarth, M.A. & Wise, R.A. (1981) *Life Sci.* **29**, 1881–1886.

Breese, G.R., Criswell, H.E., McQuade, R.D., Iorio, L.C. & Mueller, R.A. (1990) *J. Pharmacol. Exp. Ther.* **252**, 558–567.

Bunzow, J.R., Van Tol, H.H.M., Grandy, D.K., Albert, P., Salon, J., Christie, M., Cachida, C.A., Neve, K.A. & Civelli, O. (1988) *Nature* **336**, 783–787.

Byrne, J.H. & Berry, W.O. (eds) (1989) *Neural Models of Plasticity.* San Diego, Academic Press.

Cador, M., Taylor, J.R. & Robbins, T.W. (1991) *Psychopharmacology* **104**, 377–385.

Carey, R.J. (1987) *Biol. Psychiatry* **22**, 269–277.

Carey, R.J. (1990) *Brain Res.* **515**, 292–298.

Carey, R.J. & Kenney, S. (1987a) *Pharmacol. Biochem. Behav.* **28**, 203–208.

Carey, R.J. & Kenney, S. (1987b) *Neuropsychobiology* **18**, 199–204.

Carr, G.D. & White, N.M. (1983) *Life Sci.* **33**, 2551–2557.

Carr, G.D. & White, N.M. (1984) *Psychopharmacology* **82**, 203–209.

Carr, G.D. & White, N.M. (1986) *Psychopharmacology* **89**, 340–346.

Carr, G.D., Fibiger, H.C. & Phillips, A.G. (1989) In *The Neuropharmacological Basis of Reward* (eds Liebman, J.M. & Cooper, S.J.), pp 264–319. Oxford, Oxford University Press.

Chipkin, R.E., Iorio, L.C., Coffin, V.L., McQuade, R.D., Berger, J.G. & Barnett, A. (1988) *J. Pharmacol. Exp. Ther.* **247**, 1093–1102.

Church, W.H., Sabol, K.E., Justice, J.B. & Neill, D.B. (1986) *Pharmacol. Biochem. Behav.* **25**, 865–871.

Clark, D. & White, F.J. (1987) *Synapse* **1**, 347–388.

Clifton, P.G., Rusk, I.N. & Cooper, S.J. (1989) *Pharmacol. Biochem. Behav.* **33**, 21–26.

Cooper, J.R., Bloom, F.E. & Roth, R.H. (1982) *The Biochemical Basis of Neuropharmacology.* Oxford, Oxford University Press.

Cooper, S.J., Francis, J. & Rusk, I.N. (1990) *Psychopharmacology* **100**, 182–187.

Corrigall, W.A. & Coen, K.M. (1991) *Pharmacol. Biochem. Behav.* **39**, 799–802.

Coulombe, D. & White, N. (1980) *Physiol. Behav.* **25**, 267–272.

Coulombe, D. & White, N. (1982) *Can J. Psychol.* **36**, 57–66.

Daly, S.A. & Waddington, J.L. (1992) *J. Psychopharmacol.* **6**, 50–60.

Dearing, M.E. & Branch, M.N. (1981) *Psychopharmacology* **73**, 281–285.

Dearry, A., Gingrich, J.A., Falardeau, P., Fremeau, R.T., Bates, M.D. & Carson, M.G. (1990) *Nature* **347**, 72–76.

de Wit, H. & Wise, R.A. (1977) *Can. J. Psychol.* **31**, 195–203.

Di Chiara, G. & Imperato, A. (1985) *J. Pharmacol. Exp. Ther.* **235**, 487–494.

Di Chiara, G. & Imperato, A. (1988) *Proc. Natl Acad. Sci. USA* **85**, 5274–5278.

Divac, I., Öberg, G.E. & Rosenkilde, C.E. (1987) In *Basal Ganglia and Behaviour: Sensory Aspects of Motor Functioning* (eds Schneider, J.S. & Lidsky, T.I.), pp 61–67. Toronto, Hans Huber.

Doucet, G., Descarries, L. & Garcia, S. (1986) *Neuroscience* **19**, 427–445.

Drew, K.L. & Glick, S.D. (1990) *Psychopharmacology* **101**, 465–471.

Fabre, M., Rolls, E.T., Ashton, J.P. & Williams, G. (1983) *Behav. Brain Res.* **9**, 213–235.

Faustman, W.O. & Fowler, S.C. (1981) *Pharmacol. Biochem. Behav.* **15**, 327–329.

Faustman, W.O. & Fowler, S.C. (1982) *Pharmacol. Biochem. Behav.* **17**, 987–993.

Fenton, H.M. & Liebman, J.M. (1982) *Pharmacol. Biochem. Behav.* **17**, 1207–1212.

Ferrer, J.M.R., Sanguinetti, A.M., Vives, F. & Mora, F. (1983) *Pharmacol. Biochem. Behav.* **19**, 211–217.

Fibiger, H.C., Zis, A.P. & Phillips, A.G. (1975) *Eur. J. Pharmacol.* **30**, 309–314.

Fouriezos, G. & Wise, R.A. (1976) *Brain Res.* **103**, 377–380.

Fouriezos, G., Hansson, P. & Wise, R.A. (1978) *J. Comp. Physiol.* **92**, 661–671.

Fouriezos, G., Bielajew, C. & Pagotto, W. (1990) *Behav. Brain Res.* **37**, 1–7.

Franklin, K.B.J. (1978) *Pharmacol. Biochem. Behav.* **9**, 813–820.

Franklin, K.B.J. & McCoy, S.N. (1979) *Pharmacol. Biochem. Behav.* **11**, 71–75.

Freed, C.R. & Yamamoto, B.K. (1985) *Science* **229**, 62–65.
Gallistel, C.R. (1986) *Behav. Brain Res.* **22**, 97–105.
Gallistel, C.R. & Davis, A.J. (1983) *Pharmacol. Biochem. Behav.* **19**, 867–872.
Gallistel, C.R. & Karras, D. (1984) *Pharmacol. Biochem. Behav.* **20**, 73–77.
Gallistel, C.R., Boytim, M., Gomita, Y. & Klebanoff, L. (1982) *Pharmacol. Biochem. Behav.* **17**, 769–781.
Garcia-Rill, E. (1986) *Brain Res. Rev.* **11**, 47–63.
Gerber, G.J., Sing, J. & Wise, R.A. (1981) *Pharmacol. Biochem. Behav.* **14**, 201–225.
Goeders, N.E. & Smith, J.E. (1983) *Science* **221**, 773–775.
Goeders, N.E. & Smith, J.E. (1986) *Pharmacol. Biochem. Behav.* **25**, 191–199.
Goeders, N.E., Dworkin, S.I. & Smith, J.E. (1986) *Pharmacol. Biochem. Behav.* **24**, 1429–1440.
Grace, A.A. (1991) *Neuroscience* **41**, 1–24.
Gramling, S.E., Fowler, S.C. & Tizzano, J.P. (1987) *Pharmacol. Biochem. Behav.* **27**, 67–72.
Gray, T. & Wise, R.A. (1980) *Pharmacol. Biochem. Behav.* **12**, 931–935.
Graybiel, A.M. (1990) *Trends Neurosci.* **13**, 244–254.
Greengard, P., Jen, J., Nairn, A.C. & Stevens, C.F. (1991) *Science* **253**, 1135–1138.
Greenshaw, A.J., Sanger, D.J. & Blackman, D.E. (1981) *Pharmacol. Biochem. Behav.* **15**, 227–233.
Hamamura, T., Akiyama, K., Akimoto, K., Kashihara, K., Okumura, K., Ujike, H. & Otsuki, S. (1991) *Brain Res.* **546**, 40–46.
Hammond, E.O., Torok, M.L. & Ettenberg, A. (1991) *Psychopharmacology* **104**, 150–156.
Hebb, D.O. (1949) *The Organization of Behavior: A Neuropsychological Theory.* New York, John Wiley.
Heffner, T.G. & Seiden, L.S. (1980) *Brain Res.* **183**, 403–419.
Heffner, T.G., Hartman, J.A. & Seiden, L.S. (1980) *Science* **208**, 1167–1170.
Heffner, T.G., Luttinger, D., Hartman, J.A. & Seiden, L.S. (1981) *Brain Res.* **214**, 215–218.
Heimer, L. & Wilson, R.D. (1975) In *Golgi Centennial Symposium Proceedings* (ed. Santini, M.), pp 177–193. New York, Raven Press.
Heimer, L., Switzer, R.D. & Van Hoesen, G.W. (1982) *Trends Neurosci.* **5**, 83–87.
Hemmings, H.C., Walaas, S.I., Ouimet, C.C. & Greengard, P. (1987) *TINS* **10**, 377–383.
Herberg, L.J., Stephens, D.N. & Franklin, K.B.J. (1976) *Pharmacol. Biochem. Behav.* **4**, 575–582.
Herrnstein, R.J. (1970) *J. Exp. Anal. Behav.* **13**, 243–266.
Heyes, M.P., Garnett, E.S. & Coates, G. (1988) *Life Sci.* **42**, 1537–1542.
Heyman, G.M. (1983) *J. Exp. Anal. Behav.* **40**, 113–122.
Heyman, G.M., Kinzie, D.L. & Seiden, L.S. (1986) *Psychopharmacology* **88**, 346–353.
Hill, R.T. (1970) In *Amphetamine and Related Compounds* (eds Costa, E. & Garattini, S.), pp 781–795. New York, Raven Press.
Hillegaart, V., Ahlenius, S., Magnusson, O. & Fowler, C. (1987) *Pharmacol. Biochem. Behav.* **27**, 159–164.
Hiroi, N. & White, N.M. (1991) *Brain Res.* **552**, 141–152.
Hoffman, D.C. (1989) *Brain Res. Bull.* **23**, 373–387.
Hoffman, D.C. & Beninger, R.J. (1988) *Pharmacol. Biochem. Behav.* **31**, 1–8.
Hoffman, D.C. & Beninger, R.J. (1989a) *Pharmacol. Biochem. Behav.* **33**, 273–279.
Hoffman, D.C. & Beninger, R.J. (1989b) *Pharmacol. Biochem. Behav.* **34**, 923–925.
Hoffman, D.C., Dickson, P.R. & Beninger, R.J. (1988) *Neuro-Psychopharmacol. Biol. Psychiatry* **12**, 315–322.
Holmes, L.J., Smythe, G.A. & Storlien, L.H. (1989) *Brain Res.* **496**, 204–210.
Hori, Y., Fujita, A., Koike, K. & Hirose, K. (1983) *Eur. J. Pharmacol.* **88**, 37–46.
Horvitz, J.C. & Ettenberg, A. (1991) *Behav. Neurosci.* **105**, 536–541.
Huston, J.P. & Mueller, C.C. (1978) *Brain Res. Bull.* **3**, 265–270.

Huston, J.P., Mueller, C.C. & Mondadori, C. (1977) *Biobehav. Rev.* **1**, 143–150.

Imig, T.J. & Morel, A. (1983) *Annu. Rev. Neurosci.* **6**, 95–120.

Imperato, A. & Di Chiara, G. (1985) *J. Neurosci.* **5**, 297–306.

Iorio, L.C., Barnett, A., Leitz, F.H., Houser, V.P. & Korduba, C.A. (1983) *J. Pharmacol. Exp. Ther.* **226**, 462–468.

Iorio, L.C., Cohen, M. & Coffin, V.L. (1991) *J. Pharmacol. Exp. Ther.* **258**, 118–123.

Joseph, M.H. & Hodges, H. (1990) *J. Neurosci. Methods* **34**, 143–149.

Joseph, M.H., Hodges, H. & Gray, J.A. (1989) *Neuroscience* **32**, 195–201.

Joyce, J.N. (1983) *Neurosci. Biobehav. Rev.* **7**, 227–256.

Kebabian, J.W. & Calne, D.B. (1979) *Nature* **277**, 93–96.

Kebabian, J.W., Agui, T., van Oene, J.C., Shigematsu, K. & Saavedra, J.M. (1986) *Trends Pharmacol. Sci.* **7**, 96–99.

Keller, R.W., Stricker, E.M. & Zigmond, M.J. (1983) *Brain Res.* **279**, 159–170.

Kelley, A.E. & Delfs, J.M. (1991a) *Psychopharmacology* **103**, 187–196.

Kelley, A.E. & Delfs, J.M. (1991b) *Psychopharmacology* **103**, 197–203.

Kleven, M.S. & Woolverton, W.L. (1990) *Behav. Pharmacol.* **1**, 365–373.

Knapp, A.G. & Dowling, J.E. (1987) *Nature* **325**, 437–439.

Knapp, A.G., Schmidt, K.F. & Dowling, J.E. (1990) *Proc. Natl Acad. Sci. USA* **87**, 767–771.

Koob, G.F. & Goeders, N.E. *The Neuropharmacological Basis of Reward* (eds Liebman, J.M. & Cooper, S.J.), pp 214–263. Oxford, Oxford University Press.

Koob, G.F., Le, H.T. & Creese, I. (1987) *Neurosci. Lett.* **79**, 315–320.

Kurumiya, S. & Nakajima, S. (1988) *Brain Res.* **448**, 1–6.

Le Moal, M. & Simon, H. (1991) *Physiol. Rev.* **71**, 155–234.

Lidsky, T.I., Manetto, C. & Schneider, J.S. (1985) *Brain Res. Rev.* **9**, 133–146.

Liebman, J.M. & Cooper, S.J. (eds) (1989) *The Neuropharmacological Basis of Reward.* Oxford, Oxford University Press.

Liman, E.R., Knapp, A.G. & Dowling, J.E. (1989) *Brain Res.* **481**, 399–402.

Lindvall, O. (1979) In *The Neurobiology of Dopamine* (eds Horn, A.S., Korf, J. & Westerink, B.H.C.), pp 319–342. London, Academic Press.

Ljungberg, T. (1987) *Pharmacol. Biochem. Behav.* **27**, 341–350.

Ljungberg, T. (1989) *Pharmacol. Biochem. Behav.* **33**, 709–712.

Ljungberg, T. (1990) *Pharmacol. Biochem. Behav.* **35**, 111–115.

Louilot, A., Buda, M., Gonon, F., Simon, H., Le Moal, M. & Pujol, J.F. (1985) *Neuroscience* **14**, 775–782.

Louilot, A., Le Moal, M. & Simon, H. (1986) *Brain Res.* **397**, 395–400.

Louilot, A., Gonzales-Mora, J.L., Guadalupe, T. & Mas, M. (1991) *Brain Res.* **553**, 313–317.

Mackey, W.B. & van der Kooy, D. (1985) *Pharmacol. Biochem. Behav.* **22**, 101–105.

Mackintosh, N.J. (1974) *The Psychology of Animal Learning.* London, Academic Press.

Major, R. & White, N. (1978) *Physiol. Behav.* **20**, 723–733.

Martinez, J.L. & Kesner, R.P. (eds) (1991) *Learning and Menory: A Biological View.* San Diego, Academic Press.

Martin-Iverson, M.T. & McManus, D.J. (1990) *Brain Res.* **521**, 175–184.

Martin-Iverson, M.T., Ortmann, R. & Fibiger, H.C. (1985) *Brain Res.* **332**, 59–67.

Mas, M., Gonzalez-Mora, J.L., Louilot, A., Solé, C. & Guadalupe, T. (1990) *Neurosci. Lett.* **110**, 303–308.

Mason, S.T., Beninger, R.J., Fibiger, H.C. & Phillips, A.G. (1980) *Pharmacol. Biochem. Behav.* **12**, 917–923.

Maunsell, J.H.R. & Newsome, W.T. (1987) *Annu. Rev. Neurosci.* **10**, 363–401.

Mazurski, E.J. & Beninger, R.J. (1986) *Psychopharmacology* **90**, 239–243.

Mazurski, E.J. & Beninger, R.J. (1991) *Psychopharmacology* **105**, 107–112.

McQuade, R.D., Duffy, R.A., Coffin, V.L., Chipkin, R.E. & Barnett, A. (1991) *J.*

Pharmacol. Exp. Ther. **257**, 42–49.

Messier, C. & White, N.M. (1984) *Physiol. Behav.* **32**, 195–203.

Miller, J.D., Sanghera, M.K. & German, D.C. (1981) *Life Sci.* **29**, 1255–1263.

Miller, R. (1981) *Meaning and Purpose in the Intact Brain.* Oxford, Clarendon Press.

Miller, R., Wickens, J.R. & Beninger, R.J. (1990) *Prog. Neurobiol.* **34**, 143–183.

Milner, P.M. (1991) *Can. J. Psychol.* **45**, 1–36.

Mithani, S., Martin-Iverson, M.T., Phillips, A.G. & Fibiger, H.C. (1986) *Psychopharmacology* **90**, 247–252.

Mogenson, G.J. (1984) In *Modulation of Sensorimotor Activity During Alterations in Behavioral States* (ed Bandler, R.), pp 121–137. New York, Alan R. Liss.

Mogenson, G.J., Takigawa, M., Robertson, A. & Wu, M. (1979) *Brain Res.* **171**, 247–259.

Monsma, F.J., Mahan, L.C., McVittie, L.D., Gerfen, C.R. & Sibley, D.R. (1990) *Proc. Natl Acad. Sci. USA* **87**, 6723–6727.

Morency, M.A. & Beninger, R.J. (1986) *Brain Res.* **399**, 33–41.

Morley, M.J., Bradshaw, C.M. & Szabadi, E. (1984) *Psychopharmacology* **84**, 531–536.

Nakahara, D., Ozaki, N., Miura, Y., Miura, H. & Nagatsu, T. (1989) *Brain Res.* **495**, 178–181.

Nakajima, S. (1986) *Physiol. Psychol.* **14**, 111–114.

Nakajima, S. & Baker, J.D. (1989) *Psychopharmacology* **98**, 330–333.

Nakajima, S. & McKenzie, G.M. (1986) *Pharmacol. Biochem. Behav.* **24**, 919–923.

Nakajima, S. & O'Regan, N.B. (1991) *Pharmacol. Biochem. Behav.* **39**, 465–468.

Nauta, W.J.H. & Domesick, V.B. (1984) In *Ciba Foundation Symposium 107: Functions of the Basal Ganglia* (eds Evered, D. & O'Connor, M.), pp 3–23. London, Pitman.

Nielson, J.A. & Moore, K.E. (1982) *Pharmacol. Biochem. Behav.* **16**, 131–137.

Nishino, H., Ono, T., Muramoto, K., Fukuda, M. & Sasaki, K. (1987) *Brain Res.* **413**, 302–313.

O'Boyle, K.M., Molloy, A.G., Mashurano, M. & Waddington, J.L. (1986) *Psychopharmacol Bull.* **22**, 599–604.

O'Neill, R.D. & Fillenz, M. (1985) *Neuroscience* **14**, 753–763.

Packard, M.G. & White, N.M. (1989) *Pharmacol. Biochem. Behav.* **33**, 511–518.

Packard, M.G. & White, N.M. (1991) *Behav. Neurosci.* **105**, 295–306.

Pfaus, J.G., Damsma, G., Nomikos, G.G., Wenkstern, D.G., Blaha, C.D., Phillips, A.G. & Fibiger, H.C. (1990) *Brain Res.* **530**, 324–348.

Phillips, A.G. & Fibiger, H.C. (1979) *Pharmacol. Biochem. Behav.* **10**, 751–760.

Phillips, A.G. & Fibiger, H.C. (1989) In *The Neuropharmacological Basis of Reward* (eds Liebman, J.M. & Cooper, S.J.), pp 66–105. Oxford, Oxford University Press.

Phillips, A.G., Jakubovic, A. & Fibiger, H.C. (1987) *Brain Res.* **402**, 109–116.

Phillips, A.G., Blaha, C.D. & Fibiger, H.C. (1989) *Neurosci. Biobehav. Rev.* **13**, 99–104.

Phillips, A.G., Pfaus, J.G. & Blaha, C.D. (1991) In *The Mesolimbic Dopamine System: From Motivation to Action* (eds Willner, P. & Scheel-Krüger, J.), pp 200–224. New York, John Wiley.

Pleim, E.T., Matochik, J.A., Barfield, R.J. & Auerbach, S.B. (1990) *Brain Res.* **524**, 160–163.

Porter, J.H. & Villanueva, H.F. (1989) *Pharmacol. Biochem. Behav.* **31**, 779–786.

Ranje, C. & Ungerstedt, U. (1977) *Eur. J. Pharmacol.* **43**, 39–46.

Risner, M.E. & Jones, B.E. (1976) *Pharmacol. Biochem. Behav.* **5**, 477–482.

Robbins, T.W. (1975) *Psychopharmacology* **45**, 103–114.

Robbins, T.W. (1976) *Nature* **264**, 57–59.

Robbins, T.W. (1978) *Psychopharmacology* **58**, 79–87.

Robbins, T.W. & Koob, G.F. (1978) *Pharmacol. Biochem. Behav.* **8**, 219–222.

Robbins, T.W., Watson, B.A., Gaskin, M. & Ennis, C. (1983) *Psychopharmacology* **80**, 113–119.

Roberts, D.C.S. & Vickers, G. (1984) *Psychopharmacology* **82**, 135–139.

R.J. Beninger

Roberts, D.C.S. & Vickers, G. (1987) *Psychopharmacology* **93**, 526–528.
Rompré, P.-P. & Bauco, P. (1990) *Eur. J. Pharmacol.* **182**, 181–184.
Rusk, I.N. & Cooper, S.J. (1988) *Physiol. Behav.* **44**, 545–553.
Rusk, I.N. & Cooper, S.J. (1989a) *Brain Res.* **494**, 350–358.
Rusk, I.N. & Cooper, S.J. (1989b) *Pharmacol. Biochem. Behav.* **34**, 17–22.
Salamone, J.D. (1986) *Psychopharmacology* **88**, 18–23.
Sanger, D.J. (1986) *Psychopharmacology* **89**, 98–104.
Sanger, D.J. (1987) *Pharmacol. Biochem. Behav.* **26**, 509–513.
Schiff, S.R. (1982) *Biol. Psychiatry* **17**, 135–155.
Schwartz, J.H. & Greenberg, S.M. (1987) *Annu. Rev. Neurosci.* **10**, 459–476.
Seeman, P. (1981) *Pharmacol. Rev.* **32**, 230–287.
Shippenberg, T.S. (1991) *Neurosci. Lett.* **121**, 136–138.
Shippenberg, T.S. & Herz, A. (1987) *Brain Res.* **436**, 169–172.
Shippenberg, T.S. & Herz, A. (1988) *Eur. J. Pharmacol.* **151**, 233–242.
Shippenberg, T.S., Bals-Kubik, R., Huber, A. & Herz, A. (1991) *Psychopharmacology* **103**, 209–214.
Smith, A.D. & Bolam, J.P. (1990) *Trends Neurosci.* **13**, 259–265.
Sokoloff, P., Giros, B., Martres, M.-P., Bouthenet, M.-L. & Schwartz, J.-C. (1990) *Nature* **347**, 146–151.
Speciale, S.G., Miller, J.D., McMillen, B.A. & German, D.C. (1986) *Brain Res. Bull.* **16**, 33–38.
Spyraki, C. & Fibiger, H.C. (1988) *Psychopharmacology* **94**, 133–137.
Spyraki, C., Fibiger, H.C. & Phillips, A.G. (1982a) *Psychopharmacology* **77**, 379–382.
Spyraki, C., Fibiger, H.C. & Phillips, A.G. (1982b) *Brain Res.* **253**, 185–193.
Staubli, U. & Huston, J.P. (1978) *Brain Res. Bull.* **3**, 519–524.
Stellar, J.R. & Rice, M.B. (1989) In *The Neuropharmacological Basis of Reward* (eds Liebman, J.M. & Cooper, S.J.), pp 14–65. Oxford, Oxford University Press.
Stellar, J.R., Kelley, A.E. & Corbett, D. (1983) *Pharmacol. Biochem. Behav.* **18**, 433–442.
Stellar, J.R., Waraczynski, M. & Wong, K. (1988) In *Quantitative Analysis of Behavior*, Vol. VII, *Biological Determinants of Reinforcement* (eds Commons, M.L., Church, R.M., Stellar, J.R. & Wagner, A.R.), pp 31–57. New Jersey, Lawrence Erlbaum Associates.
Stewart, J. (1992) In *Learning and Memory: Behavioral and Biological Substrates* (eds Gormezano, I. & Wasserman, E.A.), pp 129–151. New Jersey, Lawrence Erlbaum.
Stewart, J. & Vezina, P. (1988) In *Sensitization in the Nervous System* (eds Kalivas, P.W. & Barnes, C.D.), pp 207–224. New Jersey, Telford Press.
Stewart, J. & Vezina, P. (1989) *Brain Res.* **495**, 401–406.
Stoof, J.C. & Kebabian, J.W. (1981) *Nature* **294**, 366–368.
Sunahara, R.K., Niznik, H.B., Weiner, D.M., Stormann, T.M., Brann, M.R., Kennedy, J.L., Gelernter, J.E., Rozmahel, R., Yang, Y., Israel, Y., Seeman, P. & O'Dowd, B.F. (1990) *Nature* **347**, 80–83.
Sunahara, R.K., Guan, H.-C., O'Dowd, B.F., Seeman, P., Laurier, L.G., Ng, G., George, S.R., Torchia, J., Van Tol, H.H.M. & Niznik, H.B. (1991) *Nature*, **350**, 1–5.
Szostak, C., Jakubovic, A., Phillips, A.G. & Fibiger, H.C. (1986) *Behav. Brain Res.* **21**, 37–46.
Szostak, C., Porter, L., Jakubovic, A., Phillips, A.G. & Fibiger, H.C. (1988) *Neuroscience* **26**, 395–401.
Szostak, C., Jakubovic, A., Phillips, A.G. & Fibiger, H.C. (1989) *Behav. Neurosci.* **103**, 678–687.
Taylor, J.R. & Robbins, T.W. (1984) *Psychopharmacology* **84**, 405–412.
Taylor, J.R. & Robbins, T.W. (1986) *Psychopharmacology* **90**, 390–397.
Timmerman, W., Rusk, I.N., Tepper, P., Horn, A.S. & Cooper, S.J. (1989) *Eur. J. Pharmacol.* **174**, 107–114.
Tombaugh, T.N., Tombaugh, J. & Anisman, H. (1979) *Psychopharmacology* **66**, 219–225.

Tombaugh, T.N., Anisman, H. & Tombaugh, J. (1980) *Psychopharmacology* **70**, 19–28.

Tombaugh, T.N., Szostak, C., Voorneveld, P. & Tombaugh, J.W. (1982) *Pharmacol. Biochem. Behav.* **16**, 67–72.

Ujike, H., Onoue, T., Akiyama, K., Hamamura, T. & Otsuki, S. (1989) *Psychopharmacology* **98**, 89–92.

Van Tol, H.H.M., Bunzow, J.R., Guan, H.-C., Sunahara, R.K., Seeman, P., Niznik, H.B. & Civelli, O. (1991) *Nature* **350**, 610–614.

Vezina, P. & Stewart, J. (1989) *Brain Res.* **499**, 108–120.

Waddington, J.L. (1989) *J. Psychopharmacol.* **3**, 54–63.

Waddington, J.L. (1992) *J. Psychopharmacol.* **6**, in press.

Waddington, J.L. & O'Boyle, K.M. (1987) *Rev. Neurosci.* **1**, 157–184.

Waddington, J.L. & O'Boyle, K.M. (1989) *Pharmacol. Ther.* **43**, 1–52.

Wang, L.-Y., Salter, M.W. & MacDonald, J.F. (1991) *Science* **258**, 1132–1135.

Weldon, D.A., Travis, M.L. & Kennedy, D.A. (1991) *Behav. Neurosci.* **105**, 450–458.

Welsch-Kunze, S., Nowak, K. & Kuschinsky, K. (1988) *Arch. Pharmacol.* **338**, 671–677.

West, M.O., Michael, A.J., Knowles, S.E., Chapin, J.K. & Woodward, D.J. (1987) In *Basal Ganglia and Behavior: Sensory Aspects of Motor Functioning* (eds Schneider, J.S. & Lidsky, T.I.), pp 27–35. Toronto, Hans Huber.

White, N.M. (1988) *Life Sci.* **43**, 7–12.

White, N.M. & Major, R. (1978) *Pharmacol. Biochem. Behav.* **8**, 565–571.

White, N.M. & Viaud, M. (1991) *Behav. Neural Biol.* **55**, 255–269.

White, N.M., Packard, M.G. & Hiroi, N. (1991) *Psychopharmacology* **103**, 271–276.

Wickens, J. (1988) *Prog. Neurobiol.* **31**, 507–528.

Wickens, J. (1990) *J. Neural Transm.* **80**, 9–31.

Willner, P., Chawla, K., Sampson, D., Sophokleous, S. & Muscat, R. (1988) *Psychopharmacology* **95**, 423–426.

Willner, P., Phillips, G., Sampson, D. & Muscat, R. (1989) *Behav. Pharmacol.* **1**, 169–176.

Willner, P., Sampson, D., Phillips, G. & Muscat, R. (1990) *Psychopharmacology* **101**, 560–567.

Wise, R.A. (1982) *Behav. Brain Sci.* **5**, 39–87.

Wise, R.A. (1991) In *Advances in Neuropsychiatry and Psychopharmacology*, Vol. 1: *Schizophrenia Research* (eds Tamminga, C.A. & Schultz, S.C.), pp 323–331. New York, Raven Press.

Wise, R.A. & Rompré, P.-P. (1989) *Annu. Rev. Psychol.* **40**, 191–225.

Wise, R.A., Spindler, J., de Wit, H. & Gerber, G.J. (1978a) *Science* **201**, 262–264.

Wise, R.A., Spindler, J. & Legault, L. (1978b) *Can. J. Psychol.* **32**, 77–85.

Wise, R.A., Murray, A. & Bozarth, M.A. (1990) *Psychopharmacology* **100**, 355–360.

Woolverton, W.L. (1986) *Pharmacol. Biochem. Behav.* **24**, 531–535.

Woolverton, W.L. & Virus, R.M. (1989) *Pharmacol. Biochem. Behav.* **32**, 691–697.

Woolverton, W.L., Goldberg, L.I. & Ginos, J.Z. (1984) *J. Pharmacol. Exp. Ther.* **230**, 678–683.

Yamamoto, B.K. & Freed, C.R. (1984) *Brain Res.* **297**, 115–119.

Yamamoto, B.K., Lane, R.F. & Freed, C.R. (1982) *Life Sci.* **30**, 2155–2162.

Yokel, R.A. & Wise, R.A. (1975) *Science* **187**, 547–549.

Yokel, R.A. & Wise, R.A. (1976) *Psychopharmacology* **48**, 311–318.

Zarevics, P. & Setler, P.E. (1979) *Brain Res.* **169**, 499–512.

Zhou, Q.-Y., Grandy, D.K., Thambi, L., Kushner, J.A., Van Tol, H.H.M., Conc, R., Pribnow, D., Salon, J., Bunzow, J.R. & Civelli, O. (1990) *Nature* **347**, 76–80.

CHAPTER 6

REGULATION OF DRUG DISCRIMINATION BEHAVIOUR BY DOPAMINE D_1 AND D_2 RECEPTORS

Erik B. Nielsen

Department of CNS Pharmacology, CNS Division, Novo Nordisk A/S, Novo Nordisk Park, DK-2760 Måløv, Denmark

Table of Contents

6.1 Introduction

Drug discrimination methodology has now been used for many years as an *in vivo* assay of what may be termed an animal counterpart of a human verbal report (White and Appel, 1982a). In a typical drug discrimination situation, a subject is trained to make a response on a designated manipulandum (e.g. pressing the left lever in an operant chamber) only when the subject is affected by a particular 'training' drug (e.g. the state induced by 0.16 mg/kg of lysergic acid diethylamide). Conversely, in the presence of no drug (or the effect of another training drug), the subject is required to make another response (e.g. pressing the right lever of an operant chamber) in order to obtain an appropriate reward (e.g. food or water after some time of food or water deprivation). After having been exposed to such conditions for a number of times (e.g. during 20–100 'training' sessions), the subject (e.g. rat, monkey, pigeon) can learn to select the 'correct' response manipulandum, presumably by having learnt to use the interoceptive effect of the training drug as a cue for selection of response manipulandum (Appel et al., 1978).

Many classes of psychoactive compounds are endowed with potent discriminable effects; however, notable exceptions exist. For example, it has been difficult to demonstrate clear effects of neuroleptics and antidepressants; see later and Schechter (1983) and Jones et al. (1980). In general, there are surprisingly few data to indicate the determining factors for when a compound can act as a strong or as a weak cue in drug discrimination situations. Furthermore, to date, there has not been described a common mechanism (neurochemical, neuroanatomical) involved in different drug discriminations (e.g. using training drugs with different mechanisms of action) (Lal, 1977; Colpaert and Slangen, 1982; Overton, 1983), although work by Nielsen and Scheel-Krüger (1986), D'Mello (1981) and Wood and Emmett-Oglesby (1989) has indicated a role for mesolimbic brain areas for at least some forms of central stimulant and hallucinogenic drug discriminations.

For several reasons, the drug cues elicited by dopaminergic drugs are of interest to the present author: dopamine (DA) is involved in both motor behaviour and in reward and learning processes and therefore plays a fundamental role in survival. DA is also involved in a variety of diseases, e.g. psychosis, Parkinsonism, depression, drug abuse and perhaps others. Thus, insights into the interoceptive pharmacology of DAergic mechanisms may help to shed light on the biology of the aforementioned diseases.

In recent years, a number of different DA receptors have been cloned. Most likely, these receptors fall into two general families: D_1, comprising the D_{1A}, D_{1B} and D_5 subtypes (Andersen et al., 1990), and the D_2 family, comprising the D_2 long and short forms, D_3 and D_4 receptors (Andersen et al., 1990; Civelli et al., 1991; Van Tol et al., 1991). At present, limited information is available on the receptor subtype selectivity of classical DAergic agonists and antagonists. Therefore, it is difficult to speculate on the relative role and importance of these receptor subtypes in controlling various DAergic drug discriminations. However, whenever possible, reference will be made to the possible significance of these divisions to the specific cues that have been described. Nevertheless, the present review is divided into three parts, focusing on D_1, D_2 and mixed D_1/D_2 cues. In parentheses, D_1 receptors here comprise the receptor sites labelled with [^{3}H]SCH 23390 (or [^{3}H]flupenthixol), whereas D_2 receptors comprise the classical [^{3}H]spiperone-labelled receptor sites (e.g. Andersen, 1988).

6.2 D_1 receptor-mediated cues

Several groups have reported on the use of the specific D_1 agonist SK & F 38393 as a discrimination training drug (see Table 1 for references). These studies have

Table 1 D$_1$ (SK & F 38393) cue.

Study	Species	Dose	Comment
Kamien and Woolverton (1985)	Rat	8 mg/kg i.p.	Central origin
Cunningham et al. (1985)	Rat	10 mg/kg i.p.	D$_1$-specific
Arnt (1988)	Rat	10 mg/kg i.p.	D$_1$-specific
			Lack of effect of d-amphetamine
Appel et al. (1988)	Rat	10 mg/kg i.p.	D$_1$-specific
			No effect of apomorphine
Kamien et al. (1987)	Rat	8 mg/kg i.p.	D$_1$-specific
Cory-Slechta et al. (1989)	Rat	8 mg/kg i.p.	D$_1$-specific
			High apomorphine generalizes

indicated that the SK & F 38393 cue is mediated by stimulation of central D_1 receptors, as the cue is only blocked by D_1 antagonists and only D_1 agonists generalize. It is also interesting to note that d-amphetamine fails to generalize with SK & F 38393 although amphetamine releases endogenous DA which non-selectively stimulates DA (Arnt, 1988). This may indicate that low levels of increased endogenous DA primarily stimulate D_2 receptors. This is supported by the fact that amphetamine, at least partially, substitutes for $(-)$-norpropylapomorphine (NPA), a D_2-mediated cue. D_2 agonists preferentially generalize with amphetamine, whereas D_1 agonists exhibit limited cue similarity to amphetamine (see later).

D_1 receptor antagonist cues have not yet been described although there have been unsuccessful attempts to train animals to discriminate SCH 23390 from saline (Kamien and Woolverton, 1989a; Nielsen, unpublished); see Table 3. It should be noted that with the prototypical benzazepine D_1 antagonist SCH 23390 (and related substances), the route of administration is rather important. Thus after intraperitoneal (or oral) administration, the compound is extensively metabolized and has a very short duration of action; in contrast, after subcutaneous administration (where much of the absorbed substance is not subject to first-pass metabolism), the compound is much more potent and may also have a protracted duration of action (Nielsen, unpublished; see also Chipkin and Latranyi, 1987; Andersen, 1988). Therefore, in future drug discrimination studies, it may be important to characterize the optimal conditions for benzazepine D_1 antagonist action with respect to route and pretreatment interval. This is further highlighted by the finding that SCH 23390, under some conditions, generalizes to other cues. Specifically, in rats trained with low (presumably 'autoreceptor'-selective) doses of quinpirole, SCH 23390 substitutes (Weathersby and Appel, 1986; Williams and Woolverton, 1990). Thus, SCH 23390 is not generally devoid of a discriminable effect. This apparently contradictory result may be explained by the ability of low autoreceptor active doses of D_2 agonists to decrease DA synthesis and, hence, D_1 tonus. In the drug discrimination situation, therefore, decreased DA levels may be mimicked by D_1 receptor antagonism. Consequently, the D_1 receptor must have physiological relevance under normal circumstances.

However, other explanations have also been possible (see later).

6.3 D_2 receptor-mediated cues

Cues elicited by stimulation of D_2 receptors also appear to be specific for that receptor, as such cues are only blocked by D_2 receptor antagonists while only D_2 agonists generalize (see Table 2). Interestingly, apomorphine, a classical mixed D_1/D_2 agonist, primarily induces a D_2-like cue (Stolerman and D'Mello, 1981; Tang and Franklin, 1987; Schechter and Greer, 1987; Woolverton et al.,

Table 2 D$_2$ cues.

Study	Species	Dose (mg/kg)	Training drug	Comment
Williams et al. (1990)	Rat	0.05 0.012	Quinpirole	Not blocked by SCH 23390
Arnt (1988)	Rat	0.04	NPA	Only blocked by haloperidol
Kamien et al. (1987)	Rat	1.0	Piribidil	Only blocked by pimozide
Woolverton et al. (1987)	Monkey	0.05	Apomorphine	D$_2$-specific
Tang and Franklin (1987)	Rat	0.1	Apomorphine	Autoreceptor activation; lack of generalization by amphetamine
Colpaert et al. (1976a)	Rat	0.16	Apomorphine	Blocked by neuroleptics
Colpaert et al. (1975)	Rat	0.16	Apomorphine	Blocked by haloperidol
Weathersby and Appel (1986)	Rat	0.025	Quinpirole	Only blocked by haloperidol SCH 23390 generalizes
Williams et al. (1990)	Rat	0.05	Quinpirole	SCH 23390 generalizes

Table 3 DA antagonist cues.

Study	Species	Dose (mg/kg)	Training drug	Comment
Kamien and Woolverton (1989a)	Rat	0.1	SCH 23390	D_1 failure
Nielsen (unpublished)		0.1	SCH 23390	D_1 failure
Weathersby and Appel (1986)	Rat	0.05	Quinpirole	D_2 generalization for SCH 23390
		0.012		
Colpaert et al. (1976b)	Rat	0.02	Haloperidol	(Extended training)
Goas and Boston (1978)	Rat	2	Chlorpromazine	D_2-mediated
Nielsen (1988)	Rat	5.76	Clozapine	Anticholinergic
Brown and Koe (1982)	Rat	3.2	Clozapine	Non-DAergic

1985, 1987; Colpaert *et al.*, 1975, 1976a) although higher doses of the compound show some D_1-like discriminable action (Cory-Schlecta *et al.*, 1989). It remains to be established whether the doses of the D_2 agonists used preferentially stimulate pre- or postsynaptic D_2 receptors. It may be speculated that the very low doses of the D_2 agonists sometimes used in drug discrimination situations (e.g. Weathersby and Appel, 1986; Holohean *et al.*, 1982; Colpaert *et al.*, 1976a) are autoreceptor selective. This is supported by the finding that amphetamine (which releases endogenous DA acting at postsynaptic receptors) generally fails to generalize with apomorphine and other D_2 agonists, e.g. Woolverton *et al.* (1987) and Tang and Franklin (1987); see, however, Arnt (1988), who found that amphetamine partially substituted for the D_2 agonist NPA.

D$_2$ antagonist cues have generally been very difficult to train (see Table 3). Colpaert *et al.* (1976b) found that haloperidol could elicit a discriminable cue, although it was only established after extensive training. Since other neuroleptics generalized, the haloperidol cue appears to be D_2 specific. As can further be seen from Table 3, discriminations based on both chlorpromazine and clozapine have been described. The discrimination based on clorpromazine seemed to be D_2 mediated as haloperidol generalized, whereas clozapine discrimination most likely is mediated by cholinergic muscarinic antagonism. Given that the haloperidol cue, established by Colpaert, required extended training (median of 80 sessions), it was surprising that the chlorpromazine cue was readily acquired (clear discrimination performance was evident after 10–15 sessions). Since haloperidol has a longer half-life than chlorpromazine (Niemegeers and Janssen, 1979), it may have been difficult to avoid the animals in Colpaert's study being affected by haloperidol under 'no-drug' conditions and, hence, it may have been more difficult for the animals to acquire the discrimination. Generally, compounds with high 'discriminability' are often rather quick-acting substances with relatively short duration of action although these issues have not been thoroughly evaluated (Schuster, 1977).

6.4 Other dopamine receptor-mediated cues

Very recently, certain classical D_2 agonists have been described as selective D_3 agonists, the D_3 receptor being a DA receptor that has only recently been cloned (Sokoloff *et al.*, 1990); notably, quinpirole is some 30 times more potent as a D_3 agonist than as a D_2 agonist (although quinpirole is still a potent D_2 agonist). This means that the quinpirole cue could be D_3 mediated; if confirmed by characterization using selective D_3 antagonists, it means that the generalization by SCH 23390 for quinpirole could be due to it acting as a specific D_3 agonist. Recently, Wachtel (1991) reported that SCH 23390 has certain DA agonist-like actions electrophysiologically. Further, Andersen and Nielsen (1986) have obtained evidence suggesting that SCH 23390 rather potently blocks [^{3}H]NPA binding *in vivo* (NPA may be a presynaptic ligand). Thus, SCH 23390 may have some D_3-like agonist actions that are shared with quinpirole.

However, although quinpirole may have D_3 agonist actions, its generalization for amphetamine (Nielsen *et al.*, 1989) is blocked by raclopride, a very specific D_2 antagonist.

6.5 $D_1:D_2$ interactions

Generally, few $D_1:D_2$ interactions have been described using agonist-mediated cues. Williams and Woolverton (1990) reported that quinpirole non-dose-dependently potentiated an SK & F 38393 discrimination, whereas SK & F 38393 failed to potentiate quinpirole discrimination (Williams *et al.*, 1990). This general lack of $D_1:D_2$ interactions may be taken to indicate that in drug discrimination, classical $D_1:D_2$ receptor interactions (e.g. synergy, enabling) are not readily seen (see also later).

6.6 Mixed D_1/D_2 cues

Many different direct and indirect 'mixed' D_1/D_2 agonists have been used as training drugs (apomorphine, lisuride and other ergots, cocaine, *d*-amphetamine, bupropion). With respect to the direct agonists, apomorphine and DAergic ergot discriminations appear mainly to be D_2 mediated; see previously and Appel *et al.* (1982, 1985, 1988), Cunningham *et al.* (1984, 1987), Appel and Cunningham (1986), Weathersby and Appel (1986), Appel and Rosecrans (1984), Hernandez *et al.* (1982), Holohean *et al.* (1982) and White and Appel (1982a, b).

With respect to indirect agonists, most studies have been carried out using amphetamine or cocaine as training drugs. Tables 4–7 summarize the studies using either cocaine or amphetamine as training compounds. It can be seen that although D_2 agonists generalize with these training drugs, D_1 agonists fail to generalize. Using antagonists, however, both D_1 and D_2 antagonists block the cue. There may be species differences between primates and rats as D_2 agonists only produce intermediate amphetamine/cocaine generalization in primates but fully generalize in rats. Further, D_2 antagonists seem not to block the amphetamine/cocaine cue fully in primates, whereas they often do in rats. However, it has sometimes been difficult to obtain complete antagonism of the cocaine cue in rats by DA D_2 antagonists, even within the same laboratory; see Colpaert (1978a, b). Cunningham and Appel (1982), Barrett and Appel (1989) and Silverman and Schultz (1989) and further discussion in Callahan *et al.* (1991). The reason for the observed discrepancies is not known but may involve subtle experimental conditions (e.g. injection route of antagonists, sensitivity of

Table 4 Amphetamine discrimination: substitution studies.

Study	Species	Dose (mg/kg)	D_1 probe	Generalization	D_2 probe	Generalization
Smith *et al.* (1989)	Rat	1.0	SK & F 38393	None	Quinpirole	Complete
Woolverton (1984)	Monkey	0.125	SK & F 38393	None	Apomorphine	Partial
		0.25			Piribidil	
					Bromocriptine	
Arnt (1988)	Rat	1.0	SK & F 38393	None	Quinpirole	Complete
					NPA	
Nielsen *et al.* (1989)	Rat	1.0	SK & F 89626	None	Quinpirole	Complete
			SK & F 81297	None	Pergolide	
			SK & F 38393	None	CH 29-717	
			SK & F 75670	None		
Kamien and Woolverton (1989b)	Monkey	0.67			Apomorphine	Complete
					Piribidil	Complete
					Bromocriptine	Complete
					Probutyl DA	Complete

Table 5 Amphetamine discrimination: antagonism studies.

Study	Species	Dose (mg/kg)	D_1 probe	Comment	D_2 probe	Comment
Smith et al. (1989)	Rat	1.0	SCH 23390	Blockade of cue	Haloperidol	Blockade of cue
Nielsen and Jepsen (1985)	Rat	1.0	SCH 23390	Blockade of cue	Haloperidol Spiroperidol Trifluperazine Perphenazine Molindone Chlorpromazine Pimozide Metoclopramide Sulpiride	Blockade of cue
Arnt (1988)	Rat	1.0	SCH 23390	Blockade of cue	YM 09151-2	Blockade of cue
Nielsen et al. (1989)	Rat	1.0	SCH 23390	Blockade of cue	Raclopride Clebopride Haloperidol	Blockade of cue
Kamien and Woolverton (1989b)	Monkey	0.67	SCH 23390	Blockade of cue	Pimozide Raclopride	Attenuation of cue
Exner et al. (1989)	Rat	0.5	SCH 23390	Blockade of cue	Haloperidol Terguride Preclamol SDZ 208911	Blockade of cue Attenuation of cue Attenuation of cue Attenuation of cue

Table 6 Cocaine discrimination: substitution studies.

Study	Species	Dose (mg/kg)	D₁ probe	Generalization	D₂ probe	Generalization
Wood and Emmett-Oglesby (1987)	Rat	10	SK & F 38393	Partial		
Callahan et al. (1991)	Rat	10	SK & F 38393	Partial	Quinpirole	Complete
Barrett and Appel (1989)	Rat	10	SK & F 38393	None	Quinpirole	Complete
Colpaert et al. (1979)	Rat	10			Apomorphine Piribidil	

Table 7 Cocaine discrimination: antagonism studies.

Study	Species	Dose (mg/kg)	D₁ probe	Comment	D₂ probe	Comment
Kleven et al. (1988)	Monkey	0.2	SCH 23390	Blockade of cue	Haloperidol	Two-fold shift
Kleven et al. (1990)	Monkey	0.2 0.4	SCH 23390	Blockade of cue 4–8 times shift		
Barrett and Appel (1989)	Rat	10	SCH 23390	Blockade of cue	Spiperone	Attenuation of cue
Callahan et al. (1991)	Rat	10	SCH 23390	Blockade of cue	Haloperidol	Blockade of cue
Vanover et al. (1989)	Monkey	0.2–0.4		Blockade of cue		
Colpaert et al. (1978a, b; 1979)	Rat	10	SCH 39166	Blockade of cue	Pimozide Haloperidol Spiperone	Blockade of cue Blockade of cue Blockade of cue

the animals to the disruptive effects of the antagonists). Nevertheless, D_1 antagonists appear to be more effective blockers of cocaine discrimination than D_2 antagonists. It can be speculated that benzazepine D_1 antagonists are biochemically selective DA antagonists, in contrast to many D_2 antagonists which commonly bind to non-DAergic receptors (Richelson, 1984; Billard *et al.*, 1984; Iorio *et al.*, 1983). Furthermore, in contrast to D_2 antagonists, D_1 antagonists apparently play a greater controlling role in DAergic neurotransmission; see also Clark and White (1987).

6.7 Conclusions

DAergic agonist action is readily discriminable in drug discrimination situations using as prototypical agents SK & F 38393 as a D_1 agonist and apomorphine or quinpirole (and analogues) as D_2 agonist. Such cues are pharmacologically specific for the DA receptor subtype involved. The basis for the specificity is presently unknown, but may involve differential localization of D_1 and D_2 receptors (post- versus presynaptic), respectively. This may have relevance in understanding why D_1 agonists fail to substitute for D_2 cues (if these are preferentially mediated by stimulation of autoreceptors which are of the D_2 family type (D_3)). However, it does not explain why D_2 agonists fail to substitute for a D_1 agonist; given that the respective agonists are only blocked by the appropriate antagonist (D_1 or D_2 type, respectively), it strongly indicates that D_1 and D_2 receptors are non-interacting in the drug discrimination model.

In the case of cues based on increased synaptic availability of DA (e.g. as induced by amphetamine or cocaine), both D_1 and D_2 receptors are apparently involved as such cues are non-selectively blocked by either type of antagonist. However, there is presently no strong demonstration of evidence of amphetamine-like effects by combining a D_1 and a D_2 agonist (Smith *et al.*, 1989; Nielsen *et al.*, 1989), although rather low (autoreceptor-sensitive) doses of quinpirole were used.

Of further relevance for understanding the inability of direct agonists to generalize with amphetamine are the results from early studies by Stolerman and D'Mello (1981). These investigators observed that the ability of apomorphine to generalize with amphetamine depended inversely on the training dose of the drug, i.e. apomorphine generalized only for amphetamine when the training dose was high; see also Nielsen and Scheel-Krüger (1988). Thus, based on this finding, it is furthermore not to be expected that a combination of a D_1 and a D_2 agonist would produce an amphetamine-like stimulus (at the presently used moderately low training dose of amphetamine).

Recently, Nielsen and Andersen (1991, 1992) attempted to theoretically account for the $D_1 : D_2$ interactions in the amphetamine discrimination model by comparing agonist and antagonist occupancies (using *in vivo* binding) necessary for obtaining induction or blockade of the amphetamine cue. Briefly, by analysing agonist– antagonist interactions under conditions of high and low levels of 'spare' receptors, respectively, these authors found that in amphetamine discrimination, there may be a low level of 'spare' D_1 receptors and a correspondingly high level of 'spare' D_2 receptors. Future studies will show if such a scenario is relevant in understanding the roles of the D_1 and D_2 receptors in controlling various DAergic drug discriminations.

References

Andersen, P.H. (1988) *Eur. J. Pharmacol.* **146**, 113–120.
Andersen, P.H. & Nielsen, E.B. (1986) *Acta Pharmacol. Toxicol (Copenh.)* **59**, 315–318.
Andersen, P.H., Gingrich, J.A., Bates, M.D., Dearry, A., Falardeau, P., Senogles, S.E. & Caron, M.G. (1990) *TIPS* **11**, 231–236.
Appel, J.B. & Cunningham, K.A. (1986) *Psychopharmacol. Bull.* **22**, 959–967.
Appel, J.B. & Rosecrans, J.A. (1984) In *Hallucinogens, Neurochemical, Behavioral and Clinical Perspectives* (ed Jacobs, B.L.), pp 77–94. New York, Raven Press.
Appel, J.B., White, F.J. & Kuhn, D.M. (1978) In *Stimulus Properties of Drugs: Ten Years of Progress* (eds Colpaert, F.C. & Rosecrans, J.A.), pp 7–29. Amsterdam, Elsevier.
Appel, J.B., White, F.J. & Holohean, A.M. (1982) *Neurosci. Biobehav. Rev.* **6**, 529–536.
Appel, J.B., Cunningham, K.A. & West, K.B. (1985) *Prog. Clin. Biol. Res.* **192**, 51–62.
Appel, J.B., Weathersby, R.T., Cunningham, K.A., Callahan, P.M. & Barrett, R.L. (1988) *Psychopharmacol. Ser.* **4**, 44–56.
Arnt, J. (1988) *Life Sci.* **42**, 565–574.
Barrett, R.L. & Appel, J.B. (1989) *Psychopharmacology* **99**, 13–16.
Billard, W., Ruperto, V., Crosby, G., Iorio, L.C. & Barnett, A. (1984) *Life Sci.* **35**. 1885–1893.
Browne, R.G. & Koe, B.K. (1982) In *Drug Discrimination: Application in CNS Pharmacology* (eds Colpaert, F.C. & Slangen, J.L.), pp 241–254. Amsterdam, Elsevier Biomedical Press.
Callahan, P.M., Appel, J.B. & Cunningham, K.A. (1991) *Psychopharmacology (Berlin)* **103**, 50–55.
Chipkin, R.E. & Latranyi, M.B. (1987) *Eur. J. Pharmacol.* **136**, 371–375.
Civelli, O., Bunzow, J.R., Grandy, D.K., Zhou, Q.-Y. & Van Tol, H.H.M. (1991) *Eur. J. Pharmacol. Mol. Pharmacol.* **207**, 277–286.
Clark, D. & White, F.J. (1987) *Synapse* **1**, 347–388.
Colpaert, F.C. & Slangen, J.L. (eds) (1982) *Drug Discrimination: Applications in CNS Pharmacology*. Amsterdam, Elsevier Biomedical Press.
Colpaert, F.C., Niemegeers, C.J., Kuyps, J.J. & Janssen, P.A. (1975) *Eur. J. Pharmacol.* **32**, 383 386.
Colpaert, F.C., Leysen, J.E., Niemegeers, C.J. & Janssen, P.A. (1976a) *Pharmacol. Biochem. Behav.* **5**, 671–679.
Colpaert, F.C., Niemegeers, C.J. & Janssen, P.A. (1976b) *Psychopharmacologia* **46**, 169–177.
Colpaert, F.C., Niemegeers, C.J. & Janssen, P.A. (1978a) *Neuropharmacology* **17**, 937–942.
Colpaert, F.C., Niemegeers, C.J. & Janssen, P.A. (1978b) *Psychopharmacology (Berlin)* **58**, 257–255.
Colpaert, F.C., Niemegeers, C.J.E. & Janssen, P.A.J. (1979) *Pharmacol. Biochem. Behav.* **10**, 535–546.

Cory-Slechta, D.A., Widzowski, D.V. & Newland, M.C. (1989) *J. Pharmacol. Exp. Ther.* **250**, 800–808.

Cunningham, K.A. & Appel, J.B. (1982) In *Drug Discrimination: Applications in CNS Pharmacology* (eds Colpaert, F.C. & Slangen, J.L.), pp 181–192. Amsterdam, Elsevier Biomedical Press.

Cunningham, K.A., Callahan, P.M. & Appel, J.B. (1984) *J. Pharmacol. Exp. Ther.* **230**, 47–52.

Cunningham, K.A., Callahan, P.M. & Appel, J.B. (1985) *Eur. J. Pharmacol.* **119**, 121–125.

Cunningham, K.A., Callahan, P.M. & Appel, J.B. (1987) *J. Pharmacol. Exp. Ther.* **241**, 147–151.

D'Mello, G.D. (1981) *Psychopharmacology (Berlin)* **75**, 184–192.

Exner, N., Furmidge, L.J., White, F.J. & Clark, D. (1989) *Behav. Pharmacol.* **1**, 101–111.

Goas, J.A. & Boston, J.E. Jr (1978) *Pharmacol. Biochem. Behav.* **8**, 235–241.

Hernandez, L.L., Holohean, A.M. & Appel, J.B. (1982) *Eur. J. Pharmacol.* **78**, 287–294.

Holohean, A.M., White, F.J. & Appel, J.B. (1982) *Eur. J. Pharmacol.* **81**, 595–602.

Iorio, L.C., Barnett, A., Leitz, F.H., Houser, V.P. & Korduba, C.A. (1983) *J. Pharmacol. Exp. Ther.* **226**, 462–468.

Jones, C.N., Howard, J.L. & McBennett, S.T. (1980) *Psychopharmacology (Berlin)* **67**, 111–118.

Kamien, J.B. & Woolverton, W.L. (1985) *Psychopharmacology (Berlin)* **87**, 368–370.

Kamien, J.B. & Woolverton, W.L. (1989a) *Pharmacol. Biochem. Behav.* **34**, 337–340.

Kamien, J.B. & Woolverton, W.L. (1989b) *J. Pharmacol. Exp. Ther.* **248**, 938–946.

Kamien, J.B., Goldberg, L.I. & Woolverton, W.L. (1987) *J. Pharmacol. Exp. Ther.* **242**, 804–811.

Kleven, M.S., Anthony, E.W., Goldberg, L.I. & Woolverton, W.L. (1988) *Psychopharmacology (Berlin)* **95**, 427–429.

Kleven, M.S., Anthony, E.W. & Woolverton, W.L. (1990) *J. Pharmacol. Exp. Ther.* **254**, 312–317.

Lal, H. (ed.) (1977) *Discriminative Stimulus Properties of Drugs.* New York, Plenum Press.

Nielsen, E.B. (1988) *Psychopharmacology (Berlin)* **94**, 115–118.

Nielsen, E.B. & Andersen, P.H. (1991) *Br. Ass. Psychopharmacol.* July 21–24 (abstract).

Nielsen, E.B. & Andersen, P.H. (1992) *Eur. J. Pharmacol.* **219**, 35–44.

Nielsen, E.B. & Jepsen, S.A. (1985) *Eur. J. Pharmacol.* **111**, 167–176.

Nielsen, E.B. & Scheel-Krüger, J. (1986) *Eur. J. Pharmacol.* **125**, 85–92.

Nielsen, E.B. & Scheel-Krüger, J. (1988) In *Transduction Mechanisms of Drug Stimuli* (ed. Colpaert, F.C. & Balster, R.L.), pp 57–72. Berlin, Springer-Verlag.

Nielsen, E.B., Randrup, K. & Andersen, P.H. (1989) *Eur. J. Pharmacol.* **160**, 253–262.

Niemegeers, C.J.E. & Janssen, P.A.J. (1979) *Life Sci.* **24**, 2201–2216.

Overton, D.A. (1983) *Psychopharmacology (Berlin)* **81**, 340–344.

Richelson, E. (1984) *J. Clin. Psychiatry* **45**, 331–336.

Schechter, M.D. (1983) *Pharmacol. Biochem. Behav.* **19**, 751–754.

Schecter, M.D. & Greer, N.L. (1987) *Life Sci.* **40**, 2461–2471.

Schuster, C. (1977) In *Behavioural Pharmacology* (ed. Dews, P.), pp 1–45. London, Pergamon.

Silverman, P.B. & Schultz, K.A. (1989) *Drug Dev. Res.* **16**, 427–433.

Smith, F.L., St John, C., Yang, T.F.T. & Lyness, W.H. (1989) *Psychopharmacology* **97**, 501–506.

Sokoloff, P., Giros, B., Martres, M.-P., Bouthenet, M.-L. & Schwartz, J.-C. (1990) *Nature* **347**, 146–151.

Stolerman, I.P. & D'Mello, G.D. (1981) *Psychopharmacology (Berlin)* **73**, 295–303.

Tang, A.H. & Franklin, S.R. (1987) *Psychopharmacology (Berlin)* **91**, 61–66.

Vanover, K., Kleven, M.S., Chipkin, R.E. & Woolverton, W.L. (1989) *Soc. Neurosci. Abstr.* **15**, 802.

Van Tol, H.H.M., Bunzow, J.R., Guan, H.-C., Sunahara, R.K., Seeman, P., Niznik, H.B. & Civelli, O. (1991) *Nature* **350**, 610–614.

Wachtel, S. (1991) *Soc. Neurosci. Abstr.* **14**, 345 (abstract).

Weathersby, R.T. & Appel, J.B. (1986) *Eur. J. Pharmacol.* **132**, 87–91.

White, F.J. & Appel, J.B. (1982a) *Science* **216**, 535–537.

White, F.J. & Appel, J.B. (1982b) *J. Pharmacol. Exp. Ther.* **221**, 421–427.

Williams, J.E.G. & Woolverton, W.L. (1990) *Pharmacol. Biochem. Behav.* **37**, 289–293.

Williams, J.E.G., Sutherland, J.V. & Woolverton, W.L. (1990) *Behav. Neural Biol.* **53**, 378–392.

Wood, D.M. & Emmett-Oglesby, M.W. (1987) *Soc. Neurosci. Abstr.* **13**, 1717.

Wood, D.M. & Emmett-Oglesby, M.W. (1989) *Pharmacol. Biochem. Behav.* **33**, 453–457.

Woolverton, W.L. (1984) *Pharmacologist* **26**, 161 (abstract).

Woolverton, W.L., Kamien, J.B. & Goldberg, L.I. (1985) *Pharmacol. Biochem. Behav.* **22**, 577–581.

Woolverton, W.L., Kamien, J.B. & Goldberg, L.I. (1987) *J. Pharmacol. Exp. Ther.* **241**, 213–217.

_____ CHAPTER 7 _____

ROLE OF D_1 VERSUS D_2 RECEPTORS IN THE MODULATION OF STATES OF AROUSAL AND SLEEP

Ennio Ongini

Research Laboratories, Schering-Plough SpA, I-20060 Comazzo, Milan, Italy

Table of Contents

7.1   Introduction

Neurotransmitters are known to play an important role in the regulation of behavioural states. Acetylcholine and the monoamines, serotonin, noradrenaline and dopamine (DA), participate in mechanisms which modulate complex behavioural states such as full arousal at one end of the spectrum, and deep sleep at the other (Jouvet, 1972). The notion is supported by several studies embracing a variety of disciplines, including pharmacology, neurophysiology and neuroanatomy. The advances made over the past 40 years and the availability of sophisticated techniques have allowed the identification of the neurotransmitters and neuronal populations that are critical for the appearance of the different behavioural states. For example, pharmacological studies have shown that the administration of drugs which alter the function of specific neurotransmitters within the brain produces marked changes of the diurnal patterns of sleep and waking in both laboratory animals and human beings.

There are excellent papers which provide a comprehensive overview of the basic neural and biochemical mechanisms that play a critical role in generating and regulating each distinct behavioural state (Jouvet, 1972; Hobson *et al.*, 1986; Shiromani *et al.*, 1987; Steriade and McCarley, 1990; Jones, 1991). In this chapter, I will review the evidence available showing that DA neurones, through the D_1 and D_2 receptor population, modulate the behavioural states of sleep and waking. Progress made over the last few years in the discovery of pharmacological agents which specifically interact with the D_1 or D_2 receptor has provided important tools for understanding the physiological and behavioural responses associated with each receptor population. The pharmacological findings which have emerged seem to suggest that D_1 receptors, more than D_2, are involved in the regulation of arousal and sleep states.

7.2   Dopamine in arousal and sleep

7.2.1   The behavioural states in mammals

The biological rhythms of sleep and waking are present across a variety of animal species and can be studied by objective measures. One reliable approach is based on the measurement of large populations of cortical neurones. Recordings of electrical activity such as the electroencephalogram (EEG) may be obtained in humans from electrodes placed on the scalp and in animals through electrodes which are placed on the surface of the brain or inserted into discrete brain regions, e.g. hippocampus. The EEG is valuable in providing an overall index of the state of activation of such areas as the cerebral cortex. Characteristic changes in both the frequency and the amplitude of discharge of the EEG are known to be associated with the different states of arousal and sleep. Thus, there are EEG patterns typical of the various sleep stages, many of which can be mimicked by drugs.

By using EEG criteria, the behavioural states of mammals can be classified into three distinct phases: wakefulness, non-rapid eye movement (non-REM) sleep and REM sleep. During wakefulness, the EEG pattern is one of low amplitude and high frequency, and the level of arousal which characterizes this stage is a most important variable in determining the behavioural responses to the external environment. The sleeping period is associated with two quite distinct types of brain activity. During non-REM sleep there are varying EEG patterns of high-amplitude slow waves and spindle bursts. In humans non-REM has been divided into four stages, whereas in other mammals it is often considered a unitary element of the sleep cycle. Instead, REM, which is also called paradoxical sleep or dreaming sleep, is characterized by an EEG activation which resembles that occurring during waking, that is, low-amplitude and fast-frequency waves in the cortex. There are episodic bursts of rapid eye movements, and a substantially reduced level of the muscle tone. REM is present in most mammals and occurs in a cyclic manner following a given period of non-REM. It has been suggested that REM represents a distinct, third behavioural state of the mammalian organism, in addition to waking and non-REM sleep (Jones, 1991). Because of its particular configuration within the sleep period, the recent phylogenetic origin and the association with dreams, REM has attracted much attention from scientists who, after its discovery in the late 1950s, have studied both its function under physiological or pathological conditions and basic mechanisms underlying its generation (Jouvet, 1972; Steriade and McCarley, 1990).

7.2.2   The importance of chemical neurotransmission

The seminal work of Jouvet in the 1960s introduced the concept that sleep and waking may be regulated by specific transmitters contained within neuronal systems with widespread projections throughout the brain. The identification of serotonin-containing neurones in the raphe nuclei of the brainstem together with the knowledge that the caudal brainstem is involved in the neural mechanisms of slow-wave sleep, suggested the possibility that serotonin is a chemical transmitter implicated in the process of sleep. Subsequent findings cast some doubt on this early hypothesis and more recent critical re-examination suggests a non-essential but permissive role of serotonin in the modulation of slow-wave sleep. The discovery that several types of serotonin receptors exist in the brain and periphery has made it possible to identify the serotonin-2 ($5HT_2$) type as having a prevailing importance in the control of sleep mechanisms (Dugovic et al., 1989b).

In contrast to serotonin are the catecholamines, noradrenaline and DA, which appear to be involved in the generation of arousal and wakefulness. Pharmacological studies have shown that treatment with a variety of drugs which act on noradrenergic and DAergic pathways can produce intense arousal and prolonged wakefulness (Jouvet, 1972; Wauquier *et al.*, 1985; Nicholson and Pascoe, 1990). Thus, the administration of amphetamine-like drugs which are known to act by releasing both noradrenaline and DA in the brain, or l-DOPA, which enhances the formation of DA, will increase wakefulness, alertness and exploratory activity and secondarily suppress sleep. Conversely, reduction of synthesis or synaptic concentrations of catecholamines by drugs such as α-methyl-*p*-tyrosine or reserpine will lead to a reduction of arousal and wakefulness (Ongini and Longo, 1989).

Histochemical studies have demonstrated that both noradrenaline- and DA-containing neurones are located in regions of the brainstem reticular formation that are traditionally considered to be important to the generation of arousal (Jouvet, 1972; Jones, 1991). In turn, the ascending projections of these neuronal populations innervate other brain areas that are also critical for maintenance arousal and wakefulness (Steriade and McCarley, 1990). Collectively these findings, together with other studies utilizing specific lesion techniques of discrete brain areas, have provided evidence that both noradrenaline and DA neurones are important for the behavioural arousal and EEG activation of wakefulness.

The acetylcholine neurones which are widely distributed in the brain are also important in wakefulness and EEG activation. These functional characteristics have been deduced mainly from studies of drugs that mimic, accentuate or block the actions of acetylcholine on muscarinic receptors. Administration of physostigmine produces EEG arousal whereas atropine has the opposite effect. The relationship between this response and behaviour is confusing, however, for the EEG changes produced by stimulation of cholinergic pathways are the same as those produced by amphetamine, whereas the behavioural effects are not.

A separate comment has to be devoted to the biochemical mechanisms which underlie the occurrence and maintenance of REM sleep. A variety of findings obtained over the last 30 years clearly suggest that this state of sleep is regulated differently as compared with non-REM and wakefulness. Most findings converge in supporting a critical role of acetylcholine-containing neurones (Jouvet, 1972; Shiromani *et al.*, 1987; Jones, 1991). Pharmacological studies show that administration of cholinergic agonists or anticholinesterase agents decreases the latency and increases the duration of REM sleep episodes in both animals and man. Conversely, scopolamine and atropine block normal and cholinomimetic-induced REM sleep. In addition to the numerous pharmacological studies which implicate cholinergic mechanisms in REM sleep generation, during the past 10 years important advances have been made in identifying the cholinergic neurones histochemically (Jones, 1991). As a result, there is considerable evidence indicating that cholinergic-containing neurones in the pontine reticular formation play an important role in regulating some tonic and phasic components of REM sleep.

In turn, the activity of acetylcholine appears to be influenced by the monoaminergic system. Early pharmacological studies by Karczmar *et al.* (1970) led the way to a series of studies which allow the possibility of a model of reciprocal interaction between cholinergic and monoaminergic systems. Thus, the generation of REM appears to depend upon the activity of cholinergic neurones which are inhibited by noradrenergic and serotoninergic cells (Hobson *et al.*, 1986; Jones, 1991).

The evidence concerning a dominant role of acetylcholine and noradrenaline-containing neurones in the generation of REM sleep is strong but not conclusive. Other neurotransmitters including DA, γ-aminobutyric acid (GABA) or peptides may be implicated in the modulation of neuronal systems involved in state control (Monti, 1983; Jones, 1991). Indeed, the concept that highly localized brain centres are involved in sleep regulation has been radically revised and replaced by the more modern view that multiple neuronal populations regulate sleep states (Hobson *et al.*, 1986; Shiromani *et al.*, 1987; Steriade and McCarley, 1990). Likewise, no single neurotransmitter or neuromodulator has been identified that is essential for the generation and maintenance of sleep and waking. On the contrary, multiple factors and systems are involved in the onset and maintenance of these states.

7.3 Stimulation of dopamine receptors

Typically, drugs which stimulate DA receptors produce arousal and reduce the time spent in sleep states, including REM (Monti, 1983; Nicholson *et al.*, 1989; Ongini and Longo, 1989). For example, the DA precursor l-DOPA enhances arousal (Ongini *et al.*, 1987) and reduces the amount of REM sleep in animals and man (Gillin *et al.*, 1973; Monti, 1983). However, most of the drugs used lead to the activation of both DA receptor subtypes. Only recently, with the discovery of selective pharmacological agents for the D_1 receptor (Iorio *et al.*, 1983), have the differential effects of agonists for either D_1 or D_2 receptors been examined (Waddington and O'Boyle, 1989).

7.3.1 Stimulation of D_1 receptors

The drug SK & F 38393, a partial agonist for D_1 receptors, has been widely used as it is the only experimental tool available for elucidating biological responses to D_1 receptor stimulation (Waddington and O'Boyle, 1989). Initially, SK & F 38393 was considered to have little or no CNS effect, but was later found to induce characteristic responses such as episodes of grooming in the absence of typical stereotyped behaviour (see Chapter 3). The occurrence of grooming is necessarily associated with a certain level of arousal. In studying specifically the latter effect, the D_1 agonist was found to induce a clear EEG activation and behavioural arousal in rats and rabbits (Ongini *et al.*, 1985). Consistent with these data, in the rat SK & F 38393 produces a dose-related increase of the duration of wakefulness at the expense of the time spent in sleep (Monti *et al.*, 1990; Trampus *et al.*, 1991). Of relevance is the marked potency of the drug in suppressing REM sleep, an effect which is apparent at a dose three-fold lower than that effective in producing grooming (Trampus *et al.*, 1991). In these studies, it is, however, difficult to establish whether suppression of REM is a direct consequence of the stimulation of D_1 receptors or whether it is secondary to an increase of wakefulness.

Considering that EEG activation induced by SK & F 38393 occurs in the absence of other more typical stereotyped behaviours, these findings indicate that arousal is an important physiological effect of the stimulation of D_1 receptors. However, a limitation of the pharmacological studies conducted with SK & F 38393 is that the drug has only a partial agonist activity in terms of efficacy in stimulating adenylyl cyclase relative to DA itself. More recent studies on other compounds having full efficacy at D_1 receptors, such as the drug A68930, have confirmed that grooming but not stereotyped behaviour is a consistent response to all the agonists examined (Daly and Waddington, 1992). Moreover, in agreement with previous data, A68930 was found to enhance waking and markedly reduce REM over a low dose range (Trampus *et al.*, 1993).

Collectively, the data available indicate that arousal and wakefulness are prominent responses to the selective stimulation of D_1 receptors. It is therefore suggested that the D_1 receptors are involved in the modulation of the state of waking.

7.3.2 Stimulation of D_2 receptors

Apomorphine and some ergot alkaloids, bromocriptine, pergolide and lisuride, all produce behavioural stimulation such as stereotyped movements and hyperactivity (Joyce, 1983). None of these drugs interacts selectively with the D_2 receptors. For example, apomorphine has equal affinity for both D_1 and D_2 receptors, even though its effects have often been interpreted as the outcome of interactions with D_2 receptors only, whereas the ergot alkaloids have affinity for D_1 and other receptors as well. Moreover, in addition to stimulating DA receptors located postsynaptically, these drugs also interact with the presynaptic DA receptors which are of the D_2 type (Carlsson, 1988).

The discovery of quinpirole (LY 171555), a drug which interacts selectively with D_2 receptors, has allowed investigators to study more precisely the functional response to D_2 receptor stimulation (Stoof and Kebabian, 1984). In the rabbit, quinpirole produces a dose-related EEG activation and a variety of stimulatory behaviours (Ongini and Caporali, 1987). In the rat, quinpirole induces activation of the EEG, associated with a variety of repetitive movements and hyperactivity (Kropf and Kuschinsky, 1991), and increases the duration of waking (Monti *et al.*, 1989). At low doses, however, the drug has the opposite effect, that is, it increases duration of total sleep and induces the typical large-amplitude low-frequency waves in the EEG associated with sedation (Monti *et al.*, 1989; Kropf and Kuschinksy, 1991).

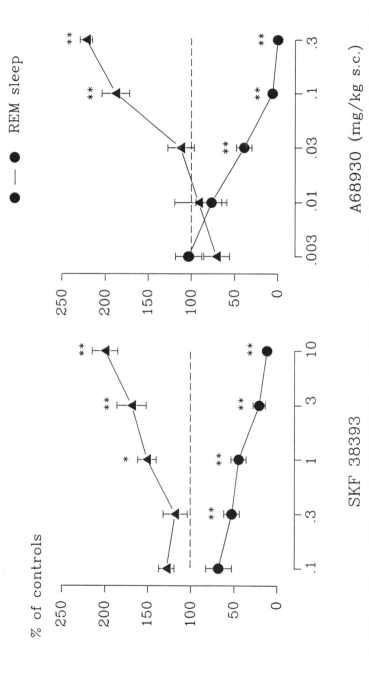

Figure 1 Effects of the partial D$_1$ agonist SK & F 38393 and the full D$_1$ agonist A 68930 on sleep–waking states in the rat. Both drugs increased curation of wakefulness (▲——▲) and reduced the amount of REM sleep (●——●). Data refer to 6-h analysis. Modified from Trampus *et al.* (1991, 1993).

Biphasic responses often occur following the administration of other drugs which interact with D_2 receptors, although with lesser selectivity than quinpirole. For example, it is known that apomorphine, when administered at low doses, induces sedation and increases total sleep in the rat (Bagetta *et al.*, 1988; Monti *et al.*, 1988; Kropf *et al.*, 1989). This apparent paradoxical effect has been explained by considering that low doses of such agonists activate only D_2 receptors located presynaptically (Bagetta *et al.*, 1988). This would lead to a reduced synthesis and release of DA, and ultimately to a decrease of the DA tone at postsynaptic sites (Carlsson, 1988). Thus, the final outcome is a series of responses, such as sedation and hypomotility, which are typically associated with the reduction of DA-mediated neurotransmission.

Further support for this interpretation comes from data obtained with drugs which have a certain degree of selectivity for presynaptic D_2 receptors. Talipexole (B-HT 920), a drug which interacts preferentially with the presynaptic D_2 receptors, has been found to produce behavioural and EEG signs of sedation (Kropf and Kuschinsky, 1991). Conversely, there are antagonists at presynaptic receptors which, by increasing release of DA, lead to activation of postsynaptic receptors and therefore produce behavioural stimulation and wakefulness (Svensson *et al.*, 1987).

The overall data therefore suggest that the D_2 receptor agonists can lead to either sleep or waking, depending on whether presynaptic or postsynaptic receptors are preferentially activated. With the stimulation of D_2 receptors located presynaptically, there is a reduction of the DA tone at both D_1 and D_2 postsynaptic receptor sites. Thus, ultimately, either receptor may well be involved in the modulation of sedation and sleep induced by interacting with presynaptic D_2 receptors. On the other hand, arousal induced by high doses of a D_2 agonist occurs concomitantly with a variety of repetitive motor behaviours. It is therefore difficult to distinguish whether or not EEG arousal and wakefulness depend directly on D_2 receptor stimulation. Indeed, these states may occur as a consequence of the excitation that accompanies motor and stereotyped responses. In general, it appears that the evidence in support of a role for D_2 postsynaptic receptors in the modulation of sleep–arousal processes is not convincing, whereas it is clear that this DA receptor type mediates various features of motor behaviour.

7.3.3   Interaction between D_1 and D_2 receptor agonists

It is an established fact that a functional interaction exists between the two DA receptors in the CNS (Chapter 3). Thus, the D_1 agonist SK & F 38393, which by itself has little behavioural effect, produces a variety of marked actions that are more additive when it is co-administered with D_2 agonists. These include DA responses such as increased locomotion, contralateral rotation, oral dyskinesia, chewing or elevated firing of DA neurones (Waddington and O'Boyle,

1989). There are no data available showing whether similar synergistic effects also occur on EEG activity and sleep–wake patterns. In the absence of such direct evidence, some conclusions can be drawn by examining the effects of non-selective agonists. The prototypic compound apomorphine, given at doses interacting with both D_1 and D_2 postsynaptic receptors, produces a variety of stimulatory behaviours that are more compulsive than those induced by other more selective D_2 agonists (Joyce, 1983; Waddington and O'Boyle, 1989). Additionally, the drug activates the EEG and enhances wakefulness at the expense of sleep stages (Ongini and Caporali, 1987; Monti et al., 1988; Kropf et al., 1989). The enhancement of wakefulness, as well as EEG activation, appears to be similar to that induced by other more selective compounds such as the D_1 agonist SK & F 38393 and the D_2 agonist quinpirole. However, these apomorphine effects are fully antagonized by the D_1 receptor blocker SCH 23390, but are weakly influenced by the D_2 receptor agonist (−)-sulpiride (Ongini and Caporali, 1987). Thus, like other behavioural responses, EEG activation and waking induced by apomorphine appear to depend upon D_1 receptor tone. Similarly, EEG arousal induced by l-DOPA is highly sensitive to blockade of D_1 receptors (Ongini et al., 1987). These findings support the view that D_1 receptors have a role in mediating EEG effects and waking state. These results also imply that D_1 and D_2 receptors function in an interactive manner since blockade of one receptor prevents the expression of the other's response. In view of the results of experiments conducted under a variety of conditions it seems possible that a synergism between D_1 and D_2 agonists may also exist for EEG arousal.

7.4   Blockade of dopamine receptors

There is evidence that blockade of DA-mediated neurotransmission by neuroleptics tends to produce sedation and reduce arousal response to sensory stimuli in both animals and man (Longo, 1978; Baldessarini, 1990; Deniker, 1990). Following the discovery of two types of DA receptors, D_1 and D_2, several studies have shown that neuroleptics commonly used in therapy either block both receptor sites or have a preferential affinity for D_2 receptors (Carlsson, 1988; Seeman, 1990). Moreover, most of them also interact with other receptor systems, such as serotonin (in particular $5HT_2$) α-adrenergic, histamine-1 and acetylcholine receptors (Peroutka and Snyder, 1980; Meltzer et al., 1989; Seeman, 1990). These observations have encouraged the search for new compounds possessing more selectivity for either the D_2 or the D_1 receptor. The efforts made have culminated in the identification of D_1 receptor antagonists (Iorio et al., 1983; Chipkin et al., 1988; Andersen et al., 1992) and substituted benzamides possessing a high degree of selectivity for D_2 receptors (Lewander et al., 1990).

7.4.1   Effects of D_1 receptor blockers

Most of the information available relies on the many studies performed on the prototype drug, the benzazepine SCH 23390. Like other neuroleptics, SCH 23390 is particularly active in suppressing conditioned avoidance responses in the rat, where the drug is effective at low doses, i.e. 0.01 mg/kg s.c. (Iorio *et al.*, 1983). At an even lower dose, SCH 23390 was found to enhance the duration of total sleep, including both non-REM and REM (Figure 2) (Trampus and Ongini, 1990). Using a higher dose range, Monti *et al.* (1990) have shown that SCH 23390 increases slow-wave sleep (in our studies, light sleep and slow-wave sleep are considered together as non-REM sleep). Other studies involving quantitative analysis of the EEG have shown that the drug enhances activity over the low-frequency range, an effect usually associated with sedation and sleep (Kropf *et al.*, 1989). Studies performed in other animal species indicate that the drug has the tendency to produce sedation. In the cebus monkey, Coffin *et al.* (1989) have observed the occurrence of sedation after once-a-week oral administration of SCH 23390 for a period of approximately 1 year. In the rabbit, the drug induces EEG signs of sedation and attenuates the arousal response to sensory stimuli, even though the effect is less marked than that induced by haloperidol (Bo *et al.*, 1988). It therefore appears that the drug influences markedly the states of sleep at doses which are believed to interact specifically with D_1 receptors.

Two other D_1 antagonists, SCH 39166 and NNC 756, also display some sedative activity. The drug SCH 39166, a benzonaphthazepine derivative of SCH 23390 (Chipkin *et al.*, 1988), which is being studied in clinical trials to assess its activity in schizophrenic patients, slightly increases total sleep, including non-REM and REM, over a low dose range (Ongini *et al.*, 1993). In keeping with these data, other studies have shown that oral administration of SCH 39166 produces sedation in cebus monkeys (Coffin *et al.*, 1992). The other D_1 antagonist, NNC 756 (Andersen *et al.*, 1992), also enhances duration of total sleep and REM at low doses (Ongini *et al.*, 1993).

The overall finding is that blockade of D_1 receptors tends to produce sedative effects in different animal species and enhances the amount of both total sleep and REM in the rat.

In pharmacology it rarely happens that drugs stimulate the generation of REM sleep (Gaillard, 1983; Monti, 1983; Nicholson *et al.*, 1989). Thus, the unique property emerging for D_1 receptor blockers appears to be interesting and worthy of further analysis. The effect on REM is observed with very low doses of the D_1 antagonists. Moreover, SCH 23390 readily prevents the REM-suppressing effects of the D_1 agonist SK & F 38393 (Trampus *et al.*, 1991). Conversely, SCH 23390 is unable to reverse the effect of desipramine, an antidepressant which rapidly suppresses REM in animals and man (Reynolds *et al.*, 1987) and acts through a mechanism involving blockade of noradrenaline uptake (unpublished data). Taken together, these data support the suggestion that the D_1 receptor system is involved in mediating REM changes.

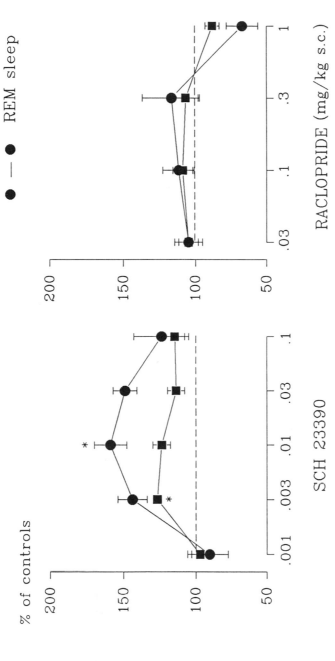

Figure 2 Effects of the D_1 antagonist SCH 23390 and the D_2 antagonist raclopride on sleep–waking states in the rat. SCH 23390 enhanced both total sleep (■——■) and REM sleep (●——●), whereas raclopride had little or no effect on sleep states. Data refer to 6-h analysis. Data on SCH 23390 are taken from Trampus and Ongini (1990).

The way the effect appears is similar for the three D_1 antagonists examined, even though the drugs differ in their potency in promoting REM. Specifically, REM changes are characterized by an increase in the number of episodes whereas the onset of the first episode remains unaltered (Figure 2) (Trampus and Ongini, 1990; Trampus et al., 1991). Moreover, enhancement of REM duration is associated with the concomitant increase of other sleep components which have been grouped as non-REM sleep.

Apparently, changes of REM stage may be viewed as an obvious consequence of the more general action on total sleep. However, this interpretation cannot be applied to the pharmacology of sleep (Nicholson et al., 1989). In fact, it is quite common that drugs which possess hypnotic or sedative properties enhance total sleep without increasing the amount of REM. For example, this is the case for barbiturates, benzodiazepines, sedating antihistamines and also neuroleptics. In contrast, there are antidepressant drugs which selectively reduce REM sleep without affecting other sleep measures (Nicholson et al., 1989). These results and other neurophysiological findings lend support to the notion that REM and non-REM sleep may be unrelated events. Nevertheless, the fact remains that the D_1 receptor blockers enhance both responses concomitantly.

Of the drugs that promote REM sleep, the best-known agents are cholinergic drugs which enhance its duration and markedly anticipate the onset of the first episode (Shiromani et al., 1987). Other drugs which instead interact with noradrenergic-mediated neurotransmission alter REM in a manner similar to D_1 receptor blockers (Monti, 1983; Nicholson et al., 1989). Considering that the interplay between cholinergic and monoaminergic systems appear to underlie the generation of REM (Jouvet, 1972; Jones, 1991), it follows that D_1 receptor systems may well be part of the monoaminergic processes which regulate this sleep state.

In the attempt to understand mechanisms underlying REM sleep, several neurophysiological and neuroanatomical studies have focused on noradrenergic pathways (Jones, 1991), but the D_1 receptor system has not been examined as yet. The availability of potent tools, such as the selective D_1 antagonists with their radiolabelled receptor-ligands and the recently discovered D_1 receptor clone (Civelli et al., 1991), provide the background for further studies devoted to a better understanding of the role played by the D_1 receptor population in the generation of REM.

7.4.2 Effects of D_2 receptor blockers

One of the most widely known antipsychotics, haloperidol, interacts preferentially with D_2 receptors, but also blocks $5HT_2$ and α-adrenergic receptors (Peroutka and Snyder, 1980; Seeman, 1990). Considerations on its pharmacological activity in relation to D_2 receptors are therefore confounded by the possible influences of other receptors.

The only drugs available which display high selectivity for the D_2 receptors are substituted benzamides (Seeman, 1990; Peselow and Stanley, 1982). Individual compounds range from sulpiride, which penetrates the brain weakly, to raclopride, which has pharmacological potency similar to that of haloperidol. A variety of findings suggest that these drugs have the common denominator of having a low potential to induce sedation. Thus, sulpiride, remoxipride and raclopride produce little effect on the EEG activity in the rabbit (Ongini and Caporali, 1987; Bo et al., 1988) and have weak sedative effects or produce minimal changes of sleep states in the rat (Bagetta et al., 1987; Ongini et al., 1993).

In selected clinical studies, sulpiride has been shown to possess effective antipsychotic properties with a spectrum of side-effects similar to that of classic antipsychotics (Peselow and Stanley, 1982). In general, it seems that there is only a low incidence of sedation in patients treated with sulpiride. Similarly, in multicentre clinical studies, Lewander et al. (1990) have demonstrated that remoxipride induces much less sedation than haloperidol. Thus, all these data on benzamides agree with the early notion that sulpiride and related compounds are low-sedative neuroleptics (Deniker, 1990).

In addition to having little or no effect on total sleep in the rat, remoxipride and raclopride do not substantially affect REM sleep (Ongini et al., 1992, 1993). Therefore, the data indicate that selective antagonists for the D_1 or D_2 receptor can be distinguished according to their differential effects on sleep states. While blockade of D_1 receptors leads to sedation and increase of both total sleep and REM, selective blockade of D_2 receptors has no clear-cut effects on such states of behaviour. These findings, together with results discussed previously, support the notion that the D_2 receptor population might not have a function in the modulation of behavioural states of sleep and wakefulness.

7.4.3 Interaction between D_1 and D_2 receptor antagonists

Selective blockade of D_1 receptors produces some behavioural effects, e.g. inhibition of conditioned avoidance response, which are indistinguishable from those induced by D_2 receptor blockers or unselective DA antagonists (Iorio et al., 1983; Barnett, 1986). The results of these studies would suggest that initially distinct mechanisms may ultimately influence the same physiological processes. However, there are other functional responses which appear to occur through independent mechanisms and which clearly distinguish selective D_1 from D_2 antagonists. For example, in rats D_2 antagonists stimulate prolactin secretion and in monkeys, following long-term administration, they produce extra-pyramidal syndrome, responses which are not induced by D_1 antagonists (Barnett, 1986; Coffin et al., 1989, 1992). Conversely, REM sleep is promoted by D_1 antagonists, but not by D_2 antagonists (Ongini et al., 1993).

In interpreting the many intriguing results obtained with selective blockade of either D_1 or D_2 receptors, it has been postulated that some common responses depend on the functional interaction between both receptor types, in a manner which remains to be clarified. Indeed, there are data showing that synergy exists between D_1 and D_2 antagonists in the induction of some typical effects such as catalepsy or inhibition of DA-mediated motor activity (Dall'Olio *et al.*, 1989; Parashos *et al.*, 1989). In parallel with the data obtained in behavioural studies, Bo *et al.* (1988) have shown that EEG synchronization, an electrophysiological marker of sedation, is more marked when SCH 23390 and raclopride are administered in combination at doses which on their own have little or no effect.

These findings are not surprising since neuroleptics which interact with both D_1 and D_2 receptors, such as the phenothiazines, display sedative properties and favour sleep in animals and man (Longo, 1978; Fornal *et al.*, 1982; Roubicek, 1980; Baldessarini, 1990). Moreover, except for chlorpromazine, neuroleptics either do not change REM or tend to reduce it. However, the data relating to currently used neuroleptics, which exert non-selective blockade of both DA receptor types, are confounded by other concomitant interactions occurring with $5HT_2$ or α-adrenergic receptors, which also have a role in mediating sedation and sleep. For example, the effect on REM of chlorpromazine has been attributed to its interaction with α-adrenergic receptors (Gaillard, 1983). Therefore, there are some indications that blockade of one of the two DA receptor types may influence the expression of the other as regards the behavioural states of sleep and waking. However, before a firm conclusion can be drawn, other experiments have to be performed to clarify the issue.

7.5   Dopamine and other neurotransmitters

7.5.1   More than two dopamine receptors

The D_1/D_2 receptor classification is widely accepted. Thus, these receptors can be differentiated on the basis of biochemical, physiological and pharmacological studies (Stoof and Kebabian, 1984). However, several findings obtained with agonists and antagonists for DA receptors are difficult to explain with the existence of only two DA receptor types. Over the last few years, the advances made in molecular biology have allowed the cloning of several receptors belonging to the superfamily of G protein-coupled receptors. So far, five types of DA receptor have been described, but it is likely that other receptor types will emerge in the future (Givelli *et al.*, 1991; Sibley and Monsma, 1992). Despite differences in the amino acid sequence or coupling with stimulation of adenylyl cyclase the DA receptor types can still be grouped as D_1/D_5 and $D_2/D_3/D_4$ on the basis of binding affinities for several DA agonists and antagonists (Civelli *et al.*, 1991; Sunahara *et al.*, 1991). There are additional variations, however. For example, like the classic D_1 receptor type, D_5 is linked to stimulation of adenylyl cyclase, whereas the existence of a D_1-like receptor which is not linked to adenylyl cyclase has emerged from a series of biochemical studies (Andersen *et al.*, 1990).

Despite the discoveries that have been made, little is known of the functional role of each receptor type and the major pharmacological properties of DAergic agents are still attributed to preferential interactions with either the D_1 or the D_2 receptor.

From an examination of the effects of partial and full D_1 receptor agonists, it seems clear that the grooming response is unrelated to their efficacy in stimulating adenylyl cyclase (Daly and Waddington, 1991; Trampus *et al.*, 1993). Likewise, when the two different D_1 agonists SK & F 38393 and A 68930 are compared for their ability to induce arousal and reduce REM sleep, it emerges that the two compounds induce effects that are qualitatively similar (Figure 1). Therefore, according to the results, functional responses to the different D_1 agonists available appear to depend only on the activation of the classic D_1 receptor.

Also, the results obtained with the D_2-selective agonist quinpirole need to be re-evaluated in the light of the compound's greater affinity for the D_3 receptor type (Civelli *et al.*, 1991). However, this profile of activity does not help towards a better understanding of the specific role of each receptor type in the modulation of arousal. In fact, such drug effects are confounded by the concomitant activation of other motor behaviours.

Theoretically, the existence of different DA receptor types should help to clarify the different pharmacological properties of the antipsychotic agents, in particular of the so-called atypical drugs. However, most of these drugs exert actions on receptors different from DA and this makes it difficult to determine the function of the newly discovered DA receptor subtypes. For example, the effects of clozapine on sleep can not be solely attributed to its preferential interaction with the putative D_4 receptor because the drug also has anticholinergic properties and it interacts with other receptors (Seeman, 1990).

There are, however, differential data on the new D_1 antagonists which can be interpreted by considering possible interactions with other DA receptor types, e.g. D_4 or D_5. In fact, the three D_1 receptor blockers previously discussed have equal D_1-receptor selectivity, but the drug SCH 39166 is less effective in promoting REM sleep (Ongini *et al.*, 1993). This finding leads us to postulate that other mechanisms, yet to be explored, might be involved for SCH 39166.

Therefore, in the absence of new compounds which possess a significant selectivity for each of the newly discovered DA receptor types, it appears that their respective functional response remains unclarified.

7.5.2 Acetylcholine

There is known to be a relationship between DA-mediated neurotransmission and muscarinic cholinergic mechanisms in the striatal neurones. Stimulation of postsynaptic DA neurones by non-selective drugs such as l-DOPA selective D_2 agonists leads to inhibition of acetylcholine release, whereas blockade of D_2 receptors increases it. In contrast, D_1 receptors appear to play little or no part in regulating acetylcholine release, but there are contradictory findings in the literature (Waddington and O'Boyle, 1989). For example, in some studies it has been shown that D_1-selective drugs interact with acetylcholine mechanisms in a manner opposite to that of D_2-selective agents (Consolo et al., 1987; Bertozelli and Consolo, 1990).

Recently, the results of biochemical studies supporting the hypothesis that D_1 receptors are involved in the regulation of acetylcholine release have been confirmed by a variety of behavioural studies. Iorio et al. (1991) have demonstrated that the anticholinergic drugs atropine and scopolamine potentiate the effects of D_1 but not of D_2 antagonists in the conditioned avoidance response model. It has also been suggested that the cholinergic system may be involved in arousal induced by the D_1 agonist SK & F 38393, whose effects are blocked by atropine (Horita et al., 1991). Conversely, under the same experimental conditions, no interaction is observed between the D_2 agonist quinpirole and atropine. Also, studies concerning convulsions, which can be considered at the upper end of the spectrum of excitatory events, are consistent with the view that D_1 and D_2 receptors interact differently with cholinergic mechanisms (Chapter 9). For example, convulsions induced by the cholinergic agonist pilocarpine are facilitated by SK & F 38393 and prevented by the D_1 receptor blocker SCH 23390. In the same model, D_2-selective agents display opposite effects (Al-Tajir et al., 1990; Barone et al., 1991).

Thus, according to recent findings, D_1 receptors can be distinguished from D_2 receptors in the way they modulate functional responses which involve cholinergic mechanisms. In view of the role of acetylcholine in regulating states of sleep and waking, it may well be that D_1 receptors exert some influence on cholinergic neurones in regulating forms of behaviour such as arousal. Other studies may lead to a better understanding of this issue. Certainly it is of interest to determine through direct approaches whether the $D_1 : D_2$ interaction also occurs in the regulation of responses in which acetylcholine is implicated.

7.5.3   Serotonin (5HT) receptors

The drug SCH 23390 blocks the D_1 receptor with about 900-fold selectivity compared with the D_2 receptor, but it retains a substantial affinity for the $5HT_2$ receptor subtype (Chipkin et al., 1988). This is also true for a series of analogues of SCH 23390, all having in common the benzazepine moiety, for which McQuade et al. (1988) have found a strong correlation between the affinities for the D_1 and the serotonin receptors.

Several other neuroleptics have elevated affinity for $5HT_2$ receptors and there is currently a debate as to the role of 5HT in both the pathophysiology of schizophrenia and the mechanism of action of antipsychotic agents (Meltzer et al., 1989). Apart from this, it is an established notion that 5HT is involved in mediating the states of sleep–wakefulness, especially of the slow-wave sleep component (Jouvet, 1972). More recent work has attributed an important function to the $5HT_2$ receptor subtype (Dugovic *et al.*, 1989b). Thus, risperidone, a new antipsychotic drug which interacts with both D_2 and $5HT_2$ receptors, dose-dependently increases the amount of slow-wave sleep in the rat (Dugovic *et al.*, 1989). Ritanserin, a selective $5HT_2$ antagonist, produces slow-wave sleep in animals and humans, whereas the respective agonists DOM (1-(2,5-dimethoxy-4-methylphenyl)-2-aminopropane) and DOI (1-(2,5-dimethoxy-4-iodophenyl)-2-aminopropane) enhance wakefulness in the rat (Dugovic *et al.*, 1989b; Monti *et al.*, 1990). However, independent of whether the $5HT_2$ receptors are stimulated or antagonized, the net result on REM sleep is a reduction of its amount.

With this background, the property of SCH 23390 of inducing sedation and enhancing total sleep may be in part attributed to its interaction with the $5HT_2$ receptor. Conversely, there is no support for a role of $5HT_2$ receptors in the modulation of REM sleep by SCH 23390. There are additional findings which strengthen the latter concept. In studies with SCH 23390 and the $5HT_2$ agonist DOI, Monti *et al.* (1990) have found that the two drugs display interaction for slow-wave sleep but not for REM. In our laboratory we performed experiments using the selective $5HT_2$ antagonist ketanserin (0.1 and 1 mg/kg, s.c.) and SCH 39166. This D_1 receptor blocker is particularly interesting because *in vitro* it has a relatively low affinity for $5HT_2$ receptors (about 90-fold separation versus D_1 (Chipkin *et al.*, 1988) but *in vivo* it appears not to interact with $5HT_2$ (about 1000-fold separation) (McQuade *et al.*, 1991). Using a threshold dose of SCH 39166 (0.03 mg/kg, s.c.) we expected to have interactions with ketanserin but we found that REM remains unaltered whereas non-REM sleep increases (unpublished results). Thus, these data, too, lend support to the suggestion that the $5HT_2$ receptor system may facilitate the sedative properties of D_1 receptor blockers but does not underlie their effects on REM sleep.

7.6   Discussion

The intense research interest stimulated by the discovery of selective agents for the D_1 receptor has provided important information on the role of one or other of the two DA receptor types. One area of interest regards the function of DA receptors in the regulation of states of the behaviour, ranging from arousal to sleep. The results of the studies generated over the past years have made it possible to draw some conclusions on the differential profile of D_1 versus D_2-selective drugs.

It is, however, difficult to establish which specific neural mechanism underlies the different responses to activation or blockade of the D_1 and D_2 receptors. Studies on the anatomical distribution of the two DA receptors in the animal and human brain indicate that D_1 and D_2 receptors are often concentrated in the same areas of the CNS (Cortés *et al.*, 1989). Moreover, there appears to be a low density of the D_1 (and D_2) receptor in brain regions, such as the brainstem, which are known to play an important part in the control of states of sleep and arousal (Steriade and McCarley, 1990), but no specific studies have been performed. Traditionally, most of the investigations have been devoted to understanding the link between function and anatomical localization of other neurotransmitters, such as noradrenaline and acetylcholine (Jones, 1991), whose effects on sleep and waking has been established since the early work of Jouvet (1972). With the availability of tools such as the D_1 receptor clone, it is likely that more information will become available.

7.6.1 D_1 versus D_2 agonists

The most evident effects of representative D_1 and D_2 agonists on sleep and waking are outlined in Table 1. As shown, the major finding is that the selective D_1 agonists examined produce arousal at the expense of sleep stages, especially REM. This is consistent with the response obtained with a variety of drugs which stimulate the DAergic system. Thus, the data further support the notion that DA is involved in mechanisms underlying arousal. There are, however, additional aspects which are worthy of further discussion.

Several studies with D_1 agonists have demonstrated that these drugs produce neither stereotyped behaviours nor hyperactivity, but promote a limited number of motor responses, such as grooming in the rat (Waddington and O'Boyle, 1989; Trampus et al., 1993). Grooming induced by D_1 agonists has been widely studied and has certainly led to a better understanding of the functional interaction between D_1 and D_2 receptors (Waddington and O'Boyle, 1989). It must be underlined, however, that although this effect is evident in the rat, a better insight into the function of D_1 receptors can only be achieved with the identification of behavioural responses which are present in a wide range of laboratory animals and are also part of human behaviour. In this regard, drug effects on sleep and waking are often found to be consistent across various animal species, including humans. This holds true for drugs interacting with DA-mediated neurotransmission since its stimulation or blockade leads to arousal or sleep in a variety of animal species (Longo, 1978; Wauquier et al., 1985). In view of this, it may be inferred that D_1 agonists are likely to stimulate wakefulness and reduce REM also in humans. With the clinical development of new D_1 agonists, this pharmacological profile will certainly be clarified.

In contrast to D_1 agonists, compounds which interact both selectively and non-selectively with D_2 receptors produce, in addition to arousal, a variety of stereotyped behaviours and hyperactivity (Joyce, 1983). It is therefore difficult to establish whether D_2 receptor-mediated neurotransmission is also directly involved in mechanisms underlying arousal. It remains the case, however, that activation of arousal and wakefulness is a common response to the stimulation of either one of the two receptors. But the overall results lead to the suggestion that the D_1 receptors have a prominent role in the regulation of arousal (Ongini and Longo, 1989). A specific feature which characterizes D_2 agonists, but not

Table 1 Effects on states of sleep and waking produced by selective stimulation of D_1 and D_2 receptors.

Receptor type	Wakefulness/arousal	Total sleep	REM sleep	Prominent behaviour
D_1	Increase	Reduction	Marked reduction	Grooming
D_2	Increase	Reduction	Reduction	Hyperactivity/stereotyped responses
D_2 (presynaptic)	Reduction	Increase	Little or no change	Hypomotility/sedation
D_1 and D_2*	Increase	Reduction	Reduction	Marked stereotypy/hyperactivity

All data obtained from the rat.
* Studies conducted with the reference non-selective DA agonist apomorphine.

D_1 agonists, is their ability to produce biphasic responses on sleep and waking (Bagetta *et al.*, 1988; Monti *et al.*, 1989; Kropf and Kuschinsky, 1991). The activation of presynaptic D_2 receptors by low doses of selective and non-selective D_2 agonists, which leads to a reduction of DA synthesis and release (Carlsson, 1988), appears to be responsible for the final behavioural outcome, namely sedation and hypomotility. This finding strengthens the view that the DA tone at synapses, with the consequent stimulation of postsynaptic D_1 and D_2 receptor sites, is critical for the generation of arousal.

7.6.2 D_1 versus D_2 antagonists

As shown in Table 2, there are differences between D_1 and D_2 antagonists with regard to their effects on sleep and waking. In particular, D_1 antagonists, but not D_2, increase the duration of total sleep, including the amount of REM. This is a remarkable finding in view of the many studies showing that selective D_1 antagonists reproduce the action of D_2 antagonists in most experimental paradigms (Iorio *et al.*, 1983; Chipkin *et al.*, 1988; Waddington and O'Boyle, 1989).

One of the effects, namely sedation and increase of total sleep by D_1 antagonists, may also depend on interactions with serotoninergic ($5HT_2$) mechanisms (McQuade *et al.*, 1988), which are known to have an important role in the regulation of slow-wave sleep (Jouvet, 1972; Dugovic *et al.*, 1989b). Conversely, selective D_2 antagonists, such as substituted benzamides, produce little or no sedation and do not change sleep stages. Other DA antagonists, such as clozapine, haloperidol and chlorpromazine, tend to produce sedation, but their effects have been interpreted mostly as a consequence of interactions with neurotransmitters different from DA (Peroutka and Snyder, 1980; Baldessarini, 1990; Seeman, 1990). Although many different neurochemical systems ultimately produce the same effect, the data sustain the conclusions that the selective blockade of D_1 receptors by itself is involved in inducing sedation and changes of the sleep state. For example, the D_1 antagonist SCH 39166 does not interact with $5HT_2$ receptors (McQuade *et al.*, 1991) but retains effects on sleep stages (Ongini *et al.*, 1993) and induces sedation in monkeys (Coffin *et al.*, 1992). Therefore, the results suggest that selective D_1 antagonists appear to have a prominent role compared with D_2 antagonists in influencing mechanisms underlying the behavioural states of sedation and sleep.

The other finding that only D_1, but not D_2, antagonists enhances REM sleep is rather uncommon. In general, with very few exceptions, DA antagonists neither change nor reduce REM sleep in animals and man (Baldessarini, 1990). An increase in the amount of REM has been observed with drugs such as chlorpromazine, but it has been attributed to interactions with α-adrenergic receptors rather than DA receptors (Gaillard, 1983). Thus, the results of studies in the rat support the suggestion that only the D_1 receptor is involved in the

Table 2 Effects on states of sleep and waking produced by selective blockade of D_1 and D_2 receptors.

Receptor type	Wakefulness/arousal	Total sleep	REM sleep	Prominent behaviour
D_1	Reduction	Increase	Increase	Hypomotility/sedation
D_2	Little or no change	Little or no change	No change	Hypomotility
D_1 and D_2*	Reduction	Increase	No change	Hypomotility/sedation

All of the data have been obtained in the rat.

* Studies conducted with non-selective DA antagonists, such as haloperidol or phenothiazine neuroleptics. It is worth noting that these drugs also interact with other non-DAergic receptor systems.

modulation of REM sleep. This is an unexpected finding when one considers that theories on REM mechanisms are based on models of reciprocal influence between monoaminergic, mostly noradrenaline, and cholinergic neuronal populations (Hobson et al., 1986; Jones, 1991). Regarding the way REM is enhanced by D_1 antagonists, it seems that D_1 receptors may be part of the monoaminergic system which is inhibitory to cholinergic mechanisms. This speculation could be a stimulus to further neurophysiological and anatomical studies which will make it possible to explore the function of D_1 receptors within the established neurochemistry of REM sleep.

In the attempt to relate the effects on REM to other aspects of the complex behavioural effects of D_1 and D_2 blockers, differences and similarities between the two drug classes have been critically reviewed. One effect which appears to be intriguing is the ability of D_1 antagonists to protect animals from chemically induced convulsions, which contrasts with the propensity of D_2 antagonists to facilitate convulsions in experimental models and epileptic patients (Al-Tajir et al., 1990; Baldessarini, 1990; Barone et al., 1991). This peculiar effect may be in part related to the D_1-mediated effect on REM. A strong basis for this association is provided by a variety of data showing that during REM sleep there is a protection against seizures in animals and man (Shouse et al., 1989). Thus, considering that D_1 antagonists have the ability to both suppress some forms of seizures and enhance REM in the rat, it is plausible to suggest that the two effects may occur through a common mechanism. Certainly, specific studies are needed in order to establish whether this hypothesis holds true.

From the studies available it seems that the D_1 receptor system is involved in the modulation of the arousal–sedation continuum, including REM sleep mechanisms. Thus, the two DA receptors can be clearly distinguished by their role on the modulation of the states of sleep and waking. Functional interactions between the D_1 and D_2 receptor systems can become operative for some effects, e.g. sedation induced by the concomitant blockade of both D_1 and D_2 receptors. But a firm conclusion concerning the effect of $D_1:D_2$ interactions on these functional responses is still to be drawn.

7.6.3 Clinical implications

While the clinical effects of selective D_2 agents have been investigated, the clinical potential of selective D_1 drugs remains to be established. There is now a considerable interest in the utility of D_1 agonists for the treatment of Parkinson's disease. On the basis of the results in animal models it is expected that these drugs will also induce arousal or enhance wakefulness in patients. In this regard, effects should be similar to those produced by l-DOPA since this drug also induces arousal in animals with a mechanism depending on the D_1 receptor tone (Ongini et al., 1987). Thus, irrespective of the effectiveness of a D_1 agonist in Parkinsonian patients, the arousing effects should be similar to that occurring with the currently used therapy.

Recently, studies conducted in animal models have led to the suggestion that D_1 receptor agonists may also have potential in the therapy of depression (Serra et al., 1990). The rationale for this approach is provided by studies suggesting that DA receptors, in particular the D_1 receptors, are involved in the mechanism of action of antidepressants (Serra et al., 1990). Moreover, there is evidence that all the antidepressants have the ability to reduce the amount of REM sleep both in animals and man, an effect which appears to be critical for the action of this class of therapeutic agents (Gillin and Borbély, 1985; Reynolds et al., 1987). In view of this, it is noteworthy that the two D_1 agonists examined potently suppress REM in the rat (Figure 1). The overall results with D_1 agonists therefore suggest that depression can be another area of therapy that merits investigation when the drugs are available for clinical studies.

As for D_1 antagonists, during 1993 the results of clinical studies on SCH 39166 will make it possible to understand whether selective blockade of D_1-mediated neurotransmission offers advantages over D_2 receptor blockers, or other less selective DA antagonists, in the treatment of psychosis. Additionally, it will become apparent whether D_1 antagonists possess a much lesser propensity to induce extrapyramidal motor symptoms than other DA antagonists, as suggested by the results of animal studies (Coffin et al., 1989, 1992). On the basis of the results discussed in this chapter, it is also expected that SCH 39166 will produce some degree of drowsiness in man. The overall effect of D_1 antagonists appears to be similar to that induced by haloperidol in the rat and monkey (Ongini et al., 1993; Coffin et al., 1989, 1992) but less so in the rabbit (Bo et al., 1988). Considering that haloperidol has an intermediate potency in inducing sedation in man (Baldessarini, 1990; Deniker, 1990), it is expected that D_1 antagonists, like most neuroleptics, will also produce a moderate level of sedation in patients.

But more interesting are the effects of D_1 antagonists on REM sleep. If this finding is confirmed in man, it will certainly stimulate further progress, in addition to an interesting debate, on the relationship between REM sleep and schizophrenia (Weiler et al., 1990; Tandon et al., 1992). Sleep alterations are often associated with psychiatric disorders (Reynolds et al., 1987). In particular, there is evidence that disturbances of REM sleep represent an important feature in depressive patients and the rapid suppression of REM appears to be critical for successful response to antidepressant treatments (Gillin and Borbély, 1985; Reynolds et al., 1987). With regard to schizophrenia, several studies have been done to identify whether specific REM sleep changes are associated with the disease, but a firm conclusion has not been drawn (Weiler et al., 1990; Tandon et al., 1992). Thus, sleep disturbances which occur in psychotic patients still need to be explained. With the availability of a D_1 antagonist which influences mechanisms underlying sleep, it may well be that further advances will be made towards understanding how REM sleep and schizophrenia relate to each other. Moreover, the unique effect of D_1 antagonists on sleep processes may also lead to a therapeutic activity in patients which so far has not emerged with the currently used antipsychotic agents.

7.7 Summary and conclusions

Evidence has been presented that the D_1 and D_2 receptor systems have different functions in the modulation of the behavioural states of sleep and waking. The D_1 receptors appear to be more involved in the regulation of changes of the sleep–waking continuum. Thus, in animal studies D_1 agonists induce EEG arousal and enhance wakefulness, whereas D_1 antagonists tend to induce sedation and increase the time spent in sleep. Interestingly, these drugs either reduce or increase the amount of REM sleep, showing that this important sleep stage is modulated by the specific stimulation or blockade of the D_1 receptors. These effects contrast with those of selective D_2 drugs. In fact, D_2 agonists induce arousal which may be secondary to the marked stereotyped behaviours which occur concomitantly and D_2 antagonists have little or no effect on sleep states. Only with the specific stimulation of D_2 receptors located presynaptically is there an increase of sedation and sleep, but this response may ultimately depend on the reduced DA tone at both D_1 and D_2 postsynaptic receptors. The two receptor systems do not function independently. An interaction between the D_1 and D_2 receptors appears to be operative in the induction of arousal and sedation, whereas REM sleep appears to be regulated by the D_1 receptors only. More studies are, however, needed to better understand the issue of $D_1 : D_2$ interaction. The results are often confounded by drug interactions with other non-DAergic receptor systems, such as acetylcholine and serotonin, which are also involved in the control of sleep states. Instead, in the absence of compounds having a significant selectivity for each of the newly discovered D_3, D_4 and D_5 receptor types, their functional roles remain unclarified.

While the clinical effects of selective D_2 drugs have been investigated, the potential of D_1 drugs has to be established. Based on the data available, it is expected that D_1 agonists, like other DAergic drugs such as l-DOPA, will induce arousal and reduce REM sleep also in man. As for D_1 antagonists, it is likely that they will induce a moderate level of drowsiness in patients as observed with most of the currently used neuroleptics. The more unusual ability of D_1 antagonists to promote REM sleep is instead worthy of further attention, since sleep alterations represent an important feature of psychiatric disorders.

References

Al-Tajir, G., Chandler, C.J., Starr, B.S. & Starr, M.S. (1990) *Neuropharmacology* **29**, 657–661.

Andersen, P.H., Gingrich, J.A., Bates, M.D., Dearry, A., Falardeau, P., Senogles, S.E. & Caron, M.G. (1990) *Trends Pharmacol. Sci.* **11**, 231–236.

Andersen, P.H., Grønvald, F.C., Hohlweg, R., Hansen, L.B., Goddal, E., Bødestrop, C. & Nielsen, E.K. (1992)*Eur. J. Pharmacol.* **219**, 45–52.

Bagetta, G., Corasaniti, M.T., Strongoli, M.C., Sakurada, S. & Nisticò, G. (1987) *J. Psychiat. Res.* **21**, 93–99.

Bagetta, G., De Sarro, G., Priolo, E. & Nisticò, G. (1988) *Br. J. Pharmacol.* **95**, 860–866.

Baldessarini, R.J. (1990) In *The Pharmacological Basis of Therapeutics* (eds Goodman Gilman, A., Goodman, L.S., Rall, T.W., Nies, A.S. & Taylor, P.), 8th edn, pp 383–435. New York, Pergamon Press.

Barnett, A. (1986) *Drugs of the Future* **11**, 49–56.

Barone, P., Palma, V., DeBartolomeis, A., Tedeschi, E., Muscettola, G. & Campanella, G. (1991) *Eur. J. Pharmacol.* **195**, 157–162.

Bertotelli, R., & Consolo, S. (1990) *J. Neurochem.* **54**, 2145–2148.

Bo, P., Ongini, E., Giorgetti, A. & Savoldi, F. (1988) *Neuropharmacology* **27**, 799–805.

Carlsson, A. (1988) *Neuropsychopharmacology* **1**, 179–203.

Chipkin, R.E., Iorio, L.C., Coffin, V.L., McQuade, R., Berger, J.G. & Barnett, A. (1988) *J. Pharmacol. Exp. Ther.* **247**, 1093–1102.

Civelli, O., Bunzow, J.R., Grandy, O.K., Zhou, Q.-Y. & Van Tol, H.H.M. (1991) *Eur. J. Pharmacol.* **207**, 277–286.

Coffin, V.L., Latranyi, M.B. & Chipkin, R.E. (1989) *J. Pharmacol. Exp. Ther.* **249**, 769–774.

Coffin, V.L., McHugh, D., Chipkin, R.E. & Barnett, A. (1992) *Neurochem. Int.* **20**, 141S–145S.

Consolo, S., Wu, C.F. & Fusi, R. (1987) *J. Pharmacol. Exp. Ther.* **242**, 300–305.

Cortés, R., Gueye, B., Pazos, A., Probst, A. & Palacios, J.M. (1989) *Neuroscience* **28**, 263–273.

Dall'Olio, R., Roncada, P., Vaccheri, A., Gandolfi, O. & Montanaro, N. (1989) *Psychopharmacology* **98**, 342–346.

Daly, S.A. & Waddington, J.L. (1991) *Br. J. Pharmacol.* **104**, 60P.

Deniker, P. (1990) *Acta Psychiat. Scand.* **82** (supplement 358), 83–87.

Dugovic, C., Wauquier, A. & Janssen, P.A.J. (1989a) *Neuropharmacology* **28**, 1431–1433.

Dugovic, C., Wauquier, A., Leysen, J.E., Marranes, R. & Janssen, P.A.J. (1989b) *Psychopharmacology* **97**, 436–442.

Fornal, C., Wojcik, W.J. & Radulovacki, M. (1982) *Neuropharmacology* **21**, 323–325.

Gaillard, J.-M. (1983) *Br. J. Clin. Pharmacol.* **16**, 230S–250S.

Gillin, J.C. & Borbély, A.A. (1985) *Trends Neurosci.* **8**, 537–542.

Gillin, J.C., Post, R.M., Wyatt, R.J., Goodwin, F.K., Snyder, F. & Bunney, W.E. (1973) *Electroencephal. Clin. Neurophysiol.* **35**, 181–186.

Hobson, J.A., Lydic, R. & Baghdoyan, H.A. (1986) *Behav. Brain Sci.* **9**, 371–448.

Horita, A., Carino, M.A. & Nishimura, Y. (1991) *Life Sci.* **49**, 595–601.

Iorio, L.C., Barnett, A., Leitz, F.H., Houser, V.P. & Korduba, C.A. (1983) *J. Pharmacol. Exp. Ther.* **226**, 462–468.

Iorio, L.C., Cohen, M. & Coffin, V.L. (1991) *J. Pharmacol. Exp. Ther.* **258**, 118–123.

Jones, B.E. (1991) *Neuroscience* **40**, 637–656.

Jouvet, M. (1972) *Ergebn. Physiol.* **64**, 165–307.

Joyce, J.N. (1983) *Neurosci. Biobehav.* **7**, 227–256.

Karczmar, A.G., Longo, V.G. & Scotti de Carolis, A. (1970) *Physiol. Behav.* **5**, 175–182.

Kropf, W. & Kuschinsky, K. (1991) *Neuropharmacology* **30**, 953–960.

Kropf, W., Kuschinsky, K. & Krieglstein, J. (1989) *Naunyn Schmiedeberg's Arch. Pharmacol.* **340**, 718–725.

Lewander, T., Westerbergh, S.E. & Morrison, D. (1990) *Acta Psychiat. Scand.* **82** (supplement 358), 92–98.

Longo, V.G. (1978) In *Principles of Psychopharmacology* (eds Clark, W.G. & Del Giudice, J.), pp 247–260. New York, Academic Press.

McQuade, R.D., Ford, D., Duffy, R.A., Chipkin, R.E., Iorio, L.C. & Barnett, A. (1988) *Life Sci.* **43**, 1861–1869.

McQuade, R.D., Duffy, R.A., Coffin, V.L., Chipkin, R.E. & Barnett, A. (1991) *J. Pharmacol. Exp. Ther.* **257**, 42–49.

Meltzer, H.Y., Matsubara, S. & Lee, J.-C. (1989) *J. Pharmacol. Exp. Ther.* **251**, 238–246.

Monti, J.M. (1983) *Life Sci.* **32**, 1401–1415.

Monti, J.M., Hawkins, M., Jantos, H., D'Angelo, L. & Fernàndez, M. (1988) *Psychopharmacology* **95**, 395–400.

Monti, J.M., Jantos, H. & Fernàndez, M. (1989) *Eur. J. Pharmacol.* **169**, 61–66.

Monti, J.M., Fernàndez, M. & Jantos, H. (1990) *Neuropsychopharmacology* **3**, 153–162.

Nicholson, A.N. & Pascoe, P.A. (1990) *Neuropharmacology* **29**, 411–417.

Nicholson, A.N., Belyavin, A.J. & Pascoe, P.A. (1989) *Neuropsychopharmacology* **2**, 131–143.

Ongini, E. & Caporali, M.G. (1987) *Neuropharmacology,* **26**, 355–360.

Ongini, E. & Longo, V.G. (1989) *Int. Rev. Neurobiology* **31**, 239–244.

Ongini, E., Caporali, M.G. & Massotti, M. (1985) *Life Sci.* **37**, 2327–2333.

Ongini, E., Caporali, M.G. & Longo, V.G. (1987) *Neurosci. Lett.* **82**, 206–210.

Ongini, E., Bo, P., Dionisotti, S., Trampus, M. & Savoldi, F. (1992) *Psychopharmacology,* **107**, 236–247.

Ongini, E., Bonizzoni, E., Ferri, N., Milani, S. & Tranpus, H. (1993) *J. Pharmacol. Exp. Ther.,* in press.

Parashos, S.A., Marin, C. & Chase, T.N. (1989) *Neurosci. Lett.* **105**, 169–173.

Peroutka, S.J. & Snyder, S.H. (1980) *Am. J. Psychiat.* **137**, 1518–1522.

Peselow, E.D. & Stanley, M. (1982) In *The Benzamides: Pharmacology, Neurobiology and Clinical Aspects* (eds Rotrosen, J. & Stanley, M.), pp 163–194, New York, Raven Press.

Reynolds, C.F., Gillin, J.C. & Kupfer, D.J. (1987) In *Psychopharmacology: The Third Generation of Progress* (ed. Meltzer, H.Y.), pp 467–654. New York, Raven Press.

Roubicek, J. (1980) In *Handbook of Experimental Pharmacology* (eds Hoffmeister, F. & Stille, G.), vol. 55/I, pp 177–192. Berlin, Heidelberg, Springer-Verlag.

Seeman, P. (1990) *Acta Psychiat. Scand.* **82** (supplement 358), 14–20.

Serra, G., Collu, M., D'Aquila, P.S., De Montis, G.M. & Gessa, G.L. (1990) *Brain Res.* **527**, 234–243.

Shiromani, P.J., Gillin, J.C. & Henriksen, S.J. (1987) *Ann. Rev. Pharmacol. Toxicol.* **27**, 137–156.

Shouse, M.N., Siegel, J.M., Wu, H.F., Saymusia, K.R. & Morrison, A.R. (1989) *Brain Res.* **505**, 271–282.

Stoof, J.C. & Kebabian, J.W. (1984) *Life Sci.* **35**, 2281–2296.

Sunahara, R.K., Guan, H.-C., O'Dowd, B.F., Seeman, P., Laurier, L.G., Ng, G., George, S.R., Torchia, J., Van Tol, H.M.M. & Niznik, H.B. (1991) *Nature* **350**, 614–619.

Svensson, K., Alföldi, P., Najòs, M., Rubicsek, G., Johansson, A.M., Carlsson, A. & Obàl, F. Jr (1987) *Pharmacol. Biochem. Behav.* **26**, 123–129.

Steriade, M. & McCarley, R.W. (1990) *Brainstem Control of Wakefulness and Sleep.* New York, Plenum Press.

Trampus, M. & Ongini, E. (1990) *Neuropharmacology* **29**, 889–893.

Trampus, M., Ferri, N., Monopoli, A. & Ongini, E. (1991) *Eur. J. Pharmacol.* **194**, 189–194.

Trampus, M., Ferri, N., Adami, M. & Ongini, E. (1993) *Eur. J. Pharmacol.*, in press.

Waddington, J.L. & O'Boyle, K.M. (1989) *Pharmacol. Ther.* **43**, 1–52.

Wauquier, A., Clincke, G.H.C., Van den Broek, W.A.E. & DePrints, E. (1985) In *Sleep—Neurotransmitters and Neuromodulators* (eds Wauquier, A., Gallard, J.M., Monti, J.M. & Radulovacki, M.), pp 107–120. New York, Raven Press.

Weiler, M.A., Buchsbaum, M.S., Gillin, J.C., Tafal-la, R. & Bunney, W.E. Jr (1990) *Neuropsychobiology* **23**, 109–118.

CHAPTER 8

D₁ : D₂ DOPAMINE RECEPTOR INTERACTIONS IN RELATION TO FEEDING RESPONSES AND FOOD INTAKE

Steven J. Cooper and Hessah A. Al-Naser

Laboratory of Psychopharmacology, School of Psychology, University of Birmingham, Edgbaston, Birmingham B15 2TT, UK

Table of Contents

8.1   Introduction

The distinction between two dopamine receptor subtypes, D_1 and D_2 (Kebabian and Calne, 1979), coupled with the availability of agonists and antagonists selective for the two subtypes (Stoof and Kebabian, 1984), provided a great impetus for the study of central dopaminergic functions. By that stage, an interest had already been established in the relations between dopamine activity and the control of ingestional responses, although the nature of the relations was poorly understood.

In one early study, Barzaghi *et al.* (1973) showed that apomorphine, a directly acting dopamine agonist, produced dose-related (0.25–2.0 mg/kg, i.p.) decreases in the food intake of 20-h food-deprived rats. Its anorectic effect was blocked by pimozide, a dopamine receptor antagonist, and, therefore, they proposed that brain dopamine plays an inhibitory role in feeding behaviour. At the same time, Kruk (1973) reported that i.c.v. (intracerebroventricular) administration of apomorphine, dopamine or *d*-amphetamine produced dose-dependent decreases in food intake in food-deprived rats. Since pimozide blocked these effects too, he also suggested an inhibitory role for dopamine. Later work confirmed these results and indicated that at least one site of action for dopaminergic anorectic activity was the perifornical lateral hypothalamus (Heffner *et al.*, 1977; Leibowitz, 1975).

Drawing a distinction between D_1 and D_2 receptor subtypes raises the question of their respective contributions to the observed dopaminergic anorectic effect. Studying the effects of indirectly acting agonists, like *d*-amphetamine or cocaine, or a non-selective dopamine agonist like apomorphine, provides no immediate insight into the possible *individual* contributions of effects mediated by the two receptor subtypes. For that, we must turn to selective dopamine D_1 receptor agonists, like SK & F 38393 (Setler *et al.*, 1978), and selective D_2 receptor agonists like N-0437 (van der Weide *et al.*, 1986), (+)-PHNO (Martin *et al.*, 1984), or quinpirole (Itoh *et al.*, 1985). Nevertheless, if we assume that endogenous dopamine acts as both receptor subtypes to produce its effects on feeding behaviour, we should proceed with three kinds of comparisons: (i) between the individual effects of selective D_1 and D_2 receptor agonists (do both types of drug affect feeding, and, if so, are their effects similar or not?); (ii) between the individual effects and the effects of dopamine agonists given in combination (are effects of D_1 and D_2 agonists in combination additive or antagonistic or are there emergent effects specific to the drugs in combination?); (iii) between effects of non-selective directly and indirectly acting dopamine agonists, on the one hand, and selective dopamine agonists, on the other (can the effects of *d*-amphetamine or cocaine, for example, be predicted from the individual effects of D_1 and D_2 receptor agonists or from their joint effects when given in combination?).

This chapter cannot pretend to address each of these issues in depth, but the way to proceed is clear enough. It is an aim of this chapter, however, to show that careful behavioural analysis of the effects of dopaminergic compounds on feeding behaviour is necessary if these issues are to be addressed satisfactorily.

8.1.1 Dopamine D_1 : D_2 receptor interactions

The important functional theme of the present volume is the nature of interactions between D_1 and D_2 receptor-mediated effects (Waddington, 1989). A good deal of the behavioural work in this field has focused upon well-characterized dopamine-mediated behaviour, e.g. stereotyped behaviour associated with D_1 receptor stimulation (Waddington *et al.*, 1990). Several authors reported that the stereotyped responses induced by quinpirole were enhanced by co-administration of SK & F 38393 (Braun and Chase, 1986; Arnt *et al.*, 1987; Longoni *et al.*, 1987; White *et al.*, 1988; Meller *et al.*, 1988). Interactions were also discovered when D_1 and D_2 agonists were jointly injected into the ventral striatum (Bordi and Meller, 1989) or nucleus accumbens (Plaznik, 1989).

   In addition to these instances of apparent cooperativity or synergism between the effects of D_1 and D_2 agonists, there are two further possibilities (Waddington, 1989). First, D_1 and D_2 agonists may act in opposition to each other, and, second, they may act independently in ways that do not interact. Feeding behaviour is not a single response, but has many aspects to it, and therefore it is impossible to predict in advance how D_1 and D_2 receptor agonists will interact in their effects on the several components of feeding behaviour. As a first step, we can address the question of whether or not D_1 and D_2 agonists interact in their effects on *food intake*, and we shall report results which bear on this issue. Nevertheless, the food intake measure is not a behavioural measure and therefore detailed behavioural analysis is required to understand the mechanisms underlying dopamine agonists' activities and their effects on feeding.

8.2   Behavioural methods in feeding research

Early psychopharmacological studies of food ingestion invariably used food-deprived animals, and limited their data to measures of food intake. Food deprivation was believed to cause hunger, and this provided the motivation to ingest the food. Nowadays we are much more clearly aware that animals can be highly motivated to eat certain foods, even if they are not food-deprived. Thus, rats will consume highly palatable foods such as sweetened mash or sucrose solutions in the absence of hunger caused by food deprivation. Furthermore, the normal free-feeding behaviour of animals can be studied; rats are nocturnal in their habits, and much of their normal feeding occurs at night. Consequently, if free-feeding is measured at night there will be an appreciable intake, but if measurement is restricted to the daytime, then the levels of food consumption may be very low. Of course, a comprehensive approach to the study of a drug treatment, or treatments, on feeding behaviour would include comparisons across several of these paradigms.

Inevitably, the measurement of feeding (and drinking) responses became automated, and microcomputers are now used to log a great deal of detailed information that can be generated. An important innovation in feeding research was the introduction of *meal pattern analysis* to analyse free-feeding and free-drinking in animals (review: Clifton, 1987). Feeding and drinking can be studied continuously over complete 24-h periods; in this case the periodicity of ingestion is manifestly apparent, and rats feed almost entirely at night in their homecages and sleep through much of the day. Since feeding is discontinuous, the sizes of meals can be measured, as well as their frequency, the intervals between meals, and the rate of eating within meals. With this kind of detailed analysis, it is clear that drug treatments may affect one or more of these behavioural measures of feeding.

At the level of a single meal, an observational method called *microstructural analysis* yields very informative data, which can greatly assist in the interpretation of drug effects (Blundell and Latham, 1978; Blundell and McArthur, 1981). Within a meal, feeding occurs in discrete bouts, separated by pauses. Hence, one can measure bout durations and frequencies, pause lengths, and rates of eating within bouts. At this level of detailed analysis, subtle as well as gross differences between drug treatments become apparent.

8.3 Psychomotor stimulants

Before considering the effects of selective dopamine receptor subtype agonists on feeding behaviour, it will be interesting to consider the effects of two indirectly acting agonists, amphetamine and cocaine, and of the non-selective agonist apomorphine. Experiments with these drugs have provided important sources of evidence linking dopamine mechanisms with appetite. Moreover, a significant amount of behavioural data has accumulated for these drugs, which can be used in comparison with recent data available for selective dopamine D_1 and D_2 receptor agonists. It should be noted, however, that these drugs not only reduce food consumption but also have pronounced behavioural stimulant effects, producing increases in activity and stereotyped behaviour (Cooper and Dourish, 1990).

8.3.1 Amphetamine

Lesses and Myerson (1938) were the first to suggest that amphetamine could be useful as an aid in the treatment of human obesity. Amphetamine quickly found favour as an aid to successful slimming, but it was not until the experiments of Harris *et al.* (1947) that it was demonstrated that the loss of body weight induced by amphetamine was due to a decrease in food consumption. Silverstone and Stunkard (1968) noted the extensive clinical use of amphetamine to treat obesity, and provided the first controlled laboratory evidence that *d-*

amphetamine could reduce hunger ratings and caloric intake in human volunteer subjects.

Amphetamine also attracted attention because its site of action was thought to be central; one idea to gain ground was that amphetamine inhibited the activity of a lateral hypothalamic 'hunger centre' (Stellard, 1954). Thus, amphetamine was less effective in rats with lateral hypothalamic lesions (Carlisle, 1964; Blundell and Leshem, 1974), while injections of d-amphetamine into the lateral hypothalamus reduced food intake (Booth, 1968; Leibowitz, 1975).

When the microstructural approach was adopted to study amphetamine's anorectic effect, it was discovered that, in rats, amphetamine increased the latency before eating, reduced the duration of eating (eating occurred in short bouts), but increased the local rate of eating (Blundell and Latham, 1980; Cooper and Sweeney, 1980; Towell et al., 1988). When meal patterns over a 24-h period were investigated in rats, it was found that d-amphetamine increased the latency to meal onset and thereafter reduced meal size and duration (Leibowitz et al., 1986). Similarly, studies with baboons over 22-h daily sessions revealed that d-amphetamine decreased food intake by increasing the latency to the first meal, decreased the size of the first meal, and decreased the number of meals (Foltin and Fischman, 1989). A common feature in all of these results is that d- amphetamine increased the latency before eating; this delay in feeding appears to be a major contributor to amphetamine's anorectic action. An interesting issue to arise from this is the extent to which feeding is normal once it has been initiated following the delayed start. Some of the results just cited suggest that amphetamine has effects on feeding behaviour itself, in addition to the delay in the onset of feeding.

A recent study by Foltin et al. (1990), carried out with human volunteers in a residential laboratory, throws further light on this question. The volunteers lived in the laboratory for 15 days, and their behaviour, and food intake, were continuously recorded. They had a wide variety of food items available and could consume any item, or number of items, at any time during the day. Twice-daily administration of d-amphetamine reduced total caloric intake to about 70% of control levels. The study provided valuable information on the means by which the drug achieved this reduction in food intake. The majority of subjects who responded to d-amphetamine did so because of the increased latency before eating after each dose of the drug. The average caloric intake during each meal (meal size) and snack, when they did occur, were not affected by d-amphetamine. In this naturalistic study, therefore, d-amphetamine appeared to have a specific effect in delaying meal initiation.

The reduction in food intake produced by amphetamine is dopamine-dependent. Early studies showed that amphetamine's effects on feeding could be blocked by dopamine antagonists (Barzaghi et al., 1973; Kruk, 1973). However, Burridge and Blundell (1979) drew a distinction between the anorectic effect of a small dose of d-amphetamine (0.5 mg/kg) in rats, and those of larger doses (1.0 and 2.0 mg/kg). They found that the effects of the larger doses were blocked by dopamine antagonists, whereas the effect of the smaller dose was not. Other data, however, do not support such a distinction, and Heffner *et al.* (1977), for example, reported that the dose-dependent anorectic effect of *d*-amphetamine, at each dose level (0.4–4.0 mg/kg), was reversed by dopamine antagonists. Towell *et al.* (1988a) showed that pimozide blocked *d*-amphetamine's anorectic effect, at 0.5 and 1.0 mg/kg of *d*-amphetamine. Gilbert and Cooper (1985) observed that the anorectic effect of a small dose of *d*-amphetamine (0.3 mg/kg) was reversed by the selective dopamine D_1 receptor antagonist SCH 23990, thus providing the first evidence for dopamine D_1 receptor involvement in *d*-amphetamine's effect on feeding.

8.3.2 Cocaine

In the past, rather little attention has been paid to the effects of cocaine on feeding responses. Van Rossum and Simons (1969) noted that cocaine (9.6 mg/kg) reduced food intake in rats by 33% in a 2-h test, while *d*-amphetamine (0.4 mg/kg) reduced food intake by 43%. In another early study, intravenous injection of cocaine (3 mg/kg) reduced food intake in food-deprived rats by 65% in a 30-min test conducted immediately post-injection (Groppetti *et al.*, 1973). The effects of cocaine on feeding are short-lived, and Balapole *et al.* (1979) found that they occurred only in the first hour post-injection (10–25 mg/kg cocaine, i.p.). Cocaine is also effective in non-deprived rats, and Foltin *et al.* (1983) found that, over a dose range of 4–32 mg/kg, cocaine produced dose-dependent reductions in sweetened milk consumption.

An anorectic effect of cocaine has therefore been demonstrated, but the results provide no behavioural analysis of the effect. Therefore, van der Hoek and I carried out an experiment applying a microstructural analysis to cocaine's effect on palatable food consumption in non-deprived male rats (Cooper and van der Hoek, 1993). We confirmed a dose-dependent effect of cocaine (5.6–30 mg/kg, i.p.) in reducing food intake, over a test period lasting 60 min (Figure 1, left panel). This anorectic effect was not due to any significant reduction in the rate of eating, which ranged from 1.5 to 2.0 g/min of eating time (Figure 1, right panel). Instead, the reduction in food consumption could be accounted for in terms of a dose-dependent reduction in the time devoted to feeding (Table 1). With the exception of a significant effect at 30 mg/kg, cocaine did not affect the mean bout duration. Ultimately the anorectic effect of cocaine depended on large reductions in the number of feeding bouts during the period of the test (Table 1). Such reductions could be distributed uniformly throughout the test, or could be particularly concentrated at the beginning or the end of feeding. Examination of the time-course of feeding indicated that cocaine (10–30 mg/kg) completely suppressed ingestion initially, and the recovery from this suppressant effect was related to its dose (Figure 2A). Thus, the essential effect of cocaine was to delay initiation of feeding, which resulted in a reduction of the frequency of eating episodes; once feeding had begun, however, the

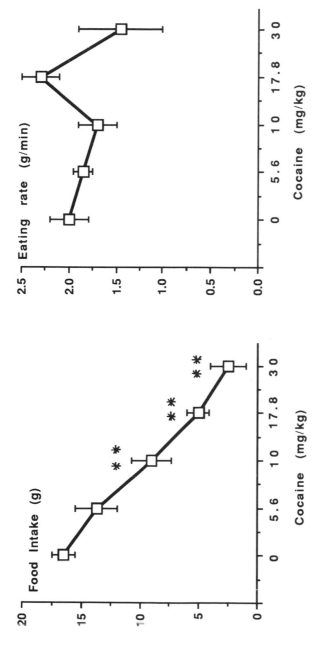

Figure 1 *Left panel*: Cocaine (5.6–30 mg/kg, i.p.) dose-dependently reduced palatable food intake (g) in a 60 min test. Non-deprived rats were used. *Right panel*: cocaine did not significantly affect the local rate of eating (g/min) in the test. Results are shown as mean ± SEM, $n = 7$ per group. Levels of significance for comparisons between individual groups and vehicle control: * $P < 0.05$; ** $P < 0.01$ (Dunnett's t-test) (Cooper and van der Hoek, 1993).

Table 1 Microsctructural analysis of the effects of cocaine hydrochloride (5.6–30 mg/kg, i.p.) on feeding and grooming behaviour in a 60-min test. Non-deprived male rats had been trained to consume a high-palatability sweetened diet.

	Cocaine (mg/kg)				
	0	5.6	10	17.8	30
Feeding					
Total duration (min.)	8.17 ± 0.56	7.53 ± 1.10	5.81 ± 0.87	2.33 ± 0.27**	1.48 ± 0.87**
Bout duration (min.)	0.37 ± 0.08	0.29 ± 0.07	0.40 ± 0.06	0.26 ± 0.03	0.12 ± 0.05*
Bout frequency	26.43 ± 4.58	28.29 ± 2.71	15.14 ± 1.87*	9.86 ± 1.46*	8.29 ± 3.9**
Grooming					
Total duration (min.)	12.28 ± 1.09	5.67 ± 1.05**	5.22 ± 1.47**	1.60 ± 0.33**	0.16 ± 0.09**
Bout duration (min.)	0.27 ± 0.02	0.11 ± 0.01**	0.10 ± 0.01**	0.05 ± 0.01**	0.025 ± 0.01**
Bout frequency	47.43 ± 4.6	53.29 ± 9.53	49.57 ± 10.84	34.57 ± 8.09	3.71 ± 1.6**

Results are shown in terms of mean ± SEM ($n = 7$ per group). Levels of significance for individual dose comparisons against control values: * $P < 0.05$; ** $P < 0.01$ (Dunnett's t-test) (Cooper and van der Hoek, 1993).

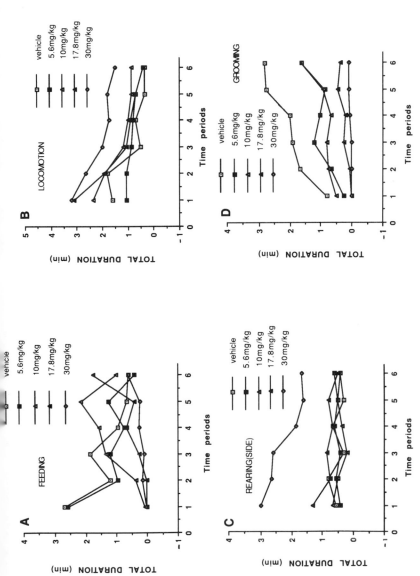

Figure 2 Time-courses for the behavioural effects of cocaine (5.6–30 mg/kg, i.p.). (A) Cocaine (10–30 mg/kg) suppressed feeding initially, although there was recovery later in the test. (B) Locomotor activity was stimulated by cocaine, particularly at the highest dose tested (30 mg/kg). (C) Rearing to the side was stimulated by cocaine at the 30 mg/kg dose. (D) Grooming was markedly suppressed by cocaine at all doses, and virtually abolished at 17.8 and 30 mg/kg. The data are plotted as mean duration for each behavioural category within consecutive time periods of a 60-min test (Cooper and van der Hoek, 1993).

duration of feeding bouts and the rate of eating within those bouts appeared to be comparatively normal. The psychomotor stimulant effects of cocaine were observed in the test; locomotor activity and rearing were increased, especially at 30 mg/kg (Figures 2B and C). The most striking behavioural change, however, apart from the effect on feeding, was the marked suppression of grooming (Figure 2D). Under baseline conditions, the time spent grooming increased throughout the test period, as the level of feeding declined. Cocaine (5.6 and 10 mg/kg) reduced grooming throughout the 60-min test period, and completely suppressed it at 17.8 and 30 mg/kg (Figure 2D). In contrast to its effect on feeding, cocaine reduced grooming by shortening quite considerably the mean bout duration (except at 30 mg/kg, when bout frequency was almost eliminated). This illustrates, quite clearly, that changes in the overall duration of behaviour during a test can be due to dissimilar changes in the level of bouts. Cocaine reduced the frequency of feeding bouts but reduced the duration of grooming bouts.

Cocaine binds to the dopamine transporter and inhibits dopamine uptake, in dopamine terminal regions, which include the striatum, nucleus accumbens and olfactory tubercle (Boja and Kuhar, 1989; Izenwasser et al., 1990; Ritz et al., 1987). Associated with these effects, cocaine increases extracellular dopamine in the striatum and the nucleus accumbens (Church et al., 1987; Pettitt and Justice, 1989, 1991). The behavioural effects of cocaine, including its effects on feeding behaviour, may therefore depend upon dopaminergic neurotransmission. Heffner et al. (1977) found that cocaine's anorectic effect at 10 mg/kg was antagonized by spiperone, a dopamine receptor antagonist. Similarly, we found that cocaine's effect at 15 mg/kg was reversed by haloperidol (Cooper and van der Hoek, unpublished data). Recently, Rapoza and Woolverton (1991) examined the effects of a selective D_1 receptor antagonist, SCH 23390, and of a selective D_2 receptor antagonist, raclopride, on milk consumption in rats. Cocaine (4–32 mg/kg, i.p.) dose-dependently decreased consumption, and both antagonists attenuated cocaine's effect for at least one of its effective doses. Stimulation of both D_1 and D_2 receptors, therefore, may be involved in cocaine's suppressant effect on milk ingestion.

There appear to be close similarities between the anorectic effects of d-amphetamine and cocaine. Both drugs delay the initiation of feeding, and this may be an important, if not the most important, factor in determining the anorectic effects of these drugs. At a neurochemical level, dopaminergic transmission is involved and, in both cases, the anorectic effect can be blocked by dopamine receptor antagonists. Effects of dopamine at D_1 receptors are involved in both cases, and the anorectic effect may depend upon the stimulation of D_1 and D_2 receptors.

8.3.3 Apomorphine

Apomorphine provides the first example of a directly acting dopamine agonist that reduces food intake, although it is not selective for either D_1 or D_2 receptor subtypes (Barzaghi *et al.*, 1973; Eichler and Antelman, 1977; Heffner *et al.*, 1977; Kruk, 1973). A microstructural analysis of its anorectic effect has been carried out by Willner *et al.* (1985). Apomorphine (0.04–0.64 mg/kg, s.c.) was administered to 21-h food-deprived rats, and their feeding behaviour was recorded over 30-min sessions. The dopamine receptor agonist dose-dependently reduced food intake, and this effect was due in part to a reduction in the rate of eating and also in the duration of bouts of feeding. As the section above makes clear, neither *d*-amphetamine nor cocaine reduced the rate of eating, so that this feature of apomorphine's anorectic effect is quite novel.

Pharmacological experiments confirm that the anorectic effect of apomorphine is dopaminergically mediated. It has been shown that its feeding-suppressant effect is blocked by pimozide, haloperidol and sulpiride (Barzaghi *et al.*, 1973; Kruk, 1973; Willner *et al.*, 1985; Muscat *et al.*, 1986; Duterte-Boucher *et al.*, 1989). These results indicate that dopamine D_2 receptors have a part to play in apomorphine's effects, but to date there appears to have been no analysis of whether D_1 receptors are involved or not. Nevertheless, it seems highly likely that the effects of apomorphine on feeding behaviour depend upon its actions at both D_1 and D_2 receptor subtypes. The best approach to this issue, though, is to investigate the effects of selective D_1 or D_2 receptor agonists on feeding to determine whether or not anorectic effects can be elicited separately by drug action at the separate receptor subtypes.

8.4 Dopamine receptor subtype agonists

8.4.1 Dopamine D_2 receptor agonists

Evidence clearly indicates that selective stimulation of D_2 receptors leads to reduction in feeding behaviour. N-0437 is a potent and selective D_2 receptor agonist (van der Weide *et al.*, 1986; 1987, 1988), and we found that it significantly reduced palatable food consumption in non-deprived rats and mice, and that this effect was blocked by the selective D_2 receptor antagonist YM 09151-2 (Rusk and Cooper, 1988). Moreover, it reduced food intake and lever pressing for food reward in food-deprived rats (Rusk and Cooper, 1988). A study of the enantiomers of N-0437 showed that (−)-N-0437 was more potent than (+)-N-0437 in reducing palatable food consumption in non-deprived rats (Timmerman *et al.*, 1989). The effects of both enantiomers on feeding were antagonized by the D_2 receptor antagonist YM 09151-2.

Martin-Iverson and Dourish (1988) investigated the effects of (+)-PHNO, a potent and selective D_2 receptor agonist (Martin *et al.*, 1984), on the 1 h food intake of non-deprived rats during the daytime. They discovered that (+)-PHNO increased the consumption of food pellets in this test, and that this apparent hyperphagic effect could be blocked, either by haloperidol or by the selective D_1 receptor antagonist SCH 23390. In addition, $(+)$-PHNO over the same range of doses $(7.5-120 \mu g/kg)$ decreased consumption of a liquid diet. Martin-Iverson and Dourish (1988) postulated that the increase in consumption of the solid food may have been a consequence of an increase in chewing responses.

We have also examined the effects of $(+)$-PHNO in freely feeding rats, but investigated its effects on nocturnal feeding as distinct from daytime feeding. Rats were first adapted to a reversed-lighting schedule, and trained to consume powdered food from spill-proof jars. Figure 3 shows the cumulative intake of food over a 6 h test period; following the vehicle injection the animals consumed about 6 g of the food in the first 2-h period, and another 6 g in the following 4-h period. There was no significant effect of $(+)$-PHNO during the first 2-h period, although by the end of 4 h $(+)$-PHNO (0.1 and 0.3 mg/kg) had produced a significant reduction in intake which was maintained until the end of the test. Other selective D_2 receptor agonists reduced food intake in the same nocturnal feeding model. Figure 4 shows that N-0437 did not affect food intake during the first 2-h period, but significantly reduced consumption at each dose level $(0.1-3.0 \text{ mg/kg})$ by the end of the 4-h period. The selective D_2 receptor agonist quinpirole (LY 171555) (Itoh et al., 1985) was also effective in this test (Figure 5). At 1 and 3 mg/kg, it significantly reduced food intake within the first 2-h period, and by the 4-h point, all doses $(0.1-3 \text{ mg/kg})$ were effective in reducing intake. So far as nocturnal free-feeding is concerned, therefore, the common effect of selective dopamine D_2 receptor agonists is to reduce food intake dose-relatedly. Providing animals with powdered food made the issue of drug-induced chewing irrelevant, and therefore we did not expect to see any apparent hyperphagic effect.

8.4.2 Dopamine D_1 receptor agonists

Gilbert and Cooper (1985) were first to demonstrate that the selective D_1 dopamine receptor agonist SK & F 38393 $(3-30 \text{ mg/kg})$ produced a dose-related suppression of palatable food consumption in non-deprived rats. Its anorectic effect was confirmed by Martin-Iverson and Dourish (1988), who reported that SK & F 38393 (5 mg/kg) reduced solid food consumption in freely feeding animals tested during the daytime. In a series of experiments, Rusk and Cooper (1989a) characterized its properties more fully. They confirmed that SK & F 38393 reduced palatable food consumption in non-deprived rats, and that it dose-dependently (3-30 mg/kg) reduced powdered food intake in food-deprived rats. At 30 mg/kg of SK & F 38393, deprivation-induced feeding was almost completely suppressed; however, thirst-induced drinking was only modestly reduced (by 29%) at the same dose. This comparison suggests that SK & F 38393 was probably not acting non-specifically in reducing food consumption. Rusk and Cooper (1989a) also demonstrated that SK & F 38393 reduced palatable food intake in mice, and that the effect was stereoselective since R-$(+)$-SK & F 38393 but not S-$(-)$-SK & F 38393 significantly reduced food

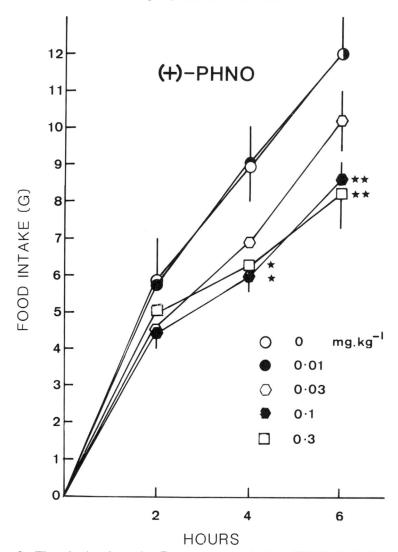

Figure 3 The selective dopamine D_1 receptor agonist (+)-PHNO (0.01–0.3 mg/kg, s.c.) significantly reduced powdered food intake in free-feeding rats during the nocturnal phase. Data are shown as mean cumulative intake (g) over a 6-h period (some SEMs are omitted for clarity). $n - 10$ rats per condition. Levels of significance for comparisons between individual treatments and vehicle control at each time-point: see legend to Figure 1 (Cooper, unpublished data).

intake. Finally, they showed that SK & F 38393 (3–30 mg/kg) dose-dependently reduced operant responding for food in food-deprived rats.

We have also carried out sham-feeding experiments in which rats with an open gastric fistula consume a 10% sucrose solution with little sign of satiety

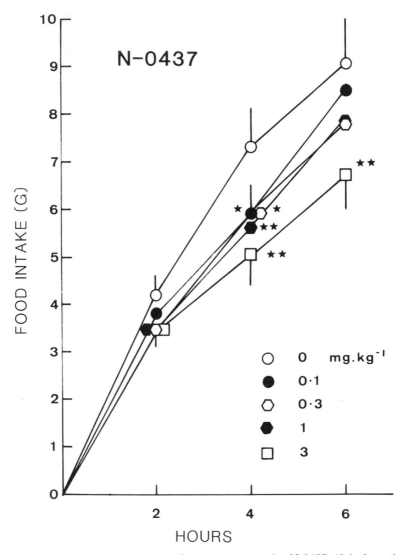

Figure 4 The selective dopamine D_2 receptor agonist N-0437 (0.1–3 mg/kg, s.c.) significantly reduced powdered food intake in free-feeding rats during the nocturnal phase. For other details, see legend to Figure 3 (Cooper, unpublished data).

over a 60-min test (e.g. Kirkham and Cooper, 1988; Neill and Cooper, 1989). Figure 6 shows that 10 mg/kg SK & F 38393 suppressed sucrose sham-feeding over the entire test period. In addition, as shown in Figure 7, the dopamine D_1 receptor agonist CY 208-243 (Foote *et al.*, 1988; Temlett *et al.*, 1988; Murray and Waddington, 1990; Abbott *et al.*, 1991) significantly reduced sucrose sham-feeding at 1 and 3 mg/kg.

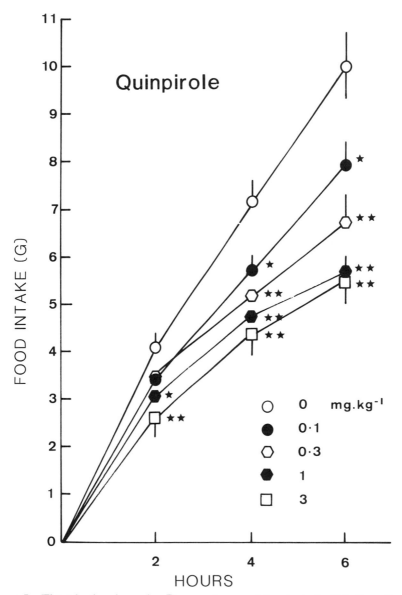

Figure 5 The selective dopamine D_2 receptor agonist quinpirole (0.1–3 mg/kg, s.c.) significantly reduced powdered food intake in free-feeding rats during the nocturnal phase. For other details, see legend to Figure 3 (Cooper, unpublished data).

In a further demonstration of the anorectic effects of selective dopamine D_1 receptor agonists, we have recently begun to investigate the potent and selective compound, A 68930 (DeNinno *et al.*, 1990, 1991; Britton *et al.*, 1991; Kebabian *et al.*, 1990). Figure 8 shows that 0.3 mg/kg (s.c.) A 68930 significantly reduced

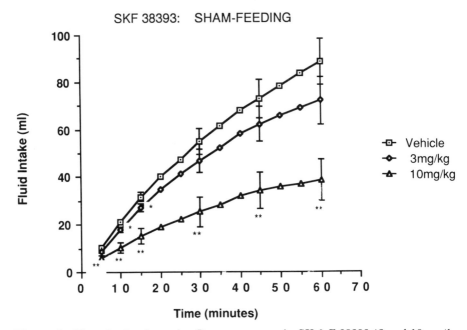

Figure 6   The selective dopamine D_1 receptor agonist SK & F 38393 (3 and 10 mg/kg, s.c.) significantly reduced 10% sucrose sham-feeding in 4-h food-deprived gastric-fistulated rats. Data are shown as mean cumulative fluid intake (ml) at 5-min intervals over the 60-min test period. Some SEMs are omitted for clarity. $n = 9$ per group. Levels of significance for comparisons between individual treatments and vehicle control at each time-point: see legend to Figure 1 (adapted from Cooper, Francis and Barber, 1993).

the ingestion of a 3% sucrose solution in a 30-min test using non-deprived rats. At 1.0 mg/kg A 68930, sucrose consumption was completely abolished. These data provide the first evidence for a potent anorectic effect of this novel dopamine D_1 receptor agonist.

8.4.3   Evidence for $D_1 : D_2$ interactions in feeding

So far, we have reviewed evidence which shows that indirectly acting dopamine agonists, like *d*-amphetamine and cocaine, as well as the directly acting agonist, apomorphine, reduce food consumption. With the distinction drawn between dopamine D_1 and D_2 receptor subtypes (Kebabian and Calne, 1979), we have been able to show that either selective D_1 receptor agonists (SK & F 38393, CY 208-243, A 68930) or selective D_2 receptor agonists (N-0437, (+)-PHNO, quinpirole) reduce food consumption. We now consider evidence which indicates that some form of *potentiation* can occur between the anorectic effects of dopamine D_1 and D_2 agonists.

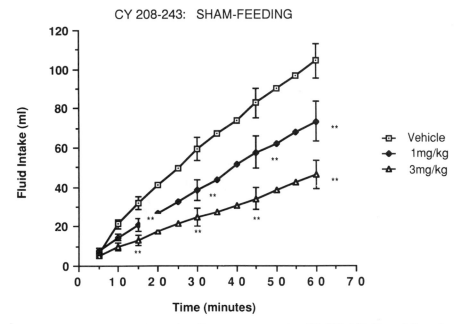

Figure 7 The selective dopamine D_1 receptor agonist CY 208-243 (1 and 3 mg/kg, s.c.) significantly reduced 10% sucrose sham-feeding in 4-h food-deprived gastric-fistulated rats. For other details, see legend to Figure 1 (adapted from Cooper, Francis and Barber, 1993).

Earlier, we referred to the anorectic effects of dopamine D_2 receptor agonists on nocturnal free-feeding in rats. Figure 9 shows that the D_1 receptor agonist SK & F 38393 (10 mg/kg) can also significantly reduce nighttime feeding. The potentiation effect emerged when a smaller dose of SK & F 38393 (3 mg/kg) was injected in conjunction with either (+)-PHNO or quinpirole in the same feeding model. As Figure 10 shows, (+)-PHNO at 0.03 mg/kg did not affect food intake over the first 4-h period of the test. Given in combination with SK & F 38393, however, it is clear that this dose of (+)-PHNO enhanced the feeding-suppressant effect of SK & F 38393. This was not an isolated example, since 0.1 mg/kg quinpirole had little effect when given alone, but in combination with SK & F 38393 there was a pronounced anorectic effect present throughout the test period (Figure 11).

Recent data provide another example of a potentiation, in this instance between the effect of quinpirole and that of the novel dopamine D_1 receptor agonist A 68930. The anorectic effect of A 68930 has been described above (Figure 8). The D_2 receptor agonist quinpirole also significantly suppressed the consumption of a 3% sucrose solution (Figure 12). In the drug-combination experiment, a dose of A 68930 (0.1 mg/kg) and a dose of quinpirole

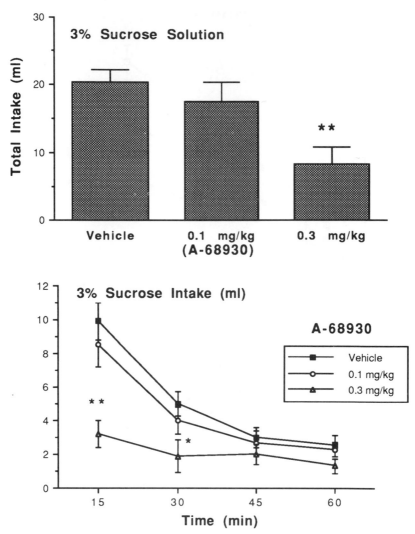

Figure 8 The potent, selective dopamine D_1 receptor agonist A 68930 (0.3 mg/kg) significantly reduced the consumption of 3% sucrose solution (ml) in non-deprived rats. *Upper panel:* mean total intake + SEM. *Lower panel:* Time-course of drinking over the 60-min test. A 68930 suppressed sucrose drinking during the first 15-min period. $n = 10$ per condition. Levels of significance for comparisons between individual doses and the vehicle control: see legend to Figure 1 (Al-Naser and Cooper, unpublished data).

(0.03 mg/kg), neither of which alone affected sucrose ingestion, produced a marked suppression of intake when administered together (Figure 13).

There is clearly some generality in this phenomenon of potentiation, since it has been demonstrated in two dissimilar feeding paradigms: nocturnal

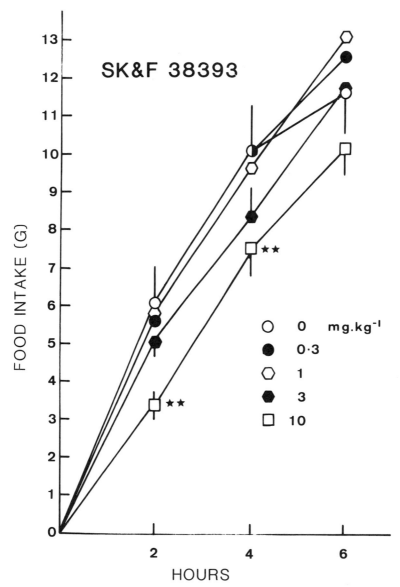

Figure 9 The selective dopamine D_1 receptor agonist SK & F 38393 (0.3–10 mg/kg, s.c.) significantly reduced powdered food intake in free-feeding rats during the nocturnal phase. For other details, see legend to Figure 3 (Cooper, unpublished data).

free-feeding and 3% sucrose consumption. Moreover, it has been demonstrated between either SK & F 38393 or A 68930 on the one hand, and quinpirole or (+)-PHNO on the other. However, it should be clearly recognized that drug interactions can be complex, and the outcomes of their interacting effects not

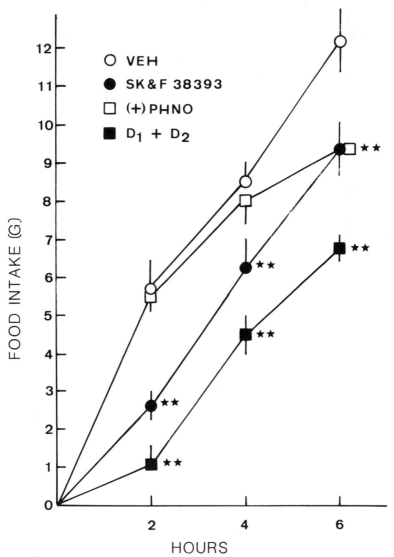

Figure 10 The combination of SK & F 38393 (10.0 mg/kg) and (+)-PHNO (0.3 mg/kg) produced a marked suppression of food intake in free-feeding rats tested during the nocturnal phase. For other details, see legend to Figure 3 (Cooper, unpublished data).

easy to predict (Cooper, 1979). In the present examples, relatively small doses of each drug in the pair were used, possibly favouring the occurrence of potentiation. Larger doses were not investigated, so that it is not possible to rule out antagonistic interactions, which may occur at other dose levels in combination. Even when doses of the two constituent drugs of a mixture are

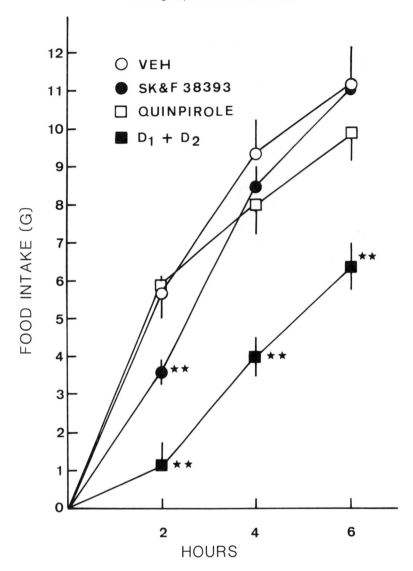

Figure 11 The combination of SK & F 38393 (10.0 mg/kg) and quinpirole (0.3 mg/kg) produced a marked suppression of food intake in free-feeding rats tested during the nocturnal phase. For other details, see legend to Figure 3 (Cooper, unpublished data).

fixed, potentiation may occur with regard to one type of behavioural response, but antagonism with regard to another (Cooper, 1979).

Nevertheless, we have been able to show that, under some circumstances at least, small doses of a D_1 receptor agonist and a D_2 receptor agonist, respectively, can lead to a potentiation in their effect on food consumption. But this

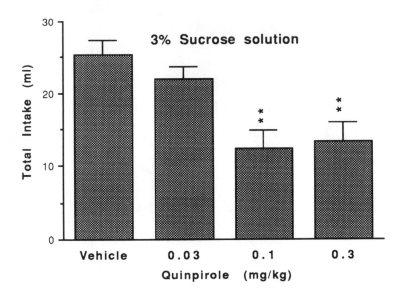

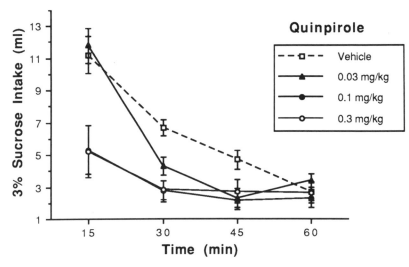

Figure 12 The selective dopamine D_2 receptor agonist quinpirole (0.1 and 0.3 mg/kg) significantly reduced the consumption of 3% sucrose solution (ml) in non-deprived rats. For other details, see legend to Figure 8 (Al-Naser and Cooper, unpublished data).

demonstration leaves open the question of the mechanisms underlying the effect. Do dopamine D_1 receptor agonists and D_2 receptor agonists, respectively, reduce food intake by the same means, or can their effects be differentiated? To answer this question, we have to go beyond simple measures of food intake and consider the effects of the drugs in question on feeding *behaviour*, in some detail.

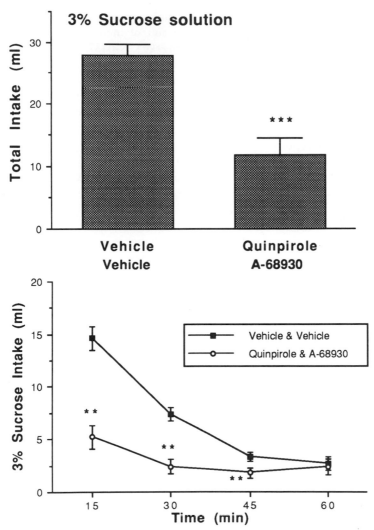

Figure 13 The combination of 0.1 mg/kg A 68930 and 0.03 mg/kg quinpirole significantly reduced the consumption of 3% sucrose solution (ml) in non-deprived rats. For other details, see legend to Figure 8 (Al-Naser and Cooper, unpublished data).

8.5 Dopamine receptor subtypes and feeding behaviour

8.5.1 Meal pattern analysis

To date, the only published report of an analysis of the effects of a dopamine D_2 receptor agonist on meal patterns is that of Clifton *et al.* (1989). Home-caged rats were continuously monitored over 24-h periods, and N-0437 (0.3–3.0 mg/kg, i.p.) was injected at the start of the night phase. Interestingly, N-0437 (0.3 mg/kg) increased food intake as a result of increases in meal size and duration. At the higher doses (1.0 and 3.0 mg/kg), N-0437 inhibited food intake for 3–6 h. This inhibition was due to a substantial reduction in meal size, with no change in the frequency of meals. In contrast to its effect on feeding, N-0437 did not affect drinking responses. Clifton *et al.* (1989) hypothesized that the increase in intake may have been due to stimulation of presynaptic dopamine autoreceptors, while the inhibition may have been due to stimulation of postsynaptic D_2 receptors.

In an unpublished study by Clifton and Cooper, (+)-SK & F 38393 (3 mg/kg) was administered to home-caged rats at the start of the night phase. Its effects on 24-h food and water intake are shown in Figure 14. The immediate effect of the D_1 receptor agonist was to increase the latency to the first meal, from a median value of 24 min in the control condition to a median value of 82 min. Subsequently, meal size was reduced, with no change in meal frequency. Drinking was relatively unaffected by the D_1 receptor agonist. Since the anorectic effect of SK & F 38393 was transient (lasting no more than 3 h), it would be advantageous to use the longer-acting compound A 68930 (DeNinno *et al.*, 1991) to gain fuller information on the effects of D_1 receptor stimulation on meal patterning.

Although there are only relatively few data from which to draw conclusions, it does appear that N-0437 (at anorectic doses) and SK & F 38393 both reduce the size of meals and meal duration, without affecting the frequency of meals. Since the meal pattern results refer essentially to nocturnal free-feeding, they may be relevant to the examples of potentiation which we have observed in nocturnal feeding rats (Figures 10 and 11). If that is the case, then D_1 and D_2 receptor stimulation may have convergent effects on feeding, i.e. to reduce meal size and duration. This leads to the prediction that the potentiation reflects a concerted effect on the size of meals; additional meal pattern studies are needed to confirm or refute this view.

8.5.2 Microstructural analysis of feeding

In further experiments, we have moved from continuous monitoring of free-feeding and drinking patterns over 24-h periods to a more detailed scrutiny of the effects of D_1 and D_2 receptor stimulation within the setting of a single meal. The paradigm we have adopted for this purpose is to train non-deprived rats to consume a palatable sweetened mash as a single meal, and to observe and record each bout of feeding. In addition, a variety of other behaviours (e.g. locomotion, rearing, grooming, sniffing) are also recorded.

8.5.2.1 The dopamine D_2 receptor agonist N-0437

In this experiment (Rusk and Cooper, 1989b), N-0437 (0.3–3.0 mg/kg, i.p.) produced a dose-dependent reduction in the consumption of the palatable food.

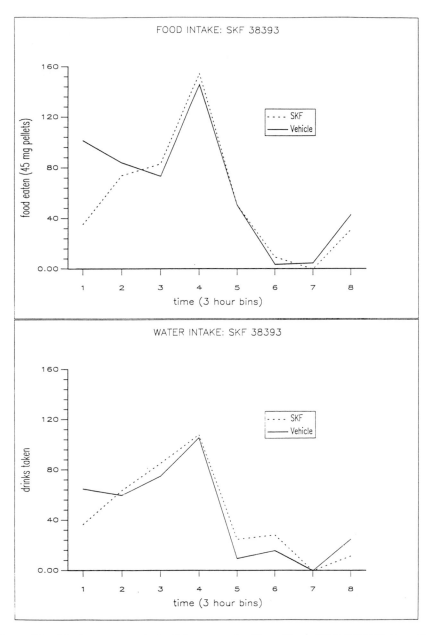

Figure 14 Meal pattern analysis of the anorectic effect of (+)-SK & F 38393 (3 mg/kg) in free-feeding and drinking rats. The experiment began at the start of the 12-h night period (night is equivalent to the first four 3-h bins), during which period most of the rats' feeding and drinking occurs. *Upper panel:* the dopamine D_1 receptor agonist substantially reduced food intake at the start of the night, but its effect was relatively short-lived. *Lower panel:* at the same time, it had little effect on drinking (Clifton and Cooper, unpublished data).

Somewhat surprisingly, it had no effect on the total duration of feeding, or on the frequency and duration of feeding bouts. Instead, its anorectic effect appeared to depend solely upon a reduction in the local rate of eating. In a recent confirmation and extension of this result, we found that quinpirole (0.03–0.3 mg/kg) dose-dependently reduced the food intake of 22-h food-deprived rats, and this was paralleled by a dose-dependent reduction in the rate of eating (Al-Naser and Cooper, unpublished data). Hence, an important consequence of selective D_2 receptor stimulation appears to be the reduction in eating rate which can lead to a reduction of food intake within a meal. Note that, earlier, we indicated that neither *d*-amphetamine nor cocaine decreased eating rate, and may, indeed, in some situations increase eating rate. In contrast, the non-selective dopamine receptor agonist apomorphine did reduce eating rate. Hence, apomorphine's anorectic effect can be linked to a reduction in eating rate, and may involve, at least in part, stimulation of D_2 receptors.

In addition to its effect on feeding, N-0437 also suppressed grooming but stimulated oral responses (licking, gnawing) and sniffing (Rusk and Cooper, 1989b). Suppression of grooming is a characteristic effect of D_2 receptor stimulation, since we have also observed it when quinpirole (0.03–3.0 mg/kg) was administered to rats (Al-Naser and Cooper, unpublished data). We noted above that cocaine is particularly effective in suppressing grooming (Cooper and van der Hoek, 1993), and its effect may depend upon D_2 receptor stimulation.

8.5.2.2   The dopamine D_1 receptor agonist SK & F 38393

Using the same microstructural approach, we have investigated the factors underlying the anorectic effect of SK & F 38393 (3 and 10 mg/kg, s.c.) (Cooper *et al.*, 1990). SK & F 38393 produced a slight reduction in eating rate, but also dose-dependently reduced the frequency of feeding bouts. It is interesting that cocaine also significantly reduced the frequency of feeding bouts (Table 1).

In contrast to the suppressant effect of the D_2 receptor agonists on grooming, SK & F 38393 significantly increased the duration of bouts of grooming (Cooper *et al.*, 1990). Moreover, SK & F 38393 did not induce oral behaviours, typical of the effects of D_2 receptor agonists. Since SK & F 38393 reduces food intake in the absence of the induction of stereotyped behaviour, it has been suggested that it may act directly on neural substrates involved in the control of feeding responses (Gilbert and Cooper, 1985; Martin-Iverson and Dourish, 1988).

8.5.2.3   The dopamine D_1 receptor agonist A 68930

We have recently carried out a microstructural analysis of the anorectic effect of A 68930 in non-deprived animals consuming a sweetened palatable diet. The results, shown in Figure 15, confirm quite strikingly the earlier data obtained with SK & F 38393. A 68930 (0.3 and 1 mg/kg, s.c.) significantly reduced food consumption, had a modest effect on eating rate but markedly reduced the

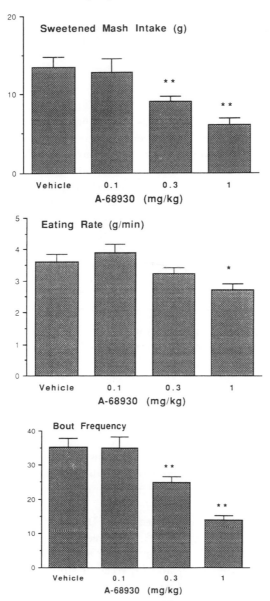

Figure 15 Microstructural analysis of the anorectic effect of the potent, selective dopamine D_1 receptor agonist A 68930 (0.1–1.0 mg/kg). *Upper panel:* A 68930 significantly reduced palatable food consumption in non-deprived animals. *Middle panel:* it slightly reduced eating rate at 1 mg/kg. *Lower panel:* it substantially reduced the frequency of eating bouts. The results are shown as mean + SEM. $n = 9$ per condition. Levels of significance for comparisons between individual dose conditions and the vehicle control: * $P < 0.05$; ** $P < 0.01$ (Dunnett's t-test) (Al-Naser and Cooper, unpublished data).

frequency of feeding bouts (Al-Naser and Cooper, unpublished data). Moreover, A 68930 (0.1–1.0 mg/kg) significantly increased grooming, but had no effect on oral behaviour.

8.5.2.4 Conclusions

While both D_1 and D_2 receptor agonists reduce the size of meals, it is quite clear that they achieve this effect by different means. D_1 receptor stimulation has comparatively little effect on the rate of eating but does reduce the frequency of feeding bouts. D_2 receptor stimulation, on the other hand, appears to achieve its main anorectic effect, within a meal, by reducing the rate of eating. Hence their effects are complementary, so that two important determinants of meal size, the frequency of feeding bouts and the rate at which food is consumed, can be affected if both D_1 and D_2 receptors are stimulated.

8.6 An interim synthesis

The experiments discussed in this chapter demonstrate quite clearly that either D_1 or D_2 receptor agonists are able to reduce food intake in a variety of feeding situations. The effects of selective dopamine D_1 agonists are, at first glance, rather easier to interpret because their anorectic effect can be obtained in the absence of induced gross stereotyped behaviour. There is some evidence, still relatively preliminary, that when small doses of a D_1 and a D_2 receptor agonist, respectively, are combined, a potentiation occurs and a profound anorectic effect may be elicited. This evidence establishes that a cooperative interaction between dopamine D_1 and D_2 receptor mechanisms may be important in our understanding of dopaminergic control of feeding. Certainly such data argue that further analysis of the nature of the interactions is of prime importance, and should be addressed.

Meal pattern experiments confirmed that a D_2 receptor agonist N-0437, and a D_1 receptor agonist, SK & F 38393, both reduced the sizes of spontaneous meals during nocturnal feeding in rats (Clifton *et al.*, 1989; Clifton and Cooper, unpublished results). Hence, D_1 and D_2 receptor stimulation may converge at the level of meal size, and produce the cooperative interaction seen when D_1 and D_2 agonists are combined. However, more detailed study using microstructural analysis reveals some interesting differences between the effects of D_1 and D_2 receptor agonists, respectively. D_2 agonists (e.g. N-0437, quinpirole) have a strong effect in reducing the rate of eating within a meal (Rusk and Cooper, 1989b; Al-Naser and Cooper, unpublished results). Conversely, a prominent effect of D_1 receptor agonists (e.g. SK & F 38393, A 68930) is to reduce the frequency of feeding bouts within a meal (Cooper *et al.*, 1990; Al-Naser and Cooper, unpublished results). Each of these effects should be examined in greater detail; for example, are both of these effects antagonized by either D_1 or D_2 receptor antagonists, or is the D_1 receptor-mediated effect on bout frequency only blocked by a D_1 receptor antagonist?. Likewise, is the D_2 receptor-mediated effect on eating rate only blocked by a D_2 receptor antagonist?

The pattern of results suggests *complementary effects* of $D_1:D_2$ receptor interaction. Release of dopamine prior to or during a meal may cause effects at both D_1 and D_2 receptors, producing distinctive effects which nevertheless complement each other. The common end result is a reduction in meal size, but achieved by different means. This kind of scheme suggests that a mixed D_1/D_2 receptor agonist like apomorphine should exert several dissociable effects on feeding behaviour. Indeed, the work of Willner and colleagues has shown that apomorphine not only reduced eating rate but also affected feeding bouts (Willner *et al.*, 1985; Muscat *et al.*, 1986). Indirectly acting dopamine agonists, like *d*-amphetamine or cocaine, reduce food consumption, but it is a feature of their actions that they do not reduce eating rate. They have a major effect in delaying the onset of feeding, and whether this represents a profound inhibition of the motivation to eat, or an interference from competing stereotyped responses, is an experimental issue that is often difficult to resolve.

The phenomenon of $D_1:D_2$ receptor interactions poses a set of problems in understanding the means by which central dopaminergic activity affects the motivation to feed, and the structure of feeding responses, across a range of feeding situations. It seems unlikely, given our present state of knowledge, that either one or other receptor is exclusively involved; instead, a useful working concept may be that of complementary interaction between the receptor subtype mechanisms determining the final outcome as it affects feeding behaviour.

Acknowledgements

We wish to thank Drs Clifton, Rusk and van der Hoek for their collaboration in some aspects of the work reviewed in this chapter. We also wish to thank John Francis and David Barber for their contributions to the work. Mrs Dorothy Trinder provided excellent assistance in preparing the manuscript.

References

Abbott, B., Starr, B.S. & Starr, M.S. (1991) *Pharmacol. Biochem. Behav.* **38**, 259–263.
Arnt, J., Hyttel, J. & Perregaard, J. (1987) *Eur. J. Pharmacol.* **133**, 137–145.
Balapole, D.C., Hansult, C.D. & Dorph, D. (1979) *Psychopharmacology* **64**, 121–122.
Barzaghi, F., Groppetti, A., Mantegazza, P & Muller, F. F. (1973) *J. Pharm. Pharmacol.* **25**, 909–911.
Blundell, J.E. & Latham, C.J. (1978) In *Central Mechanisms of Anorectic Drugs* (eds Garattini, S. & Samanin, R.), pp 83–109. New York, Raven Press.

Blundell, J.E. & Latham, C.J. (1980) *Pharmacol. Biochem. Behav.* **12**, 717–722.
Blundell, J.E. & Leshem, M.B. (1974) *Eur. J. Pharmacol.* **28**, 81–88.
Blundell, J.E. & McArthur, R.A. (1981) In *Anorectic Agents: Mechanisms of Action and Tolerance* (eds Garattini, S. & Samanin, R.), pp 19–43. New York, Raven Press.
Boja, J.W. & Kuhar, M.J. (1989) *Eur. J. Pharmacol.* **173**, 215–217.
Booth, D.A. (1968) *Nature* **217**, 869–870.
Bordi, F. & Meller, E. (1989) *Brain Res.* **504**, 276–283.
Braun, A.R. & Chase, T.N. (1986) *Eur. J. Pharmacol.* **131**, 301–306.
Britton, D.R., Kebabian, J.W. & Curzon, P. (1991) *Eur. J. Pharmacol.* **200**, 89–93.
Burridge, S.L. & Blundell, J.E. (1979) *Neuropharmacology* **18**, 453–457.
Carlisle, H.J. (1964) *J. Comp. Physiol. Psychol.* **58**, 47–54.
Church, W.H., Justice, J.B. Jr & Byrd, L.D. (1987) *Eur. J. Pharmacol.* **139**, 345–348.
Clifton, P.G. (1987) In *Feeding and Drinking* (eds Toates, F.M. & Rowland, N.E.), pp 19–35. Amsterdam, Elsevier Press.
Clifton, P.G., Rusk, I.N. & Cooper, S.J. (1989) *Pharmacol. Biochem. Behav.* **33**, 21–26.
Cooper, S.J. (1979) In *Chemical Influences on Behaviour* (eds Brown, K. & Cooper, S.J.), pp 533–597. London, Academic Press.
Cooper, S.J. & Dourish, C.T. (1990) In *Neurobiology of Stereotyped Behaviour* (eds Cooper, S.J. & Dourish, C.T.), pp 1–24. Oxford, Oxford University Press.
Cooper, S.J., Francis, J. & Barber, D.J. (1993) *Neuropharmacology* **32**, 101–102.
Cooper, S.J., Francis, J. & Rusk, I.N. (1990) *Psychopharmacology* **100**, 182–187.
Cooper, S.J. & Sweeney, K.F. (1980) *Neuropharmacology* **19**, 997–1003.
Cooper, S.J. & van der Hoek, G.A. (1993) *Brain Res.*, in press.
DeNinno, M.P., Schoenleber, R., Asin, K.E., MacKenzie, R. & Kebabian, J.W. (1990) *J. Med. Chem.* **33**, 2948–2950.
DeNinno, M.P., Schoenleber, R., MacKenzie, R., Britton, D.R., Asin, K.E., Briggs, C., Trugman, J.M., Ackerman, M., Artman, L., Bednarz, L., Bhatt, R., Curzon, P., Gomez, E., Kang, C.H., Stittsworth, J. & Kebabian, J.W. (1991) *Eur. J. Pharmacol.* **199**, 209–219.
Duterte-Boucher, D., Naudin, B. & Costentin, J. (1989) *Fundam. Clin. Pharmacol.* **3**, 337–346.
Eichler, A.J. & Antelman, S.M. (1977) *Commun. Psychopharmacol.* **1**, 533–540.
Foltin, R.W. & Fischman, M.W. (1989) *Pharmacol. Biochem. Behav.* **31**, 585–592.
Foltin, R.W., Woolverton, W.L. & Schuster, C.R. (1983) *J. Pharmacol. Exp. Ther.* **226**, 411–418.
Foltin, R.W., Kelly, T.H. & Fischman, M.W. (1990) *Appetite* **15**, 33–45.
Foote, R.W., Büscher, H.H., Römer, D., Maurer, R., Enz, A., Gähwiler, B.H., Shearman, G.T., Seiker, M.P. & Wüthrich, H. (1988) *Life Sci.* **42**, 137–152.
Gilbert, D.B. & Cooper, S.J. (1985) *Brain Res. Bull.* **15**, 385–389.
Groppetti, A., Zambotti, F., Biazzi, A. & Mantegazza, P. (1973) In *Frontiers in Catecholamine Research* (eds Usdin, E. & Snyder, S.H.), pp 917–925. New York, Pergamon Press.
Harris, S.C., Ivy, A.C. & Searle, L.M. (1947) *JAMA* **134**, 1468–1475.
Heffner, T.G., Zigmond, M.J. & Stricker, E.M. (1977) *J. Pharmacol. Exp. Ther.* **201**, 386–399.
Itoh, Y., Goldman, M.E. & Kebabian, J.W. (1985) *Eur. J. Pharmacol.* **108**, 99–101.
Izenwasser, S., Werling, L.L. & Cox, B.M. (1990) *Brain Res.* **520**, 303–309.
Kebabian, J.W. & Calne, D. (1979) *Nature* **277**, 93–96.
Kebabian, J.W., Briggs, C., Britton, D.R., Asin, K., DeNinno, M., MacKenzie, R.G., McKelvy, J.F. & Schoenleber, R. (1990) *Am. J. Hypertension* **3**, 40S-42S.
Kirkham, T.C. & Cooper, S.J. (1988) *Physiol. Behav.* **44**, 491–494.
Kruk, Z.L. (1973) *Nature New Biol.* **246**, 52–53.

Leibowitz, S.F. (1975) *Brain Res.* **84**, 160–167.
Leibowitz, S.F., Shor-Posner, G., Maclow, C. & Grinker, J.A. (1986) *Brain Res. Bull.* **17**, 681–689.
Lesses, M.F. & Myerson, A. (1938) *N. Engl. J. Med.* **218**, 119–124.
Longoni, R., Spina, L. & DiChiara, G. (1987) *Life Sci.* **41**, 2135–2145.
Martin, G.E., Williams, M., Pettibone, D.J., Yarbrough, G.G., Clineschmidt, B.V. & Jones, J.H. (1984) *J. Pharmacol. Exp. Ther.* **230**, 569–576.
Martin-Iverson, M.T. & Dourish, C.T. (1988) *Psychopharmacology* **96**, 370–374.
Meller, E., Bordi, F. & Bohmaker, K. (1988) *Life Sci.* **42**, 2561–2657.
Murray, A.M. & Waddington, J.L. (1990) *Pharmacol. Biochem. Behav.* **35**, 105–110.
Muscat, R., Willner, P. & Towell, A. (1986) *Eur. J. Pharmacol.* **123**, 123–131.
Neill, J.C. & Cooper, S.J. (1989) *Physiol. Behav.* **46**, 949–953.
Pettit, H.O. & Justice, J.B. Jr (1989) *Pharmacol. Biochem. Behav.* **34**, 899–904.
Pettit, H.O. & Justice, J.B. Jr (1991) *Brain Res.* **539**, 94–102.
Plaznik, A., Stefanski, R. & Kostowski, W. (1989) *Psychopharmacology* **99**, 558–562.
Rapoza, D. & Woolverton, W.L. (1991) *Pharmacol. Biochem. Behav.* **40**, 133–137.
Ritz, M.C., Boja, J.W., Zaczek, R., Carroll, F.I. & Kuhar, M.J. (1987) *Science* **327**, 1219–1223.
Rusk, I.N. & Cooper, S.J. (1988) *Physiol. Behav.* **44**, 545–553.
Rusk, I.N. & Cooper, S.J. (1989a) *Pharmacol. Biochem. Behav.* **34**, 17–22.
Rusk, I.N. & Cooper, S.J. (1989b) *Brain Res.* **494**, 350–358.
Setler, P.E., Sarau, H.M., Zirkle, C.L. & Saunders, H.L. (1978) *Eur. J. Pharmacol.* **50**, 419–430.
Silverstone, J.T. & Stunkard, A.J. (1968) *Br. J. Pharmacol. Chem.* **33**, 513–522.
Stellar, E. (1954) *Psychol. Rev.* **61**, 5–22.
Stoof, J.C. & Kebabian, J.W. (1984) *Life Sci.* **35**, 2281–2296.
Temlett, J.A., Chang, P.N., Oertel, W.H., Jenner, P. & Marsden, C.D. (1988) *Eur. J. Pharmacol.* **156**, 197–206.
Timmerman, W., Rusk, I.N., Tepper, P., Horn, A.S. & Cooper, S.J. (1989) *Eur. J. Pharmacol.* **174**, 107–114.
Towell, A., Muscat, R. & Willner, P. (1988a) *Pharmacol. Biochem. Behav.* **30**, 641–648.
Van der Weide, J., de Vries, J.B., Tepper, P.G. & Horn, A.S. (1986) *Eur. J. Pharmacol.* **125**, 273–282.
Van der Weide, J., Camps, M., Horn, A.S. & Palacios, J.M. (1987) *Neurosci. Lett.* **83**, 259–263.
Van der Weide, J., de Vries, J.B., Tepper, P.G., Krause, D.M., Dubocovich, M.L. & Horn, A.S. (1988) *Eur. J. Pharmacol.* **147**, 249–258.
van Rossum, J.M. & Simons, F. (1969) *Psychopharmacologia* **14**, 248–254.
Waddington, J.L. (1989) *J. Psychopharmacol.* **3**, 54–63.
Waddington, J.L., Molloy, A.G., O'Boyle, K.M. & Pugh, M.T. (1990) In *Neurobiology of Stereotyped Behaviour* (eds Cooper, S.J. & Dourich, C.T.), pp 64–90. Oxford, Oxford University Press.
White, F.J., Bednarz, L.M., Wachtel, S.R., Hjorth, S. & Brooderson, R.J. (1988) *Pharmacol. Biochem. Behav.* **30**, 189–193.
Willner, P., Towell, A. & Muscat, R. (1985) *Psychopharmacology* **87**, 351–356.

CHAPTER 9

REGULATION OF SEIZURE THRESHOLD BY D$_1$ VERSUS D$_2$ RECEPTORS

Michael S. Starr

Department of Pharmacology, School of Pharmacy, 29–39 Brunswick Square, London WC1N 1AX, UK

Table of Contents

9.1 Introduction

With an estimated 48 million sufferers worldwide, epilepsy is by far the commonest of the major neurological disorders. Many different forms of epileptic syndromes have been recognized and this heterogeneity is mirrored in the large variety of experimental models (Fisher, 1989) and in the complex classification schemes (Shorvon, 1990) that have been devised.

Children and adults suffering from epilepsy periodically experience a sudden and temporary burst of synchronous electrical activity in the limbic system or cerebral cortex, known as a seizure, which may be focal or generalized. The wide-ranging clinical manifestations that ensue (auras, arrest, confusion, loss of consciousness, convulsions etc.) are believed to reflect the different neuro-anatomical substrates and transmitter systems that are brought into play by the initial paroxysmal discharge. A better understanding of the associated neuro circuitry and its chemical transmitters not only provides a clearer insight into the aetiology of epilepsy, but also establishes a rational basis for developing new anticonvulsant drugs.

For many years noradrenaline was considered to be the catecholamine of prime importance for seizure control, with dopamine attracting only a passing interest. Historically there have been two major periods during which dopamine's status as an epileptic mediator has gained prominence. The first of these was in the 1970s, when researchers tackled the subject of dopamine in epilepsy in somewhat general terms, and an extensive literature accumulated on the effects of pharmacological manipulation of dopaminergic neurotransmission in a wide variety of seizure models. By modern standards, the compounds employed at this time lacked selectivity, and it was never entirely clear if they modified seizure susceptibility through an action on dopamine, or some other amine system (e.g. noradrenaline, 5HT). This chapter will attempt to convey a brief flavour of this early work, further information being readily available in earlier reviews of the subject (Bradford and Peterson, 1987; Jobe and Laird, 1981, 1987; Kresch *et al.*, 1987; Lamprecht, 1977; Snead, 1983).

A significant turning point came in the mid-1980s, when the concept of multiple dopamine receptors was firmly established and investigators were beginning to consider what effects the new generation of selective dopamine D_1 and D_2 receptor agonists and antagonists had on epileptic symptomatology. These studies are still very much in their infancy, but already it looks as though dopamine may have a multifaceted role in the development and spread of seizure activity, via its opposing actions at D_1 and D_2 sites, at least in some forms of epilepsy. Furthermore, there is anecdotal evidence to suggest that the D_1 and D_2 receptors that regulate epileptic behaviour are not the same as those controlling normal motor activity, and that interactions between the two sets of D_1 and D_2 receptors can take different forms. These latest findings offer new perspectives on D_1 / D_2 function in the brain and will be dealt with in some detail.

The concept of functionally discrete subgroups of D_1 and D_2 receptors may have a molecular basis in the burgeoning population of dopamine receptors recently uncovered by genetic cloning (Sokoloff *et al.*, 1990), which supports the existence of D_1 and D_2 superfamilies (Sunahara *et al.*, 1991; Van Tol *et al.*, 1991). These revelations must surely herald the start of a third era of dopamine

236

discovery with regard to epilepsy, as a result of which we may well see dopamine agonists realizing their therapeutic potential as anticonvulsants. Up till now, the anticonvulsant efficacy of drugs such as apomorphine and amphetamine has been limited by their brevity of action and/or intolerable side-effects (Anlezark et al., 1981; Quesney et al., 1981). All this could change, however, for if it can be shown that specific subcategories of dopamine receptors are localized to seizure-related neuronal pathways, it may be feasible to design novel anticonvulsants that specifically target them.

9.2 Non-specific dopaminergic influences on epilepsy

9.2.1 Mixed D_1/D_2 agonists

Much of our early appreciation of dopamine's role in epilepsy stems from investigations with the prototype D_1/D_2 dopamine agonist apomorphine. Figure 1 is a simplified view of a controversial literature on the subject. In the vast majority of experimental models of epilepsy, it will be seen that apomorphine raises the seizure threshold. There is some suggestion it does this by stimulating dopamine D_2 receptors, as several investigators have reported its antagonism by D_2 blockers such as haloperidol (Meldrum et al., 1975), spiroperidol (Dow et al., 1974) and pimozide (Farjo and McQueen, 1979). As in man (Quesney, 1981), apomorphine is particularly effective against 'reflex' forms of epilepsy and prevents the high-voltage EEG and myoclonic muscular contractions precipitated by stroboscopic light in genetically predisposed baboons (Ashton et al., 1976; Meldrum et al., 1975), and allays penicillin-induced epileptic photosensitivity in rats (Quesney, 1981). These similarities suggest a certain commonality of dopamine involvement in light-induced epileptic syndromes across different species.

Many other types of experimental seizure are amenable to inhibition by apomorphine, which is suggestive of a role for dopamine in their containment. Examples include the myoclonic jumping evoked by the administration of a high dose of 5-hydroxytryptophan (5-HTP) to guinea-pigs (Volkman et al., 1978), and the secondarily generalized seizures provoked in rats by a large systemic injection of the muscarinic cholinergic agonist pilocarpine (Turski et al., 1988). Focal seizures elicited by the chronic implantation of a cobalt-gelatine pellet, or by topical application of ouabain to the cortex, are similarly suppressed by apomorphine (Farjo and McQueen, 1979; Stach and Kacz, 1977). Apomorphine will also combine synergistically with other anticonvulsant treatments, as the latter authors found when apomorphine and aminooxyacetic acid were co-injected.

Where endogenous dopamine is thought to play a lesser or subsidiary role in controlling seizure expression, the exogenous dopaminergic influences of

237

NON-SPECIFIC ALTERATIONS IN D_1:D_2 BALANCE IN EPILEPSY MODELS

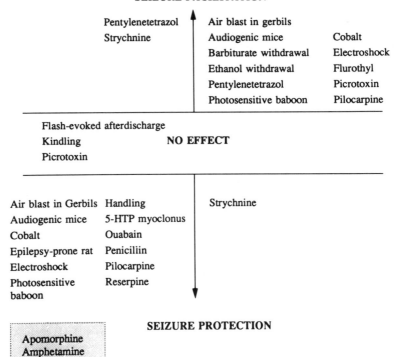

Figure 1   General effects of D_1 / D_2-unspecific drugs in experimental models of epilepsy.

apomorphine are correspondingly weaker. The fits elicited by the stress of handling, or a blast of air, in genetically epilepsy-prone gerbils, for instance, are only poorly curtailed by D_1/D_2 stimulation. A massive dose of apomorphine may be required (e.g. 16 mg/kg) (Schonfeld and Glick, 1980), which may only afford partial protection (e.g. 50%) (Cox and Lomax, 1976; Löscher, 1985). Likewise, only the clonic jerking phase of the running fit caused by a loud sound in DBA/2 strain mice, and not the subsequent tonic extension, is preventable with apomorphine (Anlezark *et al.*, 1981).

While abolition of seizures is by far the commonest result with apomorphine, it is by no means the only one. In the rat, Sandoval and Palermo-Neto (1989) noticed that apomorphine exacerbated convulsions induced by the glycine antagonist strychnine, but not by the GABA antagonist picrotoxin, pointing to a differential interaction between dopamine and the neuronal systems utilizing these two amino acids. Furthermore Anlezark *et al.* (1978) reported that apomorphine paradoxically potentiated the convulsant response to a sub-threshold dose of allylglycine in baboons, which contrasts with the beneficial effect the dopamine agonist has when administered on its own to these animals. That apomorphine can exert either pro- or anticonvulsant effects in the same species, depending on the seizure stimulus, is a positive indication of two directions of dopamine influence over epileptic symptoms.

Further evidence of a dual excitatory/inhibitory action of dopamine is seen in other models, where the actions of apomorphine are ambiguous. Some investigators have alleged that apomorphine increases seizure severity in the electroshock and pentylenetetrazol tests (Van Woert and Sethy, 1975), but this has been disputed (Kleinrok *et al.*, 1978). In a more recent analysis of the two types of epilepsy, Löscher and Czuczwar (1986) revealed an ameliorating effect of the dopamine agonist, and suggested that the disparate findings were a function of the drug dosage. The latter beneficial response was clearly a D_2 receptor-mediated phenomenon, as it was blocked with sulpiride, whereas the receptor mechanism aggravating seizures is unknown, but presumably is distinct from that conferring protection.

In yet other systems dopamine appears to be uninfluential on seizure development. The electrical afterdischarges detected in the rat's cortex after flashing light onto the retina, and which are said to mimic absence seizures (petit mal) in man, were unaffected by apomorphine (King and Burnham, 1980). As already noted, impairment of GABA-mediated inhibition with picrotoxin leads to a convulsion that is resistant to apomorphine, possibly because this occurs at a site distant from, or downstream of, apomorphine's action in the basal ganglia. The position of dopamine in electrical kindling of the amygdala is an interesting one. This much-studied method of inducing spontaneous ictal firing has traditionally been associated with noradrenergic rather than dopaminergic mechanisms (Corcoran and Mason, 1980). In agreement with this supposition, systemic apomorphine affected neither the acquisition of kindling (Callaghan and Schwark, 1979), nor the behaviour of the fully fledged kindled state (Ashton *et al.*, 1980). As we shall see later, however, a reinvestigation of the problem with selective D_2 agonists administered by microinjection directly into the nucleus accumbens disclosed a total blockade of focal and generalized seizures in half the kindled rats tested (Wahnschaffe and Löscher, 1991). This finding represents a radical departure from the long held belief in the unimportance of dopamine in the process of kindling. It also spotlights the intriguing and unanswered question of why, in so many experimental models of epilepsy, dopaminergic agents (even those selective for D_1 or D_2 receptors—see below) are often so poorly active by the systemic route as compared to intracerebral administration. The most parsimonious explanation is that dopamine regulates the induction and propagation of seizures in a complex fashion, involving different brain sites and subtypes of receptor, which are engaged indiscriminately by drugs when these are injected systemically, allowing an opportunity for opposing pro- and anticonvulsant effects to cancel each other out. If this proposal is correct, then many other types of epilepsy will clearly benefit from a systematic re-evaluation by selective dopaminergic agents applied to discrete brain structures, in order to delineate the precise role(s) of dopamine at different stages of the seizure process.

The predominantly anticonvulsant picture of dopamine, built up from the 1970s with apomorphine, is fully endorsed by parallel studies with l-DOPA and amphetamine (Figure 1). By and large, these two compounds display anticonvulsant profiles closely similar to apomorphine's. Since they also increase the synaptic availability of noradrenaline and/or 5-HT, it is not surprising that they are more effective than apomorphine in seizure models where these amines have been credited with a superior role, e.g. kindling and electroshock (Callaghan and Schwark, 1979; McKenzie and Soroko, 1972). Little can be done to improve the dopamine selectivity of amphetamine, but the selective conversion of l-DOPA into dopamine, and not noradrenaline, can be accomplished in the presence of a dopamine β-hydroxylase inhibitor. By adopting this strategy, the anti-convulsant response to l-DOPA was found to be antagonized completely by FLA-63 in mice subjected to maximal electroshock (McKenzie and Soroko, 1973), and by diethyldithiocarbamate in genetically seizure-prone rats (Ko et al., 1982) but not gerbils (Löscher, 1985). While it is hazardous to draw definitive conclusions from multiple drug treatments, these data nevertheless strongly support a preferential involvement of noradrenaline in the former two cases.

Dopamine uptake inhibitors have been used sparingly to investigate the relevance of dopamine in epilepsy. Trimble (1977) alluded to the potent anticonvulsant response to nomifensine in the baboon, but also mentioned that this might be due to the accumulation of noradrenaline as well as dopamine. Warter et al. (1988) more recently demonstrated a strong antagonism of spike-wave activity in the rat with nomifensine. The advent of newer and more selective inhibitors of the dopamine uptake carrier (e.g. GBR 12909) suggests that this approach could be used more profitably in the future.

9.2.2   Non-selective D_1 / D_2 antagonists

Complementary investigations with typical neuroleptics, the monoamine depleter reserpine or the catecholamine neurotoxin 6-hydroxydopamine (6-OHDA), collectively indicate that failure of dopaminergic neurotransmission in the brain is commensurate with an exacerbation of epileptic symptoms (Figure 1). This must mean not only that dopamine pathways have a functional input to brain centres responsible for the genesis or dissemination of ictal phenomena, but also that dopamine is released tonically to exert a predominantly stabilizing influence over these processes. Haloperidol and pimozide have come under the closest scrutiny in this regard, and through presumptive blockade of D_2 receptors they: (a) attenuate the anticonvulsant behaviour of dopamine agonists, (b) potentiate the range and severity of most seizure-promoting stimuli, and (c) are actively epileptogenic in their own right.

The latter property is sometimes quite subtle and may only be disclosed by EEG measurements, as Meldrum *et al.* (1975) demonstrated in the photosensitive baboon. Not only did haloperidol introduce an epileptiform pattern of spikes and waves into the spontaneous EEG, but it also greatly enhanced the paroxysmal EEG activity occurring as a result of photic stimulation, exactly as seen previously in psychiatric patients. All of these effects occurred with doses of haloperidol that lay within the accepted range for producing characteristic depression of motor behaviour (0.6–1.2 mg/kg), as evidenced by the severe sedation of the baboons. This is not invariably the case, however. As has already been indicated for dopamine agonists, disproportionately higher doses of neuroleptics are sometimes necessary to modulate epileptic syndromes. As an example, Turski *et al.* (1988) resorted to heroic doses of haloperidol (up to 8 mg/kg) to reliably sensitize rats to the limbic motor seizures evoked by pilocarpine. These were far in excess of the amount of drug required to produce immobility and muscle rigidity, and were quite out of character with the exquisite proconvulsant potency of the antagonist given by the intrastriatal route (ED_{50} 8.1 nmol). There is no reason to suppose that the focally injected haloperidol is working other than by occluding striatal dopamine D_2 receptors in these experiments, or that the systemically delivered drug is incapable of reaching its central site of action, which brings us back to the question of whether there are other haloperidol-sensitive receptors, in other regions of the brain, mediating an opposite effect on seizure expression. Again, one way of addressing this enigma would be to probe the likely areas with microinjections of a potent and selective D_2 antagonist.

Global depreciation of brain monoamine levels with reserpine or 6-OHDA is another way of lowering the seizure threshold and facilitating epileptic activity, and there can be little doubt that the loss of dopamine in particular is a major contributory factor in many cases (Figure 1) (Snead, 1983). Interestingly, whereas the convulsions produced by electroshock and pentylenetetrazol are facilitated by 6-OHDA pretreatment (Snead, 1983), these and strychnine-induced seizures are protected by MPTP, which depletes dopamine in the nigrostriatal system more selectively (Fariello *et al.*, 1987). As the response to strychnine and the tonic phase of maximal electroshock are thought to be mediated by bulbospinal structures, these authors suggested that a caudally projecting MPTP-sensitive dopamine system, originating in the substantia nigra, was responsible for controlling seizures that involve these hindbrain pathways. Thus while dopamine elsewhere in the brain appears to exercise an inhibitory restraint over the propagation of seizures, at the level of the nigra it would seem to act in the opposite fashion and facilitate their motor expression.

9.2.3 Interim summary

Several important inferences can be drawn thus far about dopamine's relationship with epilepsy. Firstly, and contrary to popular belief, there is abundant evidence that endogenous dopamine is tonically involved, to some degree, in the initiation and/or registration of most, if not all, types of experimental epilepsy. This usually takes a protective form, which is believed to be mediated by D_2 receptors, although a proconvulsant action mediated by an as-yet undisclosed receptor mechanism is also possible. There is some suggestion that these opposing pro- and anticonvulsant forces emanate from separate rostrocaudal sources, and are in constant competition with each other, with the anticonvulsant tendency normally prevailing. The notion that the dopamine receptors mediating epileptic influences are discrete from those regulating spontaneous motor behaviour is unproven as yet, but cannot be dismissed.

9.3 Specific D_1/D_2 influences on epilepsy

9.3.1 D_1 agonists

The behavioural properties of the benzazepine SK & F 38393, the first selective agonist of the D_1 receptor (Setler *et al.*, 1978), have been intensively studied for more than a decade, yet surprisingly little is known of SK & F 38393's effects on models of epilepsy. Ironically, with the evident expectation that SK & F 38393 might be anticonvulsant, like apomorphine before it, the first report on the subject dismissed any participation of D_1 receptors in the evolution of epilepsy (Löscher and Czuczwar, 1986). This is hardly surprising, as SK & F 38393 failed to modify amygdaloid kinding or pentylenetetrazol seizures in rats, or air blast seizures in gerbils (Figure 2). It did exhibit a species-dependent effect on the electroconvulsive threshold, however, which was increased in mice and lowered in rats (Löscher and Czuczwar, 1986). Unfortunately, the existing literature on dopamine involvement in maximal electroshock seizures was in a state of confusion at the time, and the fact that in the rat (but not in the mouse) apomorphine afforded protection against seizures via D_2 stimulation, while SK & F 38393 increased seizure severity via D_1 stimulation, did not merit special consideration.

Other inconclusive reports followed. Application of SK & F 38393 to hippocampal slices of the rat evoked a long-lasting partially SCH 23390-sensitive inhibition of spontaneously firing neurones (Smialowski and Bijak, 1987), and also powerfully suppressed the epileptiform discharges triggered by lowering the

SPECIFIC ALTERATIONS IN D_1:D_2 BALANCE IN EPILEPSY MODELS

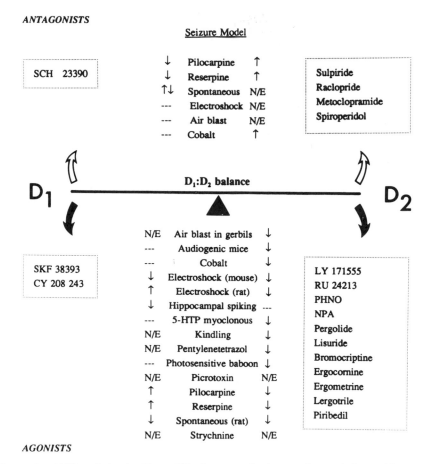

Figure 2 Ability of selective D_1 and D_2 drugs to raise (upward arrow), lower (downward arrow) or have no effect on (N/E) seizure susceptibility in experimental models of epilepsy.

external calcium concentration (Smialowski, 1990). These data are in line with the desynchronizing effects of SK & F 38393 on the hippocampal EEG reported by Ongini *et al.* (1986), which was blocked with SCH 23390 and duplicated with LY 171555, a D_2 agonist. They further suggest that the lowering of penicillin-induced epileptic bursting of CA2-CA3 neurones in the hippocampus by dopamine was also a D_1 receptor-mediated event (Suppes *et al.*, 1985). Warter *et al.* (1988) similarly discovered that SK & F 38393 dose-dependently subdued the epileptic spiking that occurred in the frontoparietal cortex of rats undergoing spontaneous, generalized non-convulsive (petit mal-like) seizures. In sharp contrast to these obviously protective effects of SK & F 38393, the D_1 agonist elicited exactly the opposite response from both hippocampal and cortical cells in rats treated with a threshold convulsant dose of pilocarpine (Barone *et al.*, 1990), where electrographic analysis revealed synchronous firing developing in both regions, eventually leading to status epilepticus. So, in the normal brain, SK & F 38393 by itself elicits EEG changes predictive of an anticonvulsant action, but whether D_1 activation accentuates or attenuates epileptogenesis in practice would seem to depend on the nature of the seizure stimulus.

The first hint that stimulating D_1 receptors might reliably evoke a proconvulsant response in the whole animal came with the serendipitous observation that reserpine-treated mice exhibited a brief running fit, culminating in a tonic and often fatal convulsion, on being treated with SK & F 38393 and then placed in a novel environment for the purposes of behavioural observation (Starr *et al.*, 1987). This effect was later shown to be dose-dependent and totally blocked by SCH 23390, confirming its mediation by D_1 receptors (Al-Tajir *et al.*, 1990a).

Reserpinized mice could also be made to convulse with the phenanthridine derivative CY 208-243, a novel agonist with unusual properties (Al-Tajir *et al.*, 1990a). In mouse striatal homogenates, CY 208–243 binds with high affinity to both D_1 and D_2 recognition sites (Jackson *et al.*, 1989), but in the whole animal it gives the appearance of being a selective D_1 agonist, with a behavioural profile indistinguishable from that of SK & F 38393 (Abbott *et al.*, 1991; Chandler *et al.*, 1990; Markstein *et al.*, 1986). It is reasonable to assume, therefore, that CY 208-243 is also convulsant through the auspices of D_1 receptor activation. Turski *et al.* (1988) later remarked that '5/7 rats receiving SK & F 38393 and pilocarpine ... died in the course of severe convulsions', which appeared to indicate that SK & F 38393 was behaving as a seizure promoter in this model. However, no quantification of the latent proconvulsant action of SK & F 38393 was possible as the compound was only administered with a maximally convulsant dose of the cholinergic agonist. Importantly, this work served to re-focus attention on the utility of muscarinic stimulation of the limbic system with pilocarpine, as a convenient means of rapidly inducing intractable generalized convulsions that mimic the secondarily generalized seizures commonly observed in man. Although these convulsions do not respond to some conventional anticonvulsant drug treatments, e.g. carbamazepine and phenytoin (Meldrum, 1988), they are open to manipulation by dopaminergic drugs. As a result, this paradigm was subsequently used to good effect to demonstrate, beyond any doubt, the existence of two opposing epileptic influences of dopamine in the brain: a protective one mediated by D_2 receptors and a facilitatory one mediated by D_1 receptors.

In 1990 reports were published by three independent research groups on the seizure-enhancing qualities of SK & F 38393 in pilocarpine-treated rats (Al-Tajir *et al.*, 1990a, b; Barone *et al.*, 1990; Turski *et al.*, 1990). A threshold convulsant amount of pilocarpine (200 mg/kg, i.p.), administered together with methyl-scopolamine to minimize peripheral autonomic effects, induced automatisms (head scratching, gustatory movements, sniffing etc.) and EEG changes. These appeared as a theta rhythm in the hippocampus and a low-voltage fast activity in the cerebral cortex, with occasional high-voltage spikes originating in the hippocampus and spreading to the cortex (Barone et al., 1990). Electrographic seizures did not usually develop and the EEG pattern returned to normal within 1–2 h. In the additional presence of SK & F 38393, however, the behavioural and electrographic manifestations were much more striking. Well-synchronized, high-voltage spiking was evident in the hippocampus and cortex, with recurrent electrographic seizures, as illustrated in Figure 3. The accompanying behavioural changes followed a strict temporal sequence of head bobbing, forelimb myoclonus, rearing and falling, which increased in frequency until they were virtually continuous and the animal was said to be in status epilepticus. In severe cases the animals convulsed tonically and fatally. Extensive brain damage was detected postmortem in limbic and basal ganglia structures (Turski et al., 1989). Essentially, SK & F 38393 did not alter the latency to onset of the seizures, but heightened their frequency, severity and lethality, with resultant electrical, behavioural and neuropathological sequelae that were identical to those described for a larger dose of the cholinomimetic injected alone. All of these SK & F 38393-induced epileptic responses were completely prevented by the D_1 antagonist SCH 23390 (Al-Tajir et al., 1990a, b; Barone et al., 1990; Turski et al., 1990). Closely similar results have been obtained with CY 208-243 versus pilocarpine-induced limbic seizures in the mouse (Figure 2) (Burke et al., 1990).

One interesting point to emerge from these studies is that both SK & F 38393 and CY 208-243 induced convulsions at dose levels that were approximately 10-fold lower than those normally required to promote hypermotility and grooming, two of the cardinal signs of D_1 receptor activation in tests of motor function (Barone et al., 1990; Chandler et al., 1990; Starr and Starr, 1986). On the basis of these potency differences, it was suggested that two functionally discrete, and possibly anatomically distinct, subpopulations of D_1 receptors were separately responsible for the transmission of seizure-related and motor-related signals in the brain.

The inability of D_1 receptor stimulation by CY 208-243 to alter the seizure threshold to picrotoxin or strychnine in the mouse (Burke et al., 1990) would seem to indicate that neither convulsion falls within the jurisdiction of the basal ganglia, where the seizure-modulating effects of dopaminergic drugs are believed to originate (see below). The result with picrotoxin was not entirely unexpected, in view of apomorphine's earlier lack of effect in this model (Sandoval and Palermo-Neto, 1989). On the other hand, since apomorphine's prominent anticonvulsant effect in many other seizure models had generally been attributed to the D_2-stimulant component of its action (Seeman, 1981), it was felt that its paradoxical ability to augment seizures in the strychnine model (Sandoval and Palermo-Neto, 1989) might be related instead to its D_1-stimulant capacity, like its effects on the EEG (Ongini et al., 1986). In the event, the matter remained unresolved, for neither the mixed D_1/D_2 agonist apomorphine nor the D_1-like

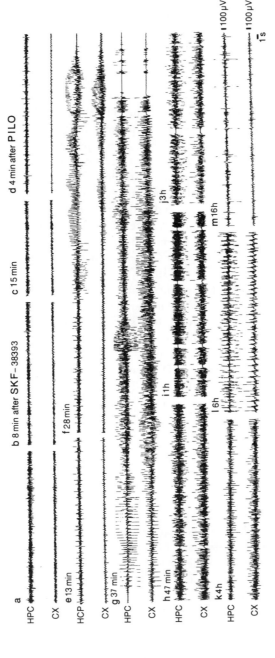

Figure 3 Bilateral intranigral SK & F 38393 (40 pmol) increases susceptibility to convulsions induced by pilocarpine (PILO, 200 mg/kg, i.p., 15 min later) in the rat. High-voltage fast activity and spiking develop in the hippocampus (HPC) which becomes progressively synchronized with the cortex (CX). Electrographic seizure is evident at 28 min, developing into status epilepticus by 47 min with gradual abatement after 4–6 h. Reproduced from Turski *et al.* (1990).

agonist CY 208-243 altered the animals' sensitivity to strychnine in the later study by Burke et al. (1990).

9.3.2 D_2 agonists

Most ergot derivatives have a complex pharmacology which includes a strong stimulant action at dopamine D_2 receptors (Seeman, 1981). Next to apomorphine and amphetamine, this class of agonists has formed the mainstay of dopaminergic D_2 investigations in epileptology. Their overriding effect in different epilepsy models is to raise the seizure threshold, but seldom to lower it (Figure 2), thereby lending credence to the notion that the historical anticonvulsant efficacies of mixed D_1/D_2 agonists are attributable to their greater affinities for D_2 rather than D_1 receptor sites.

Several ergot compounds with dopaminomimetic activity, such as bromocriptine, ergocornine and ergometrine, have the ability to inhibit reflex epilepsy, though unlike apomorphine they were more effective in the photosensitive baboon than in audiogenic epilepsy-prone mice (Anlezark et al., 1981). Such variability in the anticonvulsant potency of ergots can usually be traced to interference from non-dopamine receptors, especially those for 5HT, which have an important impact on seizure outcome depending on the species and experimental model. Lisuride, which is ostensibly one of the most potent dopamine D_2 agonists available (Cote et al., 1983), provides a classic example.

In low doses, lisuride predictably outperformed apomorphine in powerfully suppressing the focal seizures induced by cortical cobalt implants in the rat (Farjo and McQueen, 1979), as well as SK & F 38393-induced and pilocarpine-induced limbic motor seizures in the mouse (Al-Tajir et al., 1990a; Al-Tajir and Starr, 1991b). Comparable doses in the gerbil, however, never afforded greater than 30% protection against tonic–clonic convulsions, even though it was possible to abolish the air blast seizures completely with weaker dopamine agonists (Löscher and Czuczwar, 1986). The key to this anomaly lay in the attendant pattern of motor behaviour, which switched from being dopamine-like at low doses to more conspicuously 5HT-like at higher doses of lisuride. Since the 5HT precursor 5HTP was itself proconvulsant in the gerbil, it is tempting to suggest that functional antagonism from 5HT activation was the most likely factor limiting lisuride's D_2-mediated anticonvulsant effect in these experiments.

A similar dichotomy may occur in other models of epilepsy, where clear disparities are evident between the effectiveness of dopaminergic drugs in modifying seizure activity and in binding to D_2 receptors. For instance, with seizures evoked by pentylenetetrazol, kindling and electroshock (Löscher and Czuczwar, 1986), as well as spontaneous non-convulsive epilepsy (Warter et al., 1988), drugs such as lisuride, pergolide and bromocriptine often displayed no clear dose-dependency in their anticonvulsant action, which took the form of a truncated dose–response curve and toxicity at high doses. Apart from kindling, apomorphine was undeniably the more effective anticonvulsant in these situations. In the absence of substantive evidence of antagonism by selective D_2 blockers, information relating to the performance of lisuride and similar receptor-unselective ergots in seizure models must therefore be viewed with caution.

The substituted ergot LY 171555 (Tsuruta *et al.*, 1981), and other new-generation drugs such as RU 24213 (Euvrard *et al.*, 1980) and PHNO (Martin *et al.*, 1984), exhibit a much greater preference for dopamine D_2 receptors and are beginning to find application in epilepsy research. The results, however, are proving to be no less enigmatic!

In the pilocarpine model in the mouse, the order of anticonvulsant potency of assorted D_2 agonists was reported to be PHNO > pergolide > lisuride = LY 171555 ≫ RU 24213, which roughly paralleled their motor stimulant actions, i.e. PHNO > pergolide = lisuride > LY 171555 = RU 24213 (Al-Tajir and Starr, 1991b). However, other comparative studies indicated that D_2-dependent seizure protection and D_2-dependent behavioural excitation did not necessarily go hand in hand. For example, in spite of PHNO being consistently more active than lisuride in promoting hypermotility and stereotyped behaviours, the anticonvulsant profiles of these two D_2 agonists varied considerably. These were shown to range from PHNO = lisuride versus air blast convulsions in gerbils, to PHNO ≫ lisuride and lisuride ≫ PHNO against electroconvulsions in the mouse and rat respectively (Löscher and Czuczwar, 1986). A similar discrepancy was noted between the two compounds LY 17155 and RU 24213, which were invariably roughly equipotent as behavioural stimulants in the mouse and rat, yet only LY 171555 possessed anticonvulsant activity when challenged with pilocarpine in these species (Al-Tajir and Starr, 1991b). As already intimated for the D_1 agonists, these conflicting observations provide strong support for the hypothesis that D_2 agonists modulate the transmission of seizure- and motor-related signals in the brain through two pharmacologically distinct populations of D_2 receptors.

The seizure-inhibiting property of LY 171555 has been examined in some detail. The compound had no effect on the seizure threshold to picrotoxin or strychnine (Burke *et al.*, 1990), but it robustly blocked pilocarpine seizures when administered by the intracerebral (Al-Tajir and Starr, 1990, 1991a, b; Turski *et al.*, 1988) and subcutaneous routes (Al-Tajir *et al.*, 1990a; Burke *et al.*, 1990). Curiously, LY 171555 afforded no such protection if injected into the peritoneal cavity (Turski *et al.*, 1990), and it is interesting to note that the characteristic increase in locomotion occasioned by intraperitoneal LY 171555, failed to materialize in animals receiving pilocarpine shortly afterwards (Barone *et al.*, 1990). Although Ongini *et al.* (1986) described a pronounced EEG activation with systemic LY 171555, comparable to that elicited by SK & F 38393, no changes in brain electrical activity were detected with intrastriatal LY 171555 (Turski *et al.*, 1990) (Figure 4). LY 171555 applied focally to the striatum nevertheless suppressed all signs of seizure generation in the hippocampus and

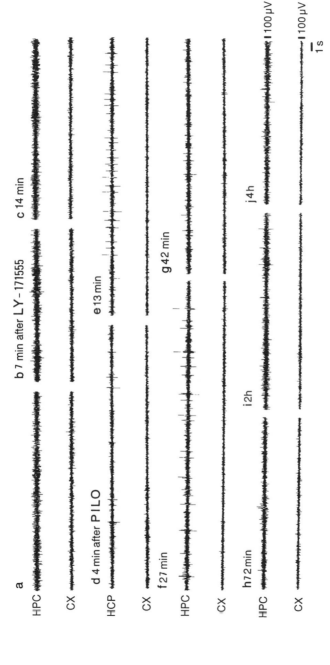

Figure 4 Anticonvulsant effect of bilateral intrastriatal LY 171555 (4 pmol) in a rat challenged 15 min later with 380 mg/kg i.p. pilocarpine (PILO). Isolated spikes appear in the hippocampus (HPC) but not cortex (CX), but these are short-lived. Reproduced from Turski *et al.* (1990).

cortex, in response to a convulsant dose of pilocarpine, and totally prevented all seizure-related damage to the neuropil in these and other susceptible brain structures, e.g. amygdala, thalamus, substantia nigra (Turski et al., 1990). The reversal of LY 171555's anticonvulsant action by haloperidol (Turski et al., 1990) and metoclopramide (Al-Tajir et al., 1990a) further attests to this being a D_2 receptor-mediated process.

From the foregoing, it will be seen that LY 171555 and SK & F 38393 behave as exact opposites in every respect, as far as their influence on the secondarily generalized seizures induced by cholinergic excitation of the limbic system is concerned. All elements of the motor seizure are enhanced by the D_1 agonist and opposed by the D_2 agonist, beginning with its initiation in the hippocampus, through to its behavioural expression via basal ganglia nuclei and its eventual widespread neurotoxicity. We may therefore deduce that endogenous dopamine also exerts a bidirectional effect on the genesis and propagation of seizures, via its opposite actions at D_1 and D_2 receptors. Whether this holds true for all seizures, irrespective of how they are evoked, remains to be determined. Nevertheless, the signs are that a D_2-mediated protective function of dopamine prevails in the majority of seizure models, given that artificial depletion of dopamine in the brain is pro- rather than anticonvulsant (Figure 1).

This raises the question of whether the dysfunction of dopamine systems in the brain is an important causative factor in the development of seizures in animals and man. Over the years, biochemical measurements of dopamine content and turnover have revealed significant reductions in these parameters in the brains of genetically epilepsy-prone, kindled and pentylenetetrazol-treated rats, as well as in epileptic chickens and following ischaemia-induced epilepsy (Snead, 1983). Similar decrements have been detected in the lumbar CSF and ictal foci removed from human patients (Hiramatsu et al., 1982; Mori et al., 1997; but see Pintor et al., 1990). There is consequently a compelling body of data which says that dopaminergic function is indeed compromised in at least some forms of artificial and congenital seizures. However, whether dopamine hypoactivity is related causally or casually to these epileptic processes remains unclear.

In the light of what has been said about dopamine exerting a dual D_1-facilitatory and D_2-inhibitory influence over ictal processes, perhaps we should be asking ourselves how the D_1/D_2 balance is altered in epilepsy, rather than looking at gross changes in the dopamine systems as a whole. Receptor measurements are already beginning to furnish us with interesting information on this issue, but the overall picture is still very much in a state of flux.

Repeated electroconvulsive shock, for instance, increased the number of D_1 receptor binding sites in the substantia nigra (Fochtmann et al., 1989) and accelerated their turnover into the striatum (Nowak and Zak, 1989), at the same time as liberating large amounts of extracellular dopamine in the striatum (Nomikos et al., 1991). Animals subjected to this procedure were found to be hyperresponsive to the behavioural effects of SK & F 38393 (Sharp et al., 1990), and so it is conceivable that their heightened D_1 receptivity will also have a bearing on their seizure susceptibility. Dopamine's role in amygdaloid kindling is also being reassessed, after finding deficits in D_1-dependent adenylyl cyclase activity in the amygdala and frontal cortex of kindled rats (Gee *et al.*, 1980), with corresponding increments in D_2 binding in the nucleus accumbens ipsilateral (but not contralateral) to the kindling electrode (Csernansky *et al.*, 1988). This knowledge has already been used to good effect by Wahnschaffe and Löscher (1991), who recently reported that stimulation of this specific D_2 receptor pool accomplished what so many other investigators had previously failed to achieve with systemic dopaminomimetics, namely a profound dopamine-dependent suppression of kindled seizures. Future topographic analyses cannot expect to be so iconoclastic, yet they could hold the key to unravelling the seizure relevance of the newly discovered dopamine receptor subtypes, all of which have close associations with limbic areas of the brain (Sokoloff *et al.*, 1990; Sunahara *et al.*, 1991; Van Tol *et al.*, 1991).

9.3.3 D_1 antagonists

We have already seen that SCH 23390 inhibits the modulatory influences of D_1 agonists in various seizure states, but what of the D_1 antagonist itself? One characteristic of the ascending dopamine systems in the brain is that they are continuously active. Thus if seizure activity is tonically regulated via dopamine released onto D_1 receptors, D_1 blockade with SCH 23390 should disclose it.

Given in small doses (<0.1 mg/kg), SCH 23390 caused a moderate and transitory increase in the duration of spontaneous spike and wave discharges from the frontoparietal cortex of generally epilepsy-prone rats, in contrast to the depressant action of SK & F 38393 (Warter *et al.*, 1988). Larger doses of SCH 23390 (0.5 mg/kg) had the reverse effect, and reduced cortical firing, but this was not considered to be mediated by D_1 receptors.

In rats and mice made to convulse with a high dose of pilocarpine, or with a low dose of pilocarpine following lithium sensitization, there is a general consensus that SCH 23390 is anticonvulsant (Al-Tajir *et al.*, 1990a, b; Al-Tajir and Starr, 1990; Barone *et al.*, 1990, 1991; Burke *et al.*, 1990). Barone *et al.* (1990, 1991) found that the D_1 antagonist was exquisitely potent in this respect, preventing the electrical seizures, but not the theta rhythm or low-voltage activity, induced by cholinergic stimulation in the hippocampus and cortex. At the same time the motor seizures, status epilepticus and death were inhibited in a dose-dependent fashion, starting with as little as 0.01 mg/kg SCH 23390. The limbic stereotypies induced by pilocarpine were resistant to SCH 23390 treatment, suggesting that D_1 receptors were primarily involved in the mechanism of epilepsy generalization. That SCH 23390 was noticeably more efficacious versus lithium/pilocarpine than pilocarpine seizures is arguably attributable to lithium's sensitization of dopamine receptors.

Work from our own laboratory supports the principle that D_1 blockade is anticonvulsant *per se,* except that much higher doses of the benzazepine were required to give effective protection, possibly due to differences in the strain and species of animals used. SCH 23390 was never 100% anticonvulsant in the mouse, even up to 0.8 mg/kg (Burke *et al.,* 1990). There was never any doubt that SCH 23390 was gaining entry to the brain in these experiments, as the severe sedation of the animals clearly demonstrated. Likewise, in the rat, SCH 23390 (0.25 mg/kg) significantly delayed the appearance of forelimb myoclonus, and diminished the severity and lethality of the seizures, but not their frequency (Al-Tajir *et al.,* 1990a). At these elevated dose levels, there was some concern that SCH 23390 owed its seizure-inhibiting effect to the blockade of $5HT_2$ receptors (McQuade *et al.,* 1988). However, the interaction of 5HT systems with epilepsy is complex and the report by Janusz and Kleinrok (1989), which pointed out that any benefits of interfering with 5HT were likely to be achieved by occluding $5HT_{1B} > 5HT_{1A}$ sites, did much to dispel this worry.

These difficulties with the apparent inefficacy of systemic SCH 23390 were reconciled by injecting the compound directly into the corpus striatum (Al-Tajir and Starr, 1990), or substantia nigra (Al-Tajir *et al.,* 1990b), from which regions a considerably greater anticonvulsant response was obtained. This finding is perhaps a tacit admission that SCH 23390 influences seizure activity at more than one point in its development. Extrapolating from the data of Warter *et al.* (1988), we could envisage that systemic SCH 23390 treatment might enhance epileptogenesis in the hippocampus, only to impair the subsequent propagation of the seizure by the basal ganglia. Targetting the drug discretely at basal ganglia nuclei would avoid any such conflict with the hippocampus, and allow it to realize its full anticonvulsant potential. Intrahippocampal delivery of the D_1 antagonist, on the other hand, should be proconvulsant. It will be interesting to see if this prophecy is fulfilled by experiment.

9.3.4 D_2 antagonists

D_2 antagonists have a much longer history of association with epilepsy, because many of the traditional neuroleptic drugs (e.g. chlorpromazine, haloperidol), which owe their clinical antipsychotic effects to D_2 receptor blockade (Seeman, 1981), also promote epilepsy (Trimble, 1977). Chlorpromazine, for instance, exacerbates existing photosensitive reflex epilepsy, and EEG measurements reveal a pattern of epileptiform activity developing in the brains of patients receiving haloperidol. There are a host of other examples of neuroleptic-enhanced epilepsy in man, supporting the idea that seizure activity in the brain is normally held in check by an underlying D_2-dependent dopaminergic tone (Lamprecht, 1977; Trimble, 1977). The seizure-enhancing property of D_2 blockers is not peculiar to chronic treatment of psychiatric patients, as it has also been amply demonstrated on many occasions with neuroleptics administered acutely in a wide variety of animal models. The actions of these compounds have already been discussed (Figure 1) and will not be elaborated further here.

The synthesis of newer, more selective D_2-blocking agents, such as the benzamide class of drugs, allows a more direct test of the above theory. In a genetic rat model of non-convulsive epilepsy, Warter et al. (1988) found that neither sulpiride nor tiapride significantly altered the electrical activity of the epileptic cortex, even at dose levels that were heavily sedating, or even toxic. These results were at variance with the potentiating effects that haloperidol fluphenazine and pimozide had in this test system. However, because the D_1 antagonist SCH 23390 was also potently proconvulsant, it looks as though the facilitation of the spontaneous seizures by these drugs was more closely related to their actions at D_1 than at D_2 recognition sites.

Sulpiride also failed to modify the seizures generated by electroshock in mice or by an air stimulus in gerbils (Löscher and Czuczwar, 1986), and together with metoclopramide was inactive against pilocarpine seizures in rats and mice (Al-Tajir et al., 1990a; Burke et al., 1990). The accompanying behavioural depression indicated that the benzamides were centrally active, while their ability to reverse the anticonvulsant responses evoked by various dopaminomimetics showed they were also capable of blocking D_2 receptors controlling the seizure threshold. It must be remembered that the capacity of neuroleptics to facilitate epileptic syndromes is clearly going to depend on the prevailing dopaminergic tone and the sensitivity of the dopamine receptors, and these in turn may change with the seizure model. Lithium treatment, as used to sensitize animals to the convulsive action of pilocarpine, is believed by some to have a profound effect on dopaminergic mechanisms, which could explain why Barone et al. (1991) were able to evoke convulsions in a large percentage of rats given lithium/pilocarpine, with modest doses (1 mg/kg) of the D_2 blockers raclopride and haloperidol. Even so, these doses were still 100-fold higher than comparable amounts of SCH 23390 giving protection, and it is a truism that D_1 receptor occlusion is by far the more efficacious of the two forms of dopamine inhibition, when it comes to modifying seizure severity.

9.4 $D_1 : D_2$ interactions in epilepsy

One of the most celebrated features of the D_1 and D_2 receptors that regulate motor behaviour is their functional interdependence. This usually takes the form of positive cooperativity, in which it is necessary to stimulate D_1 receptors in order that D_2-mediated behaviours (e.g. motility, stereotypy) are fully expressed (see Chapter 3). Occasionally, however, the reverse is true, and the blockade of D_1 receptors releases D_2-dependent responses (e.g. jerking) that are not ordinarily seen. Similarly interactions can also be shown to take place between the D_1 and D_2 receptors controlling epileptic syndromes.

The first suggestion that this might be so came from Warter et al. (1988), based on the anecdotal evidence that selective D_1 and D_2 agonists and antagonists were generally less effective than mixed $D_1:D_2$ drugs in modifying spike and wave discharges in the rat. These authors concluded that, as with motor behaviour, D_1 and D_2 stimulation worked together beneficially to modulate the epileptic firing of cortical neurones. However, no direct test of this hypothesis with combinations of selective D_1 and D_2 drugs was carried out.

From what has already been said about the opposite influences of D_1 and D_2 receptor stimulation in other models of epilepsy, we might reasonably expect D_1 and D_2 agonists, when co-injected, to cancel out each other's effects in these systems. This is precisely what occurred in the reserpine-treated mouse (Figure 5), where the convulsant action of SK & F 38393 was counteracted by the simultaneous administration of apomorphine, the more selective D_2 agonists LY 171555 and RU 24213, and of course by D_1 blockade with SCH 23390 (Al-Tajir et al., 1990a).

The intractable limbic seizures produced by pilocarpine in rodents also exhibit bimodal susceptibility to D_1 and D_2 stimulation, being accentuated by SK & F 38393 and attenuated by LY 171555 (Al-Tajir et al., 1990a; Burke et al., 1990). For reasons that are not understood, Turski et al. (1990) were unable to replicate the systemic anticonvulsant response to LY 171555, although they did find that as little as 4 pmol of the D_2 agonist was potently anticonvulsant in the striatum (Turski et al., 1988). Curiously, intraperitoneal injections of LY 171555, which by themselves were without any effect on the animals' sensitivity to pilocarpine, interacted synergistically with SK & F 38393 to facilitate seizure development (Table 1). SK & F 38393, at 0.01 mg/kg, was below the threshold for potentiating seizures to a subconvulsant dose of pilocarpine (200 mg/kg), but could be made to do so in the presence of increasing doses of LY 171555. This is therefore the first recorded case of cooperative $D_1:D_2$ synergism in a model of epilepsy. The paradoxical finding was reproduced in mice treated with a subconvulsant mixture of CY 208-243 and pilocarpine, but only at the highest dose of 4.5 mg/kg LY 171555 (Table 1) (Starr, unpublished data). Ordinarily, 4.5 mg/kg LY 171555 is sufficient to inhibit completely the development of these motor seizures in the mouse (Burke et al., 1990). In the same seizure model, then, D_2 stimulation with LY 171555 can be either beneficial or harmful, depending on the dose or route of administration.

The switch from LY 171555 being anticonvulsant at low doses to proconvulsant at high doses could simply signify the onset of non-specific toxicity unrelated to D_2 receptor stimulation, or it could mean that there are two populations of receptors with opposite functions in epilepsy and different affinities for LY 171555. Further experimentation with other D_2 agonists will be required to clarify this puzzling result. Meanwhile, our earlier tentative suggestion, that the unusually low *systemic* efficacy which many dopaminergic drugs display in models of epilepsy could be explained if the drugs were simultaneously engaging D_2 receptors mediating opposite pro- and anticonvulsant responses, begins to look more tenable.

What makes the above results doubly intriguing is that the seizure-enhancing

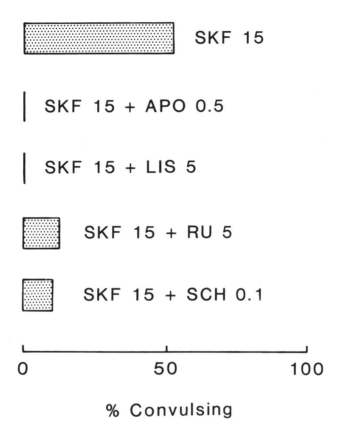

Negative D1:D2 interaction

in reserpine treated mice

SKF 15

SKF 15 + APO 0.5

SKF 15 + LIS 5

SKF 15 + RU 5

SKF 15 + SCH 0.1

0   50   100

% Convulsing

Figure 5 Antagonism of D_1-induced convulsions in reserpine-treated mice by various D_2 agonists and SCH 23390. SKF, SK & F 38393; APO, apomorphine; LIS, lisuride; RU, RU 24213; SCH, SCH 23390. Data from Al-Tajir *et al.* (1990a).

effects of D_1 stimulation in rats and mice were just as readily augmented by *blocking* D_2 receptors as they were by stimulating them. Burke *et al.* (1990) tested a number of typical (haloperidol, metoclopramide) and atypical neuroleptics (sulpiride, clozapine, thioridazine) in the pilocarpine-treated mouse, none of which facilitated limbic seizures on their own, but all of which interacted synergistically to potentiate the convulsant tendency of subthreshold D_1 receptor stimulation (Table 2). A similar positive interaction was noted between

Table 1 Potentiation of D_1-induced convulsions by D_2 stimulation in pilocarpine-treated rodents.

Treatment	Dose (mg/kg)	% convulsing to subthreshold dose of pilocarpine	
		Rats	Mice
Vehicle	—	0/4	0/8
LY 171555	2	0/4	0/8
	5	1/5	0/8
	10	4/6	0/9
	20	7/7*	5/9**

Rats received SK & F 38393 (0.1 mg/kg), methylscopolamine (1 mg/kg) and doses of LY 171555 as shown, before pilocarpine (200 mg/kg). Mice received CY 208-243 (0.1 mg/kg), methylscopolamine (1 mg/kg) and doses of LY 171555 as shown, before pilocarpine (100 mg/kg). * $p < 0.01$, ** $p < 0.025$ versus vehicle. Data from Turski *et al.* (1990) and Starr (unpublished).

Table 2 Synergism between the convulsant effects of neuroleptics and CY 208-243 in pilocarpine-treated mice.

Neuroleptic	Dose (mg/kg)	% convulsing to 100 mg/kg pilocarpine	
		Saline	CY 208-243 (0.375 mg/kg)
Vehicle	—	5.0	21.4
Haloperidol	1	0	75.0*
	4	0	100**
Sulpiride	10	0	50.0*
	50	0	75.0*
Metoclopramide	1.25	0	75.0*
	6.25	0	100**
Clozapine	0.5	0	37.5
	2	0	75.0*
	10	100	100
Thioridazine	0.5	0	75.0*
	2	0	100**
	10	100	100

All neuroleptics were injected 60 min, CY 208-243 and methylscopolamine (1 mg/kg) 30 min before pilocarpine. * $p < 0.05$, ** $p < 0.01$ versus controls ($n = 6$–14). Data from Burke *et al.* (1990).

Table 3 Lack of interaction between the anticonvulsant effects of D_2 stimulation and D_1 blockade in pilocarpine-treated mice.

Treatment	Dose (mg/kg)	% convulsing to 400 mg/kg pilocarpine		
		Saline	SCH 23390 (0.05 mg/kg)	SCH 23390 (0.2 mg/kg)
Vehicle	—	90.9	100	42.8
LY 171555	0.167	75.0	75.0	62.5
	0.5	50.0	50.0	50.0
	1.5	50.0	75.0	37.5
	4.5	0*	0*	0*

SCH 23390 was injected 60 min, methylscopolamine (1 mg/kg) and LY 171555 30 min before pilocarpine. * $p < 0.005$ versus vehicle ($n = 6-11$). Data from Burke et al. (1990).

haloperidol and SK & F 38393 in rats challenged with a subconvulsant dose of the cholinergic stimulant (Turski et al., 1990). By contrast, no functional interaction whatsoever was detected between the protective effects of the D_1 antagonist SCH 23390 and the D_2 agonist LY 171555 (Table 3).

The differential results of these various drug interaction studies provide an indirect clue that endogenous dopamine is perhaps tonically more active at D_2 than D_1 receptors, i.e. is physiologically anticonvulsant. This is illustrated in Figure 6. Let us assume that, under normal conditions, endogenous dopamine is liberated tonically and is active at both D_1 and D_2 receptors, but that the latter effect predominates and provides the animal with a modest background level of seizure resistance (i.e. $D_2 > D_1$). This D_2-anticonvulsant effect is not maximal and can therefore be intensified (i.e. $D_2 \gg D_1$) by exogenous D_2 agonists like LY 171555, whereas exogenous D_1 agonists such as SK & F 38393 and CY 208-243 will reverse the order of receptor dominance in favour of convulsions (i.e. $D_1 > D_2$). Neuroleptics block the D_2 receptors and thereby release the opposite D_1 proconvulsant tendency, but this is normally inherently weak and so convulsions do not necessarily ensue. If, however, additional D_1 stimulation is provided externally, then a supra-additive anticonvulsant response is expressed. On the other hand, since dopamine's action at the D_1 site is judged to be weak, its removal by SCH 23390 does not supplant the powerful anticonvulsant action expressed through the D_2 receptor by LY 171555, which consequently interacts non-additively with the D_1 antagonist.

Before we can assign anatomical meaning to this scheme, we first have to pinpoint the sites of action of the dopaminergic drugs referred to above. This can best be done by intracerebral infusion of the compound into a designated part of the brain immediately prior to seizure induction.

D1 and D2 actions and interactions in epilepsy

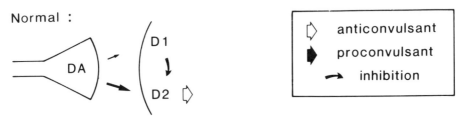

Normal :

D1 agonist :

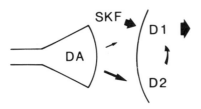

D1 agonist + D2 antagonist :

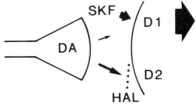

D2 agonist :

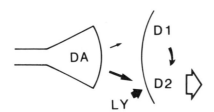

D2 agonist + D1 antagonist :

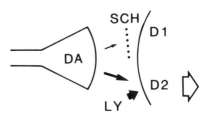

Figure 6 Schematic view of $D_1:D_2$ interactions in pilocarpine-treated mice. Abbreviations: DA, dopamine; SKF, SK & F 38393; HAL, haloperidol; LY, LY 171555; SCH, SCH 23390. Results indicate synergism between the proconvulsant effects of D_1 stimulation and D_2 agonists in this model, but non-additive anticonvulsant effects of simultaneous D_2 stimulation and D_1 blockade. Actions of endogenous dopamine are presented as being $D_2 > D_1$ dominant. Data from Burke *et al.* (1990).

9.5 Sites of D_1 and D_2 action in epilepsy

It has long been recognized that the basal ganglia in general, and the corpus striatum and substantia nigra in particular, are inhibitory towards the genesis and behavioural expression of epilepsy. Various neural circuits and transmitter systems contribute to these effects, as discussed by Meldrum (1988) and Turski *et al.* (1988, 1989). Prominent among these are the nigrostriatal dopamine and striatonigral GABA pathways. Precisely how the epileptic influences of these two systems are disseminated to other parts of the brain is still controversial, and lies outside the scope of this discussion, which will focus instead on the known sites of activity of dopaminergic drugs as revealed by their discrete stereotaxic injection into the brain (Figure 7).

One of the first intracerebral microinjection studies was performed by Farjo and McQueen (1979), who reported that unilateral or bilateral dosing of the striatum with relatively large amounts of dopamine (25 μg) or apomorphine (60 μg) significantly diminished cobalt-induced focal epilepsy. A possible striato pallidothalamocortical circuit was suggested to mediate these responses.

Turski et al. (1988) obtained similar beneficial effects against pilocarpine-induced seizures with much smaller quantities of apomorphine (ED_{50} 1.6 pmol) or the selective D_2 agonist LY 171555 deposited into the rostralmost segment (but not mid-body) of the caudate-putamen, indicating a very specific localization of this anticonvulsant function. Apomorphine was without effect in the overlying neocortex or globus pallidus, but was equiactive in the limbic areas of the nucleus accumbens and olfactory tubercle (Figure 7). These responses to apomorphine were abolished by haloperidol co-administered focally (1 nmol) or systemically (1 mg/kg). Moreover, the butyrophenone itself actively promoted pilocarpine seizures with an intrastriatal ED_{50} of 8.1 pmol. Further studies from our own laboratory confirmed that LY 171555 was anticonvulsant, but not proconvulsant, in these forebrain regions (Al-Tajir and Starr, 1990, 1991a, b), but not in the substantia nigra pars compacta or pars reticulata (Al-Tajir et al., 1991b; Turski et al., 1990). Strangely, no protection was obtained with intrastriatal RU 24213, a selective D_2 agonist structurally different from LY 171555, but nonetheless comparable to LY 171555 in its behavioural profile. The reasons for this disparity are unknown, but could further indicate that the dopamine receptors mediating motor and epileptic events are pharmacologically distinguishable.

Interestingly, the ability of striatal D_2 receptors to limit seizure propagation appears to depend on the functional integrity of the overlying cerebral cortex. Inadvertent damage to the cortex caused by cannula implantation, or the deliberate placement of punctate kainic acid lesions into the primary motor area of the cortex dorsal to the striatum, prevented seizure suppression by instrastriatal LY 171555 (Al-Tajir and Starr, 1991a).

The observation that amygdala or hippocampal kindling increased the density of accumbens D_2 receptors in the same hemisphere (Csernansky et al., 1988) led Wahnschaffe and Löscher (1991) to discover that intra-accumbens LY 171555 (4 or 40 pmol) would potently suppress all kindling parameters. A larger amount of LY 171555 (400 pmol) showed a reduced effect, reminiscent of the emergence of an opposite proconvulsant action of systemic LY 171555 at high doses (Table 1).

Intrahippocampal injection of apomorphine (0.1–1 μg) greatly attenuated the epileptogenic spiking induced by penicillin in the cat, as also did sulpiride

Sites of action of D1 and D2 drugs

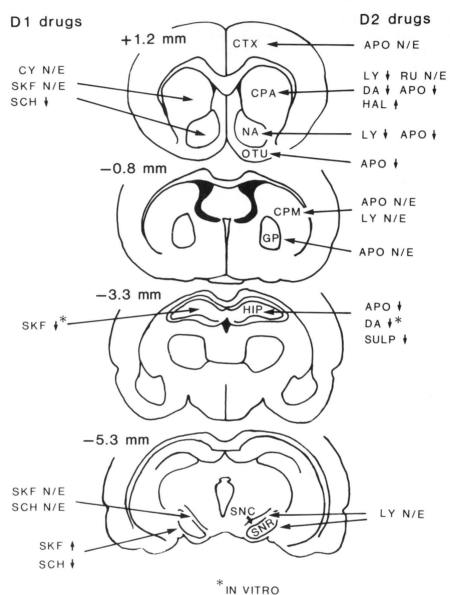

Figure 7 Schematic view of epileptic responses to D_1 and D_2 drugs microinjected into different brain areas. CTX, cortex; CPA, anterior caudate-putamen; CPM, mid-body caudate-putamen; NA, nucleus accumbens; OTU, olfactory tubercle; GP, globus pallidus; HIP, hippocampus; SNC, substantia nigra pars compacta; SNR, substantia nigra pars reticulata; APO, apomorphine; LY, LY 171555; RU, RU 24213; CY, CY 208-243; SKF, SK & F 38393; DA, dopamine; HAL, haloperidol; SULP, sulpiride; SCH, SCH 23390. Drugs shown as increasing (upward arrow), decreasing (downward arrow) or having no effect (N/E) on seizure susceptibility.

in 1/3 animals (La Grutta and Sabatino, 1990). These data are in line with hippocampal neuronal excitability being depressed by D_1 agonists (in this case apomorphine) and increased by D_2 agonists. More importantly, they show that the sphere of dopamine's influence over epileptic processes extends beyond the major dopaminergic areas of the basal ganglia, and highlight the functional relevance of lesser known dopamine systems at the site of seizure induction. Fariello et al. (1987) alluded to the control of strychnine seizures by dopamine at the level of the spinal cord, and Quesney (1981) hypothesized that the abolition of generalized photosensitive epilepsy by apomorphine could be due to its inhibitory action on neurones in the cortex. It is quite likely, therefore, that dopamine in other brain areas will be found to have a significant role in seizure control.

Dopamine D_1 receptors are distributed just as widely, and often in higher densities, than D_2 sites across the brain (Dawson et al., 1988), yet less is known of their contribution to cerebral mechanisms. Turski et al. (1988) dismissed any involvement of D_1 receptors in anticonvulsant processes in the striatum, where local injections of SK & F 38393 (4 pmol) failed to protect rats against pilocarpine convulsions. If anything, the seizures were more severe. Al-Tajir and Starr (1990) corroborated this finding with SK & F 38393 and CY 208-243 deposited into the caudate-putamen and nucleus accumbens. Similarly, intra-accumbens SK & F 38393 did not influence the duration or intensity of the motor and limbic seizures kindled from the amygdala, nor the local afterdischarges (Wahnschaffe and Löscher, 1991). It would be worth exploring the in vivo effects of SK & F 38393 injected directly into the hippocampus in these models, however, given the ability of D_1 stimulation to attenuate epileptic firing of hippocampal cells in vitro (Smialowski, 1990; Suppes et al., 1985).

Because D_1 receptors were particularly abundant in the substantia nigra, which was renowned for its role in seizure containment (Iadorola and Gale, 1982), this nucleus seemed a logical site of origin of the proconvulsant action noted with systemic D_1 agonists. Bilateral intranigral treatment with SK & F 38393 confirmed this suspicion, by lowering the convulsive threshold to pilocarpine in an SCH 23390-sensitive fashion (Al-Tajir et al., 1990b; Turski et al., 1990). Conversely, SCH 23390 delivered into the pars reticulata of both nigras was significantly anticonvulsant, a finding later reproduced with the D_1 antagonist from the nucleus accumbens and all rostrocaudal levels of the caudate-putamen (Figure 7) (Al-Tajir and Starr, 1990).

Though limited in scope, these stereotaxic studies provide a fascinating insight into the sites and possible mechanisms by which dopamine regulates epileptic activity in the brain. Three important inferences can be drawn: (a) dopamine can regulate both the induction and the propagation of seizures from many brain areas, including the hippocampus, nucleus accumbens, olfactory tubercle, caudate-putamen and substantia nigra pars reticulata; (b) D_1 influences are much more widespread than D_2, being evident in all of the aforementioned structures, whereas D_2 influences have so far only been demonstrated convincingly in a circumscribed rostral part of the striatal complex; (c) the potencies of D_1 and D_2 dopaminergic drugs (especially antagonists) in modifying pilocarpine seizures are often dramatically higher by the intracerebral route, possibly because systemic treatment gives them global access to multiple and mutually antagonistic sites of action across the brain.

9.6 Possible D_1 and D_2 mechanisms in epilepsy

Experimental evidence suggests that dopamine may affect all aspects of seizure activity, from its inception through to its behavioural expression, via its actions at D_1 and D_2 receptors located principally in the limbic system and cerebral cortex, and in executive structures such as the striatal complex, globus pallidus and substantia nigra. The cellular mechanisms of dopamine's actions in these different brain areas, however, are thought to be quite different.

9.6.1 Epileptic focus

The primary aberration at the epileptic focus (in the hippocampus, amygdala or cerebral cortex) is currently believed to be overactivity of the excitatory glutamatergic input, which synchronizes the spontaneous bursting of local neurones and initiates interictal hyperexcitability (Bradford and Peterson, 1987). Being physiologically active in these areas, dopamine must be viewed as a putative modulator of the repetitive firing process.

Dopamine has a complex effect on hippocampal epilepsy. In line with dopamine's dual D_1-inhibitory/D_2-excitatory action on hippocampal cell firing rate (Smialowski and Bijak, 1987), the D_1 agonist SK & F 38393 desynchronized the hippocampal EEG (Ongini et al., 1986) and produced a SCH 23390-sensitive antagonism of the epileptiform discharges evoked in the CA1 subfield of the rat's hippocampus by low external calcium (Smialowski, 1990). Suppes et al. (1985) documented a similar beneficial effect of dopamine versus penicillin-induced spiking in the CA2–CA3 region of the guinea-pig hippocampal slice, but did not identify the receptor mechanism with selective antagonists. Contrary to the above D_1 and D_2 neuronal actions of dopamine, however, SK & F 38393 caused synchronization of the hippocampal EEG in pilocarpine-treated rats (Barone et al., 1990). Further, the anticonvulsant effect of stimulating the nigrohippocampal dopamine pathway in penicillin-treated cats was attenuated by haloperidol and sulpiride, both D_2 antagonists (La Grutta and Sabatino, 1990). Since spontaneous bursts are thought to arise principally in CA2–CA3 'pacemaker' cells and then spread to drive the CA1 pyramidal neurones, which exhibit a different physiological responsivity to dopamine (Suppes et al., 1985), it is possible that these variations in hippocampal response to D_1 and D_2 dopaminergic drugs involve different cellular elements of the hippocampus. Dopamine lengthens the duration of the afterhyperpolarization of hippocampal cells, but this does not fully explain its anticonvulsant property, which may also result from increases in conductance and membrane potential, as well as presynaptic modulation of the release of other transmitters.

Early extracellular recordings documented a profound inhibitory effect of dopamine on cell firing in various areas of the cortex (e.g. Krnjevic and Phillis, 1963) as well as the amygdala (Ben-Ari and Kelly, 1976). Later experiments with selective D_1 and D_2 agonists failed to confirm this finding, and demonstrated instead a D_2-dependent excitatory response to LY 171555 in the rat's cerebral cortex, with SK & F 38393 being totally ineffective (Bradshaw et al., 1985). More remote electrographic measurements have further confused the issue, disclosing net inhibitory D_2 and both excitatory and inhibitory D_1 effects on cortical electrical activity of drugs whose locus of action may lie elsewhere in the brain (Barone et al., 1990; Ongini et al., 1986; Warter et al., 1988). These disparities, plus the shortage of direct information on dopamine–epilepsy interrelations in the cortex, preclude meaningful discussion of dopamine's contribution to cortical epileptogenesis at this stage.

9.6.2 Striatal complex

As well as modulating their induction at source, dopamine also interferes with the transmission of seizures via pathways connecting with the basal ganglia, and thence with principal executive centres in the globus pallidus and substantia nigra.

Focal injection of SCH 23390 or haloperiodol into the nucleus accumbens or caudate-putamen of the rat respectively raised and lowered the convulsive threshold to pilocarpine, indicating that endogenous dopamine is normally tonically active at both D_1 and D_2 receptors in these regions (Al-Tajir and Starr, 1990; Turski et al., 1988). However, since D_2 agonists and dopamine protected against seizures from these same areas, while D_1 agonists were ineffectual, we can deduce that D_2 receptors play a dominant role in seizure containment in the corpus striatum (in contrast to the hippocampus). The opposing influences on epilepsy mediated by striatal D_1 and D_2 receptors could reflect a simple interplay between their respective postsynaptic hyperpolarizing and depolarizing actions on striatal neurones. By activating D_2 receptors and exciting GABAergic striatonigral projection neurones, dopamine would enhance synaptic inhibition in the nigra and prohibit further seizure spread (Iadorola and Gale, 1982). D_1 agonism would theoretically work in the opposite direction by diminishing striatonigral GABA activity and removing the brake on seizure transmission.

The anticonvulsant action of dopamine in the striatum appears to depend on the functional integrity of corticostriatal glutamate neurones, as kainate lesions of the overlying cerebral cortex eliminated the protective action of intrastriatal LY 171555 against pilocarpine seizures (Al-Tajir and Starr, 1991a). Activation of NMDA-type glutamate receptors in the striatum is likewise anticonvulsant

(Turski *et al.*, 1987), which means the beneficial effect of D_2 agonists in this part of the brain might be due to the stimulation of presynaptic D_2 receptors on the corticostriatal axon terminals (Schwarcz *et al.*, 1978) and the consequent release of glutamate (Godukhin *et al.*, 1984). However, most investigators find that dopamine *inhibits* rather than excites glutamate output. A more plausible explanation, in line with recent behavioural data, is that the dopamine–glutamate interaction takes place postsynaptically, with glutamate facilitating the response of striatal neurones to dopamine.

9.6.3 Substantia nigra

The nigra can influence both epileptogenesis and the bilateral generalization of limbic epileptic foci, via nigrothalamocortical and nigroreticulocortical feedback circuits, as well as the behavioural expression of seizures via its nigrotectospinal connections. Dopamine released from nigral dendrites can theoretically modulate epileptic events in one of several ways. Firstly, by activating inhibitory D_2 autoreceptors present on the dopamine cells, it will diminish the amount of the catecholamine released tonically in target structures. This, as we have already seen, would tend to be epileptogenic. In practice, however, intranigral LY 171555 conspicuously failed to modify seizures at all, suggesting that D_2 mechanisms are of little importance in this respect in this nucleus.

The second possibility is that dopamine can affect seizure evolution and/or propagation via D_1 receptors located on the largely GABAergic relay neurones (Dawson *et al.*, 1988). Seizure susceptibility is inversely related to the level of synaptic inhibition in the substantia nigra pars reticulata (Iadorola and Gale, 1982), so that any procedure which increases or mimics GABA's action in this nucleus is effectively anticonvulsant. There is a well-defined population of presynaptic D_1 receptors on the axon terminals of nigrostriatal GABA neurones. Stimulating these receptors facilitates GABA outflow in nigral slices (Starr, 1987), which would be expected to decrease rather than increase seizure susceptibility, and so cannot be the mechanism of SK & F 38393's proconvulsant action *in vivo* (Al-Tajir *et al.*, 1990b; Turski *et al.*, 1990).

Postsynaptically, D_1 receptors mediate excitation and D_2 receptors mediate inhibition of nigral output neurones (Matthews and German, 1986). SK & F 38393 could therefore exacerbate epilepsy from the pars reticulata by directly activating efferent pathways to the thalamus and tectum, unlike GABA, which reduces impulse flow in these projections. Dopamine released from dendrites in the nigra is also excitatory towards these cells, both by directly stimulating their D_1 receptors (as SK & F 38393) and by activating their D_2 receptors, which in turn antagonizes GABA-mediated inhibition (as LY 171555) (Waszczak, 1990; Waszczak and Walters, 1986). Either of these two actions, as well as autoinhibition of the dopamine pathways, would suggest that hyperactivity of dopamine in the nigra invariably favours seizure development, in direct contrast to the predominantly seizure-preventative effects of dopamine in striatal and hippocampal terminal regions.

It would appear, then, that dopamine liberated from opposite ends of the nigrostriatal and nigrohippocampal axes has the potential either to lower or raise the animal's susceptibility to seizure stimuli. Which of these options is exercised under physiological conditions will depend on the factors that control the dendritic and axonal release of dopamine. As Cheramy et al. (1984) have clearly demonstrated, these processes can occur independently of each other, indicating that physiological mechanisms exist in the brain which are theoretically capable of altering the balance of dopamine's activity at proconvulsant and anticonvulsant sites.

9.7   Expanding dopamine receptor nomenclature: clinical implications

One can sense the buzz of excitement generated by the recent disclosures of further D_3, D_4 (D_2-like) and D_5 (D_1-like) receptor subtypes, with the prospect of more receptors still to come. If discriminative ligands for these different recognition sites can be found, they promise to revolutionize the clinical management of dopamine-related neurological disorders.

To begin with, the potent anticonvulsant property of D_2 agonists might be therapeutically exploitable, provided this action can be separated pharmacologically from undesirable behavioural, endocrine and emetic effects. But first, we must determine if other dopamine receptors are involved. The high density of D_3 receptor mRNA in the nucleus accumbens and olfactory tubercles (Sokoloff et al., 1990) overlaps appreciably with the limbic anticonvulsant site of action of apomorphine and LY 171555, both of which are good D_3 stimulants. However, while D_3 receptors may contribute to the regulation of seizure spread in the ventral striatum, this is evidently not the case in the caudate-putamen, which does not transcribe the D_3 gene.

Conversely, the existence of a limbic D_4 receptor showing a high selectivity for the atypical antipsychotic clozapine (Van Tol et al., 1991) provides a molecular basis for the synthesis of a new breed of neuroleptics that are devoid of D_2-mediated extrapyramidal, endocrine and proconvulsant side-effects. In certain biochemical and behavioural paradigms, clozapine has been likened to the D_1 antagonist SCH 23390 which, as we have already seen, potently suppresses limbic-derived seizures induced by pilocarpine in the rodent. If the new benzonaphthazepine SCH 39166 proves ineffectual against schizophrenia in current preclinical tests, it may be worth considering if this type of drug offers any practical advantages for the amelioration of secondarily generalized seizures, the equivalent and commonest form of human epilepsy.

265

For the time being these therapeutic considerations remain purely speculative, whereas the seizure-promoting capacity of D_1 agonists constitutes an immediate and serious problem. This class of drug is currently being explored for its antiparkinson potential, in spite of the danger signs of epileptogenesis being clearly visible with D_1 agonist treatments in both rodent and primate models of Parkinson's disease. If these harmful effects are already apparent with the relatively weak, partial D_1 agonists investigated thus far, parkinsonian patients regaining their mobility with more potent, full agonists of the D_1 receptor, are just as likely to throw a fit! This problem may not be insuperable, because the 10-fold potency separation for the convulsant and motor stimulant actions of SK & F 38393 and CY 208-243 suggests that different subcategories of the D_1 receptor might mediate these responses. Although the D_5 receptor identified by Sunahara *et al.* (1991) has a 10-fold higher affinity for dopamine, this is unlikely to be the receptor lowering the seizure threshold, as it is localized primarily within the limbic regions of the brain and is scarce in the basal ganglia. Such a pattern of distribution is inconsistent with the SK & F 38393-induced potentiation of convulsions obtained from the substantia nigra. Other D_1 receptors are known to exist (D_{1A}, D_{1B} etc.) whose role in epilepsy remains to be determined. The first pharmacological probes for these new receptors, that will allow these theories to be put to the test, are eagerly awaited.

9.8 Conclusions

Although dopamine has been dismissed for so long as being largely irrelevant to epilepsy, studies with D_1 and D_2 ligands now suggest that there is a much closer involvement of dopamine with the mechanisms of seizure induction and execution than previously thought, particularly in limbic epilepsy. The onset and development of pilocarpine-induced seizures, for example, are altered bidirectionally via D_1 and D_2 receptors. D_1 stimulation exacerbates and D_2 stimulation ameliorates the epileptic state. Whilst these two influences are mutually exclusive, the protective D_2 response generally predominates. This explains why mixed D_1/D_2 agonists gave a net, though often weak, anticonvulsant effect (and vice versa for most neuroleptics), and why the harmful effects of D_1 receptor activation have previously gone unnoticed.

Topographic mapping has disclosed a discrete D_1-dependent proconvulsant site in the substantia nigra pars reticulata, and a D_2-dependent anticonvulsant site in the anteroventral striatum and associated limbic structures, although an action of dopamine within the epileptic focus cannot be ruled out. The potencies of D_1 and D_2 dopaminergic drugs modifying seizure and motor thresholds often differ widely, contributing to the general feeling that the D_1 and D_2 receptors which control epileptic sensitivity are both pharmacologically and anatomically distinct from those which regulate motor behaviour. Moreover, there is an undercurrent of anecdotal evidence, suggesting that a further functional dichotomy may exist within the D_1 and D_2 receptor groups themselves. That is to say, certain subpopulations of D_1 receptors (e.g. hippocampal) may prevent rather than worsen the seizure condition, and the converse could also be true of D_2 receptors. The picture will become clearer as these theories are put to the test in future stereotaxic experiments, which will also have to consider the roles of D_3, D_4 and D_5 dopamine receptors in epilepsy.

From a clinical standpoint, it may be possible to exploit the above differences to produce therapeutically useful dopaminergic anticonvulsants, which are devoid of motor effects, as well as novel antiparkinson drugs and atypical antipsychotics that do not cause epilepsy as a side-effect.

References

Abbot, B., Starr, B.S. & Starr, M.S. (1991) *Pharmacol. Biochem. Behav.* **38**, 259–263.

Al-Tajir, G. & Starr, M.S. (1990) *Eur. J. Pharmacol.* **191**, 329–336.

Al-Tajir, G. & Starr, M.S. (1991a) *Neuroscience* **43**, 51–57.

Al-Tajir, G. & Starr, M.S. (1991b) *Pharmacol. Biochem. Behav.* **39**, 109–113.

Al-Tajir, G., Chandler, C.J., Starr, B.S. & Starr, M.S. (1990a) *Neuropharmacology* **29**, 657–661.

Al-Tajir, G., Starr, M.S. & Starr, B.S. (1990b) *Eur. J. Pharmacol.* **182**, 245–251.

Anlezark, G., Horton, R. & Meldrum, B. (1978) *Biochem. Pharmacol.* **27**, 2821–2828.

Anlezark, G., Marrosu, F. & Meldrum, B. (1981) In *Neurotransmitters, Seizures and Epilepsy* (eds Morselli, P.L., Lloyd, K.G., Löscher, W., Meldrum, B.S. & Reynolds, E.H.), pp 251–259. New York, Raven Press.

Ashton, C., Anlezark, G. & Meldrum, B.S. (1976) *Eur. J. Pharmacol.* **39**, 399–401.

Ashton, D., Leysen, J.E. & Wauquier, A. (1980) *Life Sci.* **27**, 1547–1556.

Barone, P., Parashos, S.A., Palma, V., Marin, C., Campanella, G. & Chase, T.N. (1990) *Neuroscience* **34**, 209–217.

Barone, P., Palma, V., De Bartolomeis, A., Tedeschi, E., Muscettola, G. & Campanella, G. (1991) *Eur. J. Pharmacol.* **195**, 157–162.

Ben-Ari, Y. & Kelly, J.S. (1976) *J. Physiol.* **256**, 1–21.

Bradford, H.F. & Peterson, D.W. (1987) *Mol. Aspects Med.* **9**, 119–172.

Bradshaw, C.M., Sheridan, R.D. & Szabadi, E. (1985) *Br. J. Pharmacol.* **86**, 483–490.

Burke, K., Chandler, C.J., Starr, B.S. & Starr, M.S. (1990) *Pharmacol. Biochem. Behav.* **36**, 729–733.

Callaghan, D.A. & Schwark, W.S. (1979) *Neuropharmacology* **18**, 541–545.

Chandler, C.J., Wohab, W., Starr, B.S. & Starr, M.S. (1990) *Neuroscience* **38**, 437–445.

Cheramy, A., Romo, R., Godehen, G. & Glowinski, J. (1984) *Neurosci. Lett.* **44**, 193–198.

Corcoran, M.E. & Mason, S.T. (1980) *Brain Res.* **190**, 473–484.

Cote, T.E., Eskay, R.L., Frey, E.A., Grewe, C.W., Munemura, M., Tsuruta, K., Brown, E.M. & Kebabian, J.W. (1983) In *Lisuride and Other Dopamine Agonists* (eds Calne, D.B., Horowski, R., McDonald, R.J. & Wuttke, W.), pp 45–53. New York, Raven Press.

Cox, B. & Lomax, P. (1976) *Pharmacol. Biochem. Behav.* **4**, 262–267.

Csernansky, J.G., Melicutin, J., Beauclair, L. & Lombrozo, L. (1988) *Biol. Psychiatry* **23**, 285–294.

Dawson, T.M., Barone, P., Sidhu, A., Wamsley, J.K. & Chase, T.N. (1988) *Neuroscience* **26**, 83–100.

Dow, R.C., Hill, A.G. & McQueen, J.K. (1974) *Br. J. Pharmacol.* **52**, 135P.

Euvrard, C., Ferland, L., Di Paolo, T., Beaulieu, M., Labrie, F., Oberlander, C., Raynaud, J.P. & Boissier, J.R. (1980) *Neuropharmacology* **19**, 379–386.

Fariello, R.G., De Mattei M., Castorina, M., Ferraro, T.N. & Golden, G.T. (1987) *Brain Res.* **426**, 373–376.

Farjo, I.B. & McQueen, J.K. (1979) *Br. J. Pharmacol.* **67**, 353–360.

Fisher, R.S. (1989) *Brain Res. Rev.* **14**, 245–278.

Fochtmann, L.J., Cruciani, R., Aiso, M. & Potter, W.Z. (1989) *Eur. J. Pharmacol.* **167**, 305–306.

Gee, K.W., Killam, E.K., Hollinger, M.A. & Giri, S.N. (1980) *Exp. Neurol.* **70**, 192–199.

Godukhin, O.V., Zharikova, A.D. & Budantsev, A.Y. (1984) *Neuroscience* **12**, 377–383.

Hiramatsu, M., Fujimoto, N. & Mori, A. (1982) *Neurochem. Res.* **7**, 1299–1305.

Iadorola, M.J. & Gale, K. (1982) *Science* **218**, 1237–1240.

Jackson, D.M., Ross, S.B. & Larsson, L.-G. (1989) *Naunyn Schmiedeberg's Arch. Pharmacol.* **340**, 355–365.

Janusz, W. & Kleinrok, Z. (1989) *Neurosci. Res.* **7**, 144–153.

Jobe, P.C. & Laird, H.E. (1981) *Biochem. Pharmacol.* **30**, 3137–3144.

Jobe, P.C. & Laird, H.E. In *Neurotransmitters and Epilepsy* (eds Jobe, P.C. & Laird, H.E.), pp 339–366. New York, Humana Press.

King, G.A. & Burnham, W.M. (1980) *Psychopharmacology* **69**, 281–285.

Kleinrok, Z., Czuczwar, S., Wojak, A. & Przegalinski, E. (1978) *Pol. J. Pharmacol. Pharm.* **30**, 513–519.

Ko, K.H., Dailey, J.W. & Jobe, P.C. (1982) *J. Pharmacol. Exp. Ther.* **222**, 662–669.

Kresch, M.J., Shaywitz, B.A., Shaywitz, S.E., Anderson, G.M., Leckman, J.L. & Cohen, D.J. (1987) In *Neurotransmitters and Epilepsy* (eds Jobe, P.C. & Laird, H.E.), pp 321–338. New York, Humana Press.

Krnjevic, K. & Phillis, J.W. (1963) *Br. J. Pharmacol.* **20**, 471–490.

La Grutta, V. & Sabatino, M. (1990) *Brain Res.* **515**, 87–93.

Lamprecht, F. (1977) *J. Neural Transm.* **40**, 159–170.

Löscher, W. (1985) *J. Pharmacol. Exp. Ther.* **233**, 204–211.

Löscher, W. & Czuczwar, S.J. (1986) *Eur. J. Pharmacol.* **128**, 55–65.

Markstein, R., Seiler, M.P., Vigouret, J.M., Urwyler, S., Enz, A. & Dixon, K. (1986) In *Progress in Catecholamine Research*. Part B. *Central Aspects* (eds Sandler, M., Dahlstrom, A. & Belmaker, R.H.), pp 59–64. New York, Liss.

Martin, G.M., Williams, M., Pettibone, D.J., Yarbrough, G.G., Clineschmidt, B.V. & Jones, J.H. (1984) *J. Pharmacol. Exp. Ther.* **230**, 569–576.

Matthews, R.T. & German, D. (1986) *Eur. J. Pharmacol.* **120**, 87–93.

McKenzie, G.M. & Soroko, F.E. (1972) *J. Pharm. Pharmacol.* **24**, 696–701.

McKenzie, G.M. & Soroko, F.E. (1973) *J. Pharm. Pharmacol.* **25**, 76–77.

McQuade, R.D., Ford, D., Duffy, R.A., Chipkin, R.E., Iorio, L.C. & Barnett, A. (1988) *Life Sci.* **43**, 1861–1869.

Meldrum, B.S. (1988) In *Recent Advances in Epilepsy* (eds Pedley, T.A. & Meldrum, B.S.), **16**, 1–19. New York, Churchill.

Meldrum, B.S., Anlezark, G. & Trimble, M. (1975) *Eur. J. Pharmacol.* **32**, 203–213.

Mori, A., Hiramatsu, M., Namba, S., Nishimoto, A., Ohmoto, T., Mayanagi, Y. & Aasakura, T. (1987) *Res. Commun. Chem. Pathol. Pharmacol.* **56**, 157–164.

Nomikos, G.G., Zis, A.P., Damsma, G. & Fibiger, H.C. (1991) *Neuropsychopharmacology* **4**, 65–69.

Nowak, G. & Zak, J. (1989) *Eur. J. Pharmacol.* **168**, 307–308.

Ongini, E., Caporali, M.G. & Massotti, M. (1986) In *Modulation of Central and Peripheral*

Transmitter Function (eds Biggio, G., Spano, P.F., Toffano, C. & Gessa, G.L.), pp 37–46. Padova, Liviana Press.

Pintor, M., Mefford, I.N., Hutter, I., Pocotte, S.L., Wyler, A.R. & Nadi, S. (1990) *Synapse* **5**, 152–156.

Quesney, L.F. (1981) In *Neurotransmitters, Seizures and Epilepsy* (eds Morselli, P.G., Lloyd, K.G., Löscher, W. & Meldrum, B.), pp 269–274. New York, Raven Press.

Quesney, L.F., Andermann, F. & Gloor, P. (1981) *Neurology* **31**, 1542–1544.

Sandoval, M.R.L. & Palermo-Neto, J. (1989) *Eur. J. Pharmacol.* **167**, 117–125.

Schonfeld, A.R. & Glick, S.D. (1980) *Neuropharmacology* **19**, 1009–1016.

Schwarcz, R., Creese, I., Coyle, J.T. & Snyder, S.H. (1978) *Nature* **271**, 766–768.

Seeman, P. (1981) *Pharmacol. Rev.* **32**, 229–313.

Setler, P.E., Sarau, H.M., Zirkle, C.L. & Saunders, H.L. (1978) *Eur. J. Pharmacol.* **50**, 419–430.

Sharp, T., Kingston, J. & Grahame-Smith, D.G. (1990) *Psychopharmacology* **100**, 110–114.

Shorvon, S.D. (1990) *Lancet* **336**, 93–96.

Smialowski, A. (1990) *Brain Res.* **528**, 148–150.

Smialowski, A. & Bijak, M. (1987) *Neuroscience* **23**, 95–101.

Snead, O.C. (1983) *Int. Rev. Neurobiol.* **24**, 93–180.

Sokoloff, P., Giros, B., Martres, M.-P., Bouthenet, M.-L. & Schwartz, J.-C. (1990) *Nature* **347**, 146–151.

Stach, R. & Kacz, D. (1977) *Epilepsia* **18**, 417–423.

Starr, M.S. (1987) *J. Neurochem.* **49**, 1042–1049.

Starr, B.S. & Starr, M.S. (1986) *Neuropharmacology* **25**, 455–463.

Starr, B.S., Starr, M.S. & Kilpatrick, I.C. (1987) *Neuroscience* **22**, 179–188.

Sunahara, A.K., Guan, H.-C., O'Dowd, B.F., Seeman, P., Laurier, L.G., Ng, G., George, S.R., Torchia, J., Van Tol, H.H.M. & Niznik, H.B. (1991) *Nature* **350**, 614–619.

Suppes, T., Kriegstein, A.R. & Prince, D.A. (1985) *Brain Res.* **326**, 273–280.

Trimble, M. (1977) *Biol. Psychiatry* **12**, 299–304.

Tsuruta, K., Frey, E.A., Grewe, C.W., Cote, T.E., Eskay, R.L. & Kebabian, J.W. (1981) *Nature* **292**, 463–465.

Turski, L., Cavalheiro, E.A., Turski, W.A. & Meldrum, B.S. (1987) In *Advances in Epileptology* (eds Wolf, P., Dam, M., Janz, D. & Dreifuss, F.F.), **16**, 115–118. New York, Raven Press.

Turski, L., Cavalheiro, E.A., Bortolotto, Z.A., Ikonomidou-Turski, C., Kleinrok, Z. & Turski, W.A. (1988) *J. Neurosci.* **8**, 4027–4037.

Turski, L., Ikonomidou, C., Turski, W.A., Bortolotto, Z.A. & Cavalheiro, E.A. (1989) *Synapse* **3**, 154–171.

Turski, W.A., Cavalheiro, E.A., Ikonomidou, C., Bortolotto, Z., Klockgether, T. & Turski, L. (1990) *Synapse* **5**, 113–119.

Van Tol, H.H.M., Bunzow, J.R., Guan, H.-C., Sunahara, R.K., Seeman, P., Niznik, H.B. & Civelli, O. (1991) *Nature* **350**, 610–614.

Van Woert, M.H. & Sethy, V.H. (1975) *Neurology* **25**, 135–140.

Volkman, P.H., Lorens, S.A., Kindel, G.H. & Ginos, J.Z. (1978) *Neuropharmacology* **17**, 947–955.

Wahnschaffe, U. & Löscher, W. (1991) *Brain Res.* **553**, 181–187.

Warter, J.-M., Vergnes, M., DePaulis, A., Tranchant, C., Rumbach, L., Micheletti, G. & Marescaux, C. (1988) *Neuropharmacology* **27**, 269–274.

Waszczak, B.L. (1990) *Brain Res.* **513**, 125–135.

Waszczak, B.L. & Walters, J.R. (1986) *J. Neurosci.* **6**, 120–126.

Weiner, W.J., Carvey, P.M., Nausieda, P.A. & Klawans, H.L. (1979) *Neurology* **29**, 1622–1625.

_____ CHAPTER 10 _____

FUTURE DIRECTIONS: THE CLINICAL SIGNIFICANCE AND THE THERAPEUTIC POTENTIAL OF $D_1 : D_2$ INTERACTIONS IN PARKINSON'S DISEASE, SCHIZOPHRENIA AND OTHER DISORDERS

John L. Waddington

Department of Clinical Pharmacology, Royal College of Surgeons in Ireland, St Stephen's Green, Dublin 2, Ireland

Table of Contents

DOPAMINE RECEPTOR INTERACTIONS
ISBN 0–12–729045–1

10.1 The nature of $D_1:D_2$ interactions as a substrate for neuropsychiatric disorder

10.1.1 Concepts of $D_1:D_2$ interaction deriving from studies in rodents

Over the past several years, our concept of the functional role of the D_1 dopamine (DA) receptor has metamorphosed from that of a neurochemical entity of uncertain functional role (other than the defining characteristic of linkage to the stimulation of adenylyl cyclase) to a physiological unit of prominent behavioural and putative therapeutic significance. As elaborated in a series of recent reviews (Waddington, 1986, 1988, 1989a, b; Breese and Creese, 1986; Arnt, 1987; Clark and White, 1987; Waddington and O'Boyle, 1987, 1989), DAergic neuroscience was to evolve rapidly from an era in which, on the basis only of indirect evidence in the absence of any selective D_1 antagonist, the D_2 receptor was held to be prepotent in essentially all aspects of DAergic function. There then followed a period of anomalous findings in initial studies with the first selective D_1 antagonists, the benzazepines SCH 23390 and SK & F 83566, which culminated in the proposal and subsequent widespread acceptance that D_1 and D_2 receptors interact critically in the regulation of numerous aspects of DAergic physiology and psychomotor function; the concept was of cooperative/ synergistic $D_1:D_2$ interactions, whereby activity through the D_1 receptor was necessary to 'enable' or 'permit' the expression of activity through the D_2 receptor, and thus to generate the totality of DAergic function in the intact, adult rodent.

Among the more prominent effects identified in such studies were the actions of selective D_1 agonists such as the benzazepine SK & F 38393 to inducing a modest stimulation of elements of behaviour (typically grooming) distinct from those induced by selective D_2 agonists such as quinpirole (typically sniffing and locomotion) when given separately, but showing synergism in the induction of classical stereotypy on their co-administration; conversely, selective D_1 antagonists readily reproduced almost all of the actions both of non-selective DA antagonists and of selective D_2 antagonists. However, in rodents in whom the function of DA neurones had been eliminated by 6-hydroxydopamine (6-OHDA) lesions (or *chronically* interrupted by reserpine/α-methyl-p-tyrosine (αMPT), this profile appeared to be altered significantly: responses to selective D_1 agonists were more typical and similar to those of their D_2 counterparts but were blocked only by selective D_1 antagonists, *and* vice versa. Thus, in animals deprived chronically of tonic DAergic activity, D_1 and D_2 receptor systems appeared to be no longer linked to the same extent, but acted more as separate systems that could be manipulated independently with their respective agonists and antagonists; yet synergistic $D_1:D_2$ interactions on the co-administration of D_1 and D_2 agonists, at least those influencing behaviour, appeared to endure in such circumstances.

The most recent studies have sustained and elaborated such concepts, but have additionally identified a number of complexities. These include evidence for oppositional $D_1:D_2$ interactions in the regulation of atypical behaviours that appear associated with selective stimulation of the D_1 receptor during concurrent blockade of tonic activity through the D_2 receptor (vacuous chewing/oral dyskinesia) and vice versa (jerking behaviour) (Chapter 3). Furthermore, molecular biological studies indicate that the number of DA receptors is much larger than envisaged originally. Currently, on the basis of their cloned sequences and known pharmacological characteristics, these might be best put into two *families*, of 'D$_1$-like' (D_{1A}, D_{1B}/D_5) and 'D$_2$-like' ($D_{2L/S}$, D_3, D_4) receptors (Sibley and Monsma, 1992); pending the identification of agents able to discriminate reliably between the individual members of either family, the above concept of $D_1:D_2$ interactions might be modified only to recognize, rather, the apparent existence of 'D$_1$-like':'D$_2$-like' interactions (Chapter 3).

10.1.2 Apparent species differences between rodents and non-human primates in profiles of $D_1:D_2$ interaction

Of particular importance for considering the putative clinical significance of $D_1:D_2$ interactions is an expanding body of evidence that there exist significant species differences in their manifestation. The great bulk of our knowledge and understanding of $D_1:D_2$ interactions derives from studies in the two most common rodent species, rats and mice; these have generated usually complementary results, though a recent comparative study suggests that, within a series of partial selective D_1 agonist analogues of SK & F 38393, a relationship between efficacy in stimulating adenylyl cyclase and extent of behavioural synergism with the selective D_2 agonist quinpirole can be demonstrated in mice but *not* in rats (Arnt *et al.*, 1992).

Among lower organisms and phylogenetically related species, stimulation of D_1 receptors with SK & F 38393 in planaria (*Dugesia gonocephala*) induced 'screw-like' hyperkinesias that were blocked by SCH 23390 but not by the selective D_2 antagonist sulpiride, while stimulation of D_2 receptors with PHNO or lisuride induced 'C-shaped' curling that was blocked by sulpiride but not by SCH 23390 (Venturini *et al.*, 1989). This profile of results suggests that D_1 and D_2 receptors have distinct motoric roles and act in a functionally independent manner in this organism; however, any such interpretation may be confounded by the ability both of D_1 *and* D_2 agonists to stimulate adenylyl cyclase (as distinct from their abilities to stimulate and inhibit, respectively, this enzyme system in rat striatum), though with these agonist responses also being sensitive to blockade only by the homologous antagonist. A profile of $D_1:D_2$ interactions comparable to that evident in rats and mice appears to regulate pecking behaviour in chicks (Zarrindast and Amin, 1992). However, in the guinea-pig, quinpirole induces locomotion, with other typical and atypical behaviours, that appears sensitive to antagonism by sulpiride and by another selective D_2 antagonist, raclopride, but not by SCH 23390; SK & F 38393 and SCH 23390 each produced little or no behavioural effect when given alone, and SK & F 38393 attenuated quinpirole-induced locomotion with release of vacuous chewing (Brent, 1991). These results, in an alternative rodent species, are considerably at variance with, and indeed appear in several respects opposite to, those evident in rats and mice.

Among phylogenetically higher species, quinpirole induced a mild increase in locomotion in cats, while SK & F 38393 induced mild sedation which occurred with emesis (classically considered a D_2 receptor-mediated response; see Seeman (1980)) at higher doses; the preferential D_2 antagonists haloperidol and spiperone, but not SCH 23390, produced some decrease in spontaneous locomotion with mild catalepsy, though interactions between these agonists and antagonists at the level of such unconditioned motor behaviours were not reported (Sweidan et al., 1990). This profile appears somewhat at variance with that evident in rats and mice and shows some overlap with that evident in the guinea-pig; there was, however, some evidence that D_1 receptor activation might play a 'permissive' role in feline affective defence behaviour elicited by electrical stimulation of the ventromedial hypothalamus. Clearly, studies of such drugs and drug combinations in non-human primates are most likely to yield results of direct relevance for predicting potential effects in humans. Initial studies were conducted in monkeys rendered parkinsonian by prior administration of 1-methyl-4-phenyl-1,2,3,6-tetrahydropyridine (MPTP) or sensitized by prior exposure to DAergic antagonists; results from such studies are important, and are considered in depth below (Sections 10.2.1, 10.2.4 and 10.3.2), but the initial focus will be on studies in the whole animal.

In intact monkeys (*Macaca fascicularis*), quinpirole readily stimulated locomotion while SK & F 38393 reduced both spontaneous activity and the locomotor response to quinpirole; SCH 23390 had no significant effect on residual activity following this combination of D_1 and D_2 agonists. Conversely, SK & F 38393 and quinpirole induced moderate and low levels of lingual dyskinesia (tongue protrusions), respectively, that showed synergism on the co-administration of these agonists; the synergistic effect of this agonist combination was blocked both by SCH 23390 and by sulpiride (Bedard and Boucher, 1989). Similarly, in normal common marmosets (*Callithrix jacchus*), quinpirole stimulated locomotor activity with some stereotypy of movement at high doses, while SK & F 38393 decreased spontaneous activity and vigilance without evidence of catalepsy or of any other form of behaviour; pretreatment with SK & F 38393 inhibited these stimulatory actions of quinpirole, with no other form of behaviour being induced. SCH 23390 and raclopride each reduced spontaneous activity, with evidence of sedation and catalepsy; while each of these antagonists also inhibited responses to quinpirole, the action of raclopride was potent while that of SCH 23390 was incomplete and weak (Loschmann et al., 1991). However, using a paradigm not usually employed in non-primate species, both PHNO and the putative, full-efficacy preferential D_1 agonist dihydrexidine produced rapid increases in the blink rate of green monkeys (*Cercopithecus aethiops sabaeus*), with the action of PHNO being blocked by the selective D_2 antagonist remoxipride but not by SCH 23390, and that of dihydrexidine being blocked by SCH 23390 but not by remoxipride; while D_1 and D_2 receptors appear to influence blink rate in a complementary yet functionally independent manner, other elements of behaviour were not reported on (Elsworth *et al.*, 1991).

The above studies suggest that in paradigms similar to those employed in intact rats and mice, resultant profiles of $D_1 : D_2$ interaction are very different in the intact non-human primate; in particular, D_1 receptor stimulation appears to exert little stimulatory effect in monkeys when given alone, with the possible exception of inducing some lingual dyskinesia, and to *inhibit* both spontaneous activity and D_2 agonist-induced hyperactivity; furthermore, selective D_1 antagonism appears to exert less prominent influences on behaviour than does D_2 antagonism. Thus, when evident, $D_1 : D_2$ interactions in these primate species, like those in the guinea-pig (Brent, 1991), appear more oppositional in nature; there is considerably less evidence (with the further exception of modest $D_1 : D_2$ agonist synergism in promoting yawning in rhesus monkeys; Code and Tang (1991)) for the prominent cooperative/synergistic $D_1 : D_2$ interactions evident in rats and mice. Clearly, effects in such rodent species cannot be considered predictive of events occurring in non-human primates.

10.2 $D_1 : D_2$ interactions and Parkinson's disease

10.2.1   Studies with SK & F 38393 in the MPTP non-human primate model

In monkeys rendered parkinsonian by systemic injection of MPTP, initial studies indicated acutely administered SK & F 38393 to be devoid of the anti-parkinsonian activity that was readily demonstrable for l-DOPA and for selective D_2 agonists; rather, SK & F 38393 appeared to *exacerbate* bradykinesia. Furthermore, in monkeys rendered hemiparkinsonian by unilateral intracarotid injection of MPTP, even high doses of SK & F 38393 produced at best a mild reduction in hypokinesia, though such hypokinesia was readily reduced by selective D_2 agonism; additionally, co-administration of SK & F 38393 with a selective D_2 agonist *diminished* the motoric effect of that D_2 agonist (Waddington, 1988).

Subsequent studies in several non-human primate species have, without exception, confirmed and extended these preliminary findings. Thus, acutely administered SK & F 38393 did not alleviate the motor deficits associated with MPTP exposure but, rather, appeared to increase such symptomatology and attenuated the antiparkinsonian efficacy of quinpirole (Nomoto *et al.*, 1988; Bedard and Boucher, 1989; Boyce *et al.*, 1990; Close *et al.*, 1990); furthermore, 25 days of chronic treatment with SK & F 38393 also failed to show antiparkinsonian activity (Falardeau *et al.*, 1988), though it did enhance, rather than attenuate, the antiparkinsonian efficacy of the D_2 agonist bromocriptine (Rouillard *et al.*, 1990).

MPTP-treated monkeys also demonstrate the serious treatment side effects of DAergic dyskinesia and dystonia, particularly on long-term l-DOPA adminis- tration, and there is now some information on the effects of D_1 and D_2 agonists and antagonists on these adverse motor phenomena. As in unlesioned monkeys, acute SK & F 38393 potentiated the dyskinetic (tongue protrusion) effect of quinpirole in their MPTP counterparts, though only sulpiride and not SCH 23390 could alleviate this combination effect in the latter situation (Bedard and Boucher, 1989); conversely, the action of SK & F 38393 in potentiating the antiparkinsonian efficacy of bromocriptine during chronic treatment was not at a cost of inducing dyskinesia (Rouillard *et al.*, 1990). However, Boyce *et al.* (1990) reported that SCH 23390 reduced l-DOPA-induced choreiform movements of the limbs and body, while SK & F 38393 reduced spontaneous dystonic movements of the lower limbs. Following establishment of l-DOPA- induced dyskinesia of the limbs, selective D_2 agonists but not SK & F 38393 reproduced these adverse phenomena; like therapeutic efficacy, dyskinesias induced by D_2 agonists were blocked completely by sulpiride, while SCH 23390 alleviated markedly such dyskinesia yet attenuated only weakly their antiparkinsonian efficacy (Gomez-Mancilla and Bedard, 1991).

10.2.2 Studies with SK & F 38393 in patients with Parkinson's disease

On the basis of studies in rats and mice as elaborated above (Section 10.1.1), and in advance of any substantial body of evidence from the MPTP non-human primate model, SK & F 38393 was given to patients with Parkinson's disease by two groups of investigators.

In a preliminary study, doses of SK & F 38393 up to 720 mg daily were administered; only in two patients receiving the largest doses was there some evidence for an antibradykinetic effect when combined with a subtherapeutic dose of l-DOPA, without any evident increase in dyskinesia or hallucinations (see Waddington, 1988). In a more systematic investigation, involving the administration of SK & F 38393 to seven patients with idiopathic Parkinson's disease in a double-blind, placebo-controlled trial at doses up to 19 mg/kg, the drug was found to be rapidly absorbed when given orally and to occur in micromolar concentrations in cerebrospinal fluid, but failed to induce any change in severity of parkinsonian symptoms, whether given alone or in combination with intravenous infusion of subtherapeutic doses of l-DOPA; however, in patients receiving l-DOPA at therapeutically supraoptimal rates, SK & F 38393 again had no significant effect on parkinsonian symptoms but tended to reduce l-DOPA-induced orofacial and/or limb-trunkal dyskinesias in those patients manifesting such involuntary movements (Braun *et al.*, 1987).

10.2.3 The nature of the anomalous effects of SK & F 38393 in primates

Following an era in which D_2 receptors were ascribed the prepotent role in regulating motor function, both in rodents (Seeman, 1980) and in humans (Schachter et al., 1980), subsequent studies in the mid-1980s provided a sound rationale for investigating the antiparkinsonian potential of the only available selective D_1 agonist, SK & F 38393; in terms of rodent models with established capacity to predict antiparkinsonian efficacy, this drug induced contralateral rotational behaviour in rats with unilateral 6-OHDA lesions of the nigrostriatal pathway and acted synergistically with D_2 agonists in the induction of such behaviour (Waddington and O'Boyle, 1989; Chapter 3). However, in primates, whether non-human species lesioned with MPTP or patients with idiopathic Parkinson's disease, SK & F 38393 has been conspicuous in terms of its failure to demonstrate any antiparkinsonian activity; furthermore, only one (chronic) study using the MPTP model has indicated that it shows any therapeutic synergism with D_2 agonist treatment, while the remainder report that it attenuates the therapeutic effects of D_2 agonism. Indeed, the negative findings under these pathophysiological conditions complement the results of studies in intact, non-human primates; there, profiles of D_1 agonist activity and of $D_1:D_2$ interaction are not only different from those evident in rats and mice, but indicate that SK & F 38393 exerts effects that seem *opposite* to those evident in these rodent species (Sections 10.1.1 and 10.2.1).

What might be the basis of what appear to be such prominent species differences in D_1 agonist response and in $D_1:D_2$ interaction? It is possible that there exist some fundamental differences in DAergic physiology between these various species. At a gross level, though the striatum of rats and mice is recognized to be heterogeneous both in structure and in function, it does not possess an internal capsule to effect the ready demarcation between the functionally and neuroanatomically discrete caudate nucleus and putamen that is evident in most higher species, including some other rodents. There exist also more subtle neuroanatomical differences between rats and non-human primates that have already been the subject of speculation as to whether they might underlie some of the more general behavioural and psychopharmacological differences between such species; for example, there is immunohistochemical evidence for the presence of neuronal cell bodies containing tyrosine hydroxylase in the caudate nucleus and putamen of the latter but not in the striatum of the former species (Dubach et al., 1987).

Alternatively (or additionally), psychopharmacological evidence in rats and mice suggests that there may be at least two distinct forms of $D_1:D_2$ interaction, cooperative/synergistic and oppositional, which can act concurrently in the regulation of distinct elements of behaviour (Waddington, 1989a; Waddington and O'Boyle, 1989; Chapter 3) (Section 10.1.1); if the overall effect of D_1 and/or D_2 agents reflects some balance between these distinct forms of interaction, there may be phylogenetic differences in that balance between primates and some rodent species. In a related manner, it has been argued, primarily on the basis of studies in rodents (Robertson, 1992) that $D_1 : D_2$ synergism may involve D_1 and D_2 receptors located in distinct brain regions (substantia nigra and striatum, respectively) rather than or in addition to those located in close proximity within the striatum; phylogenetic differences in the relative contribution of these two putative modes of $D_1 : D_2$ synergism, or in how they adapt to lesion- or disease-induced disruption of DAergic neuronal activity, might be relevant factors.

While the vast majority of studies in rats and mice indicate a two- to four-fold higher density of D_1 relative to D_2 receptors in the striatum (Waddington and O'Boyle, 1989), there is some evidence that in non-human primates (Madras et al., 1988; but see Duffy et al., 1991) and in postmortem human brain (O'Boyle and Waddington, 1987; Hall et al., 1988; Seeman et al., 1989; Rinne et al., 1990; McCauley, O'Boyle and Waddington, in preparation; but see Hess et al., 1987; De Keyser et al., 1990a; Pifl et al., 1992a) this ratio may be nearer to unity; any such diminution in the density of D_1 as opposed to D_2 receptors could constitute a reduction in extent of primate D_1 receptor reserve relative to that present in rats (Chapter 3) which might preferentially reduce responsiveness to partial D_1 agonists such as SK & F 38393. Indeed, in recent studies, the full D_1 agonist DA has been shown to stimulate adenylyl cyclase in the caudate nucleus and putamen of non-human primates to an extent indistinguishable from that evident in rat striatum; also, the sensitization characteristics of adenylyl cyclase in response to stimulation by DA both in the non-human primate lesioned with MPTP and in post-mortem brain from patients with Parkinson's disease were found to be indistinguishable from those evident in the unilateral 6-OHDA-lesioned rat. However, in caudate and putamen tissue from non-human primates, SK & F 38393 showed less than one-third of the already modest partial efficacy (and less than one-fifth of the potency) in stimulating adenylyl cyclase that it demonstrated in rat striatum; furthermore, SK & F 38393 was considerably more effective in inhibiting the stimulatory action of DA on adenylyl cyclase in the non-human primate than in the rat (Pifl et al., 1991, 1992a, b).

It is tempting to equate the unexpected lack of therapeutic effect of SK & F 38393 in the MPTP non-human primate model and in Parkinson's disease with these apparent reductions in D_1 receptor efficacy and affinity in such species. However, it should not be overlooked that there exists evidence from rodent studies (Chapter 3) and in human post-mortem brain (De Keyser et al., 1989) for some of the pharmacological actions of SK & F 38393 possibly involving a subtype of D_1 receptor not linked to the stimulation of adenylyl cyclase. Also, the unexpected, occasional induction by SK & F 38393 of emesis in cats (Sweidan et al., 1990) and in (MPTP-lesioned) monkeys (Close et al., 1990), together with its attenuation on chronic administration to non-human primates of D_2 receptor upregulation associated with MPTP lesions (Falardeau et al., 1988), is suggestive of some direct or indirect action on the D_2 receptor in these species; regarding the latter phenomenon, in rats it is selective D_1 *antagonist* treatment that has been reported to attenuate D_2 receptor upregulation, at least that associated with chronic administration of a selective D_2 antagonist (Chapter 3).

10.2.4 The effects of 'second-generation' putative selective D_1 agonists in the MPTP non-human primate model and in Parkinson's disease

One approach to clarifying the nature of these unexpected species differences in responsivity to SK & F 38393 is to examine the extent to which they do or do not generalize to other putative selective D_1 agonists. The phenanthridine CY 208-243 is another partial D_1 agonist (Markstein *et al.*, 1988) that has now been investigated in similar studies. In the MPTP-treated non-human primate, CY 208-243 but not SK & F 38393 reversed parkinsonian motor deficits and induced locomotor hyperactivity, while it induced only small increases in activity when administered to normal, drug-naive animals, and neither nausea or vomiting were apparent; this antiparkinsonian efficacy was readily antagonized by SCH 23390 and, to a lesser extent, by sulpiride (Temlett *et al.*, 1988; Markstein *et al.*, 1988). In patients with Parkinson's disease, administration of CY 208-243 resulted in therapeutic benefit at moderate doses; its efficacy appeared somewhat less than that of l-DOPA, with signs of toxicity emerging at higher doses (Temlett *et al.*, 1989; Tsui *et al.*, 1989).

More recently, Gomez-Mancilla and Bedard (1991) have confirmed the antiparkinsonian activity of CY 208-243 in the MPTP non-human primate model and its greater sensitivity to antagonism by SCH 23390 than by sulpiride; this antiparkinsonian activity was also blocked by pretreatment with the DA synthesis inhibitor αMPT and restored by a low dose of quinpirole that was subthreshold for alleviating parkinsonian symptoms in its own right. These latter results, which also include the greater antagonism of the antiparkinsonian efficacy of selective D_2 agonists by sulpiride than by SCH 23390, suggest here a profile more similar to that evident in the 6-OHDA-lesioned rat: after MPTP lesions, non-human primates show restoration of movement both by CY 208-243 and by quinpirole, with these effects being reduced preferentially by the homologous antagonist and by further depletion of residual DA with αMPT; the ability in this MPTP + αMPT model of an otherwise ineffective dose of SK & F 38393 to restore responsivity to quinpirole, and of an otherwise ineffective dose of quinpirole to restore responsivity to CY 208-243, suggests: (i) that small amounts of residual DA or stimulation of the heterologous receptor are able to influence responses to stimulation either of the D_1 *or* of the D_2 receptor, in a manner consistent with cooperative/synergistic D_1 : D_2 interactions; and (ii) that SK & F 38393 can show *some* effects similar to those evident in rats, though it seems clear that this does *not* extend to antiparkinsonian activity in its own right. It will be the task of future investigations to reconcile these results with those from the larger body of studies on SK & F 38393 and on D_1 : D_2 interactions in non-human primates. Furthermore, while CY 208-243 appears to demonstrate many of the *in vivo* and functional *in vitro* properties expected of a selective (partial) D_1 agonist, it fails to show any selectivity for the D_1 over the D_2 receptor in *in vitro* radioligand binding studies; additionally, in such studies it shows non-selective affinity for a wide range of non-DAergic receptors (Markstein *et al.*, 1988; Murray and Waddington, 1990a; Abbott *et al.*, 1991). These anomalous properties of CY 208-243 must be considered when attempting to interpret any finding with this compound, in any species.

The preferred approach to clarifying these issues is to examine in primates the properties of a full-efficacy, selective D_1 agonist. However, as recently reviewed (Daly and Waddington, 1992a), it has proved extremely difficult to identify such compounds; only recently have putative agents with appropriate properties for *in vivo* studies become available, and preliminary studies are now being reported. Dihydrexidine is a benzophenanthridine derivative which shows full-efficacy agonist activity at the rat striatal D_1 receptor; it induced grooming, sniffing and locomotion in intact rats and extensive grooming in those lesioned with 6-OHDA (Lovenberg *et al.*, 1989; Darney *et al.*, 1991). This compound has been reported to induce a marked alleviation of parkinsonian symptoms in MPTP-treated non-human primates (Taylor *et al.*, 1991). However, it has been acknowledged (Brewster *et al.*, 1990) that, for technical reasons, the original report of a 60-fold selectivity for D_1 over D_2 receptors appears to have been an overestimate, the true value being of the order of 10-fold; thus, the interpretation of these findings in the MPTP non-human primate model is confounded by the limited 'preference' of dihydrexidine for D_1 receptors, and there remains the possibility of some influence from the (lesser) D_2 agonist component of its actions.

More recently, DeNinno *et al.* (1991) have described a series of isochroman D_1 agonists which demonstrate full efficacy in rat striatum; among these, A 68930 shows not only full D_1 efficacy but also > 200-fold selectivity for D_1 over D_2 receptors and high *in vivo* potency. We have confirmed the selectivity of A 68930 and find that it induces intense grooming behaviour in the rat at extremely low doses, together with some vacuous chewing and sniffing but in the absence of locomotor stimulation even at higher doses (Daly and Waddington, 1991). Though A 68930 represents the most potent and selective full-efficacy D_1 agonist yet identified, among this or any other series of compounds, it has been reported (DeNinno *et al.*, 1991) to induce forepaw myoclonus at moderate to high doses, and this might engender some concern in relation to proceeding with this drug as a potential clinical candidate. A close analogue from this isochroman series, A 77636, is somewhat less potent and only 30-fold selective at D_1 versus D_2 receptors and shows supramaximal efficacy in stimulating adenylyl cyclase with a maximal response 35% *greater* than that induced by DA; in preliminary studies it has been reported to induce prolonged, dose-related alleviation of parkinsonian symptoms in the MPTP-treated non-human primate (Kebabian *et al.*, 1992).

The discovery of the isochromans, typified by A 68930 and A 77636, constitutes a fundamental new advance in the search for 'second-generation' full-efficacy, selective D_1 agonists; it will be important to conduct a detailed examination of their psychopharmacological effects in intact, drug-naive non-human primates, including as wide a range of $D_1 : D_2$ interaction paradigms as might prove possible, alongside studies in MPTP-treated counterparts. Evidence in rodents that A 68930 may interact additionally with a subtype of 'D_1-like' receptor which is relatively insensitive to the benzazepine D_1 agonists and antagonists (Daly and Waddington, 1992b; Chapter 3) makes it essential to examine whether comparable profiles can be identified in non-human primates. Should clinical studies proceed with one or more of the isochromans, they could provide critical, new information on the role of the D_1 receptor and of $D_1 : D_2$ interactions in human primates and in the treatment of Parkinson's disease. The data available to date on the therapeutic potential of 'second-generation' full-efficacy, selective D_1 agonists for Parkinson's disease are provocative, but are in urgent need of confirmation and elaboration.

10.3 $D_1 : D_2$ interactions and schizophrenia

10.3.1 The nature of the antipsychotic potential of 'first-' and 'second-generation' selective D_1 antagonists

Currently accepted notions that essentially all clinically available neuroleptic drugs block brain DA receptors go back some 30 years. However, the relationship of this property to therapeutic efficacy in schizophrenia and other psychoses received powerful support in the mid-1970s from data indicating that the *in vitro* affinities of a very broad range of neuroleptic drugs for DA antagonist binding sites were correlated highly with their clinical potencies in controlling psychotic symptoms. Subsequent re-evaluation of this relationship in terms of the D_1 / D_2 schema, undertaken in the absence of any known selective D_1 antagonist, indicated very high correlations between affinity for the D_2 receptor and a wide range of pharmacological actions of neuroleptics, including antipsychotic potency, that were not evident in relation to affinity for the D_1 receptor; similarly, selective or preferential D_2 antagonists such as the substituted benzamides (e.g. sulpiride) and the butyrophenones (e.g. haloperidol), respectively, reproduced the pharmacological and clinical effects of less selective or indeed of non-selective antagonists of both D_1 and D_2 receptors, such as the phenothiazines (e.g. chlorpromazine, fluphenazine) or thioxanthenes (e.g. flupenthixol, clopenthixol) (Waddington, 1989b, 1993a).

However, over the past decade it has become apparent that selective D_1

antagonists can produce effects very similar to those of D_2 antagonists, via the $D_1 : D_2$ interactions that are the subject of this volume. In the above analysis, this was exemplified in terms of classical DAergic responses such as stereotyped behaviour. However, the first selective D_1 antagonists, SCH 23390 and its benzazepine congener SK & F 83566, not only inhibit DA agonist-induced motor behaviour in rats and mice; they also inhibit conditioned avoidance responding, intracranial self-stimulation and the amphetamine cue in drug discrimination responding, and are therefore active in those rodent models currently believed to predict clinical antipsychotic efficacy. These properties do not appear to be idiosyncratic effects of the benzazepines, as they are also evident in recent studies with new, 'second-generation' selective D_1 antagonists that are chemically distinct (NNC 756, a benzofuranylbenzazepine; SCH 39166, a benzonaphthazepine; A 69024 and BW 737C, isoquinolines) (Waddington, 1988, 1993a; Daly and Waddington, 1992c; Chapter 3).

An important, related matter is whether selective D_1 antagonists might be more or less likely to induce the adverse effects that can be encountered during therapy with classical or selective D_2 antagonist neuroleptics, and whether any different problems might be encountered. Selective D_1 antagonists can induce catalepsy in rodents, suggesting some likelihood of inducing typical extrapyramidal side-effects such as parkinsonism; however, they are active at low doses in models predictive of antipsychotic efficacy, and these properties might prove dissociable by dose (Waddington, 1988, 1992; Chipkin et al., 1988). Furthermore, in a new rodent model which purported to distinguish atypical neuroleptics (i.e. those with reduced propensity to induce acute extrapyramidal side-effects and, ideally, with greater antipsychotic efficacy) from typical agents, SCH 23390 more closely resembled the atypical antipsychotic clozapine and the atypical neuroleptic thioridazine than the typical neuroleptics haloperidol or chlorpromazine (Ellenbroek et al., 1987; but see Hietala et al., 1990). Of critical importance is the extent to which selective D_1 antagonists might be more or less likely to induce tardive dyskinesia. The weaknesses of the DA receptor hyperfunction (supersensitivity) hypothesis appear so profound (Waddington, 1989c) as to vitiate any attempt to predict such propensity on the basis of their known interactions with brain DAergic systems, whether on acute or following 'chronic' administration; they have yet to be examined in rodents over much more prolonged periods in putative phenomenological models of tardive dyskinesia (Waddington, 1990).

It should be noted that clozapine, the only available atypical antipsychotic which appears to show both a low propensity to induce acute extrapyramidal side-effects *and* additional efficacy in alleviating psychotic symptoms in a significant minority of those schizophrenic patients who fail to respond to typical neuroleptics (Kane et al., 1988), is a weak and non-selective antagonist of both D_1 and D_2 receptors; it does, however, appear to exert some preferential attentuation of D_1 receptor-mediated function (Murray and Waddington, 1990b;

Ellenbroek *et al.*, 1991; Waddington and Daly, 1992), and may particularly attenuate function mediated via a subtype of D_1 receptor (Daly and Waddington, 1992d).

10.3.2 Studies with selective D_1 antagonists in non-human primates

The great bulk of our knowledge of the therapeutic potential and side-effects liability of selective D_1 antagonists derives from studies in the common rodent species; thus, studies in non-human primates are more likely to provide phylogenetically relevant information on these issues.

In terms of predictors of antipsychotic efficacy, SCH 23390 and SCH 39166 have been reported to inhibit conditioned avoidance responding in non-human primates at doses which, relative to those of haloperidol, produced few signs of any acute extrapyramidal syndrome(s); however, these studies were carried out in animals with prior exposure to psychotropic medication(s), which in one instance included DA antagonist 'sensitization' (see below) by repeated prior exposure to haloperidol, and thus the extent to which such findings may be relevant to the drug-naive state is unclear (Waddington, 1988, 1993a; Chipkin *et al.*, 1988). Stereotypy and social isolation induced in non-human primates by *d*-amphetamine have been proposed to constitute both symptomatological and psychopharmacological models of positive and negative schizophrenic symptoms, respectively; while typical neuroleptic drugs can suppress stereotypy, these have less effect on social isolation, perhaps in accordance with the perspective that negative symptoms may be less responsive to such agents, and it may be of note that preliminary data suggest that SCH 23390 can antagonize *both* phenomena (Ellenbroek *et al.*, 1989). Such studies, if confirmed and generalized to other similar agents, would suggest that selective D_1 antagonists could constitute a potentially new approach to the treatment of psychotic disorders.

Regarding potential substrates of any such atypical actions of selective D_1 antagonists, these might involve important differences in the microscopic functional localization of D_1 versus D_2 receptors within region(s) that contain (macroscopically) both subtypes, or might reflect the more extensive distribution of D_1 receptors to include cerebral regions that show relative impoverishment of their D_2 counterparts. In relation to the latter possibility, one might speculate particularly on the considerably more widespread cortical (including prefrontal) distribution of D_1 than of D_2 receptors in non-human primates, as determined both *in vitro* by autoradiography (Richfield *et al.*, 1989; Lidow *et al.*, 1991) and *in vivo* by positron emission tomography (PET) (Sedvall *et al.*, 1991); furthermore, at least in the rabbit, there are both considerably higher ratios of D_1 to D_2 receptor density and elevations in DA turnover in the hippocampus and parahippocampal gyrus (entorhinal cortex) than in the caudate nucleus or putamen (Dewar and Reader, 1989). It may be relevant that such prefrontal cortical and medial temporal lobe structures are to the forefront in contemporary theorizing on the pathobiology of schizophrenia (Waddington, 1993b).

A critical, complementary issue concerns the potential for extrapyramidal side-effects of selective D_1 antagonists. In non-human primates, it is well established that repeated prior administration of haloperidol results in progressive sensitization (priming) to neuroleptic-induced extrapyramidal dysfunction, particularly dystonia, and that subsequent parenteral challenge with a selective antagonist either of D_1 or of D_2 receptors will then induce such a syndrome (Waddington, 1988, 1992; Peacock et al., 1990; Christensen, 1990); on the basis of such studies, however, it is not clear whether selective D_1 antagonists might or might not share the liability of their D_2 antagonist counterparts in the unprimed situation. Provocatively, studies by Coffin et al. (1989, 1992) have indicated that neither acute nor repeated oral administration of SCH 23390 or SCH 39166 to the drug-naive, non-human primate results in any form of motor symptomatology, other than sedation, while comparable treatment with haloperidol was associated with the emergence of a multifaceted dyskinetic/ dystonic extrapyramidal syndrome; indeed, these authors (McHugh and Coffin, 1991) have suggested that subsequent daily oral administration of SCH 39166 to such previously haloperidol-sensitized animals results in a progressive *diminution* of the resultant extrapyramidal syndrome over several days; see also Christensen (1990).

Conversely, *parenteral* administration of SCH 23390 to (apparently or explicitly) drug-naive non-human primates has been reported by other investigators to induce catalepsy/akinesia/parkinsonism (Ellenbroek et al., 1991; Loschmann et al., 1991; Lawrence et al., 1991) with dystonia (Casey, 1992); though of somewhat briefer duration, these extrapyramidal reactions to SCH 23390 were qualitatively similar to those induced by typical neuroleptics such as haloperidol. It will be important to determine whether these parenteral administration studies are in fundamental contradiction with those utilizing oral administration, or else represent extremes along a continuum of possible extrapyramidal response(s) as determined by considerations of species, dose and route of administration.

There is little in the way of studies that involve the long-term continuous (as opposed to the repeated intermittent) administration of selective D_1 antagonists to non-human primates that might throw some light on their relative liability to induce tardive dyskinesia. The most recent studies in such animals withdrawn from long-term treatment with typical neuroleptics (Peacock et al., 1990) continue to suggest a role for acute D_1 hyperfunction/D_2 hypofunction in the expression of some oral hyperkinesias (with, additionally, inhibition by selective D_1 agonism of the dystonic response to acute SCH 23390 but not of that to acute raclopride); though such data (Section 10.1.2) might be interpretable as consistent with the D_1 hyperfunction/D_2 hypofunction hypothesis of tardive dyskinesia that derives primarily from studies in rodents (Rosengarten et al., 1991), the dangers in generalizing from acute DA agonist paradigms to a disorder that occurs spontaneously during long-term administration of DA antagonists are considerable (Waddington, 1990).

10.3.3 Studies with selective D_1 antagonists in human subjects

To suggest, on the basis of comparable activities of a non-selective D_1/D_2 antagonist and of a preferential D_2 antagonist in exerting both antipsychotic efficacy (Ehmann et al., 1987) and acute diminution of tardive dyskinesia (Lubin et al., 1991), that selective D_1 antagonists should be clinically inert is a flawed argument (Waddington, 1989b); critically, such notions ignore the concept of $D_1:D_2$ interactions, for which a substrate has been proposed in human postmortem brain (and noted to be deficient in patients with schizophrenia; Seeman et al. (1989)). Furthermore, the location of D_1 and D_2 receptors in the human brain, whether assessed in vitro by autoradiography (De Keyser et al., 1988; Cortes et al., 1989; Camps et al., 1989) or in vivo by PET (Farde et al., 1987), does not differ fundamentally from that described for non-human primates (Section 10.3.2). However, it has not yet proved possible to address the vast majority of the above issues directly in humans, as controlled, clinical studies with selective D_1 antagonists are in their relative infancy (Chipkin, 1990).

In an initial, open study (Gessa et al., 1991), 0.5–4.0 mg SCH 23390 was given acutely by intramuscular injection to seven patients with affective or schizoaffective disorder; neither any acute therapeutic effect nor any adverse effects were noted. However, Casey (1991) has offered cogent criticisms on the extremely limited capacity of such an exploratory study to clarify the likely antipsychotic efficacy, or otherwise, of such agents: none of the patients had a diagnosis of schizophrenia, and even typical neuroleptic drugs fail to display therapeutic efficacy following acute, parenteral administration. SCH 23390 has also been given to normal, volunteer subjects in PET studies utilizing [^{11}C]SCH 23390 (Farde, 1992). Intravenous doses of 0.6–0.8 mg were associated with perceived unease/restlessness and observed motor restlessness, i.e. akathisia, that was transient and occurred only when [^{11}C]SCH 23390 binding in the basal ganglia was at a high level, indicative of a brain D_1 receptor occupancy of 45–59%; no signs or symptoms of dystonia or parkinsonism were reported or observed. These phenomena were qualitatively similar to those recorded following similar injections to schizophrenic patients of 0.2–0.5 mg raclopride, which gave a brain D_2 receptor occupancy of 46–73%; thus, such data indicate that selective blockade of D_1 and D_2 receptors can each produce comparable psychomotor phenomena, in accordance with cooperative $D_1:D_2$ interactions in the living human brain. In the light of its atypical antipsychotic properties (Section 10.3.1), it remains unexplained why clozapine demonstrates in humans the highest relative occupancy of D_1 to D_2 receptors (approximately 1:1) among those neuroleptics examined by PET (Farde et al., 1989). The results of controlled clinical trials with the new, 'second-generation' selective D_1 antagonists SCH

39166 (Chipkin, 1990) and NNC 687 in schizophrenia will be necessary to throw further light on these critical issues.

10.4 $D_1 : D_2$ interactions and other neuropsychiatric disorders

The oral administration in a placebo-controlled trial of 3.2–32.0 mg/kg SK & F 38393 to small numbers of patients with Huntington's disease, Gilles de la Tourette's syndrome, tardive dyskinesia or torsion dystonia neither exacerbated nor ameliorated these movement disorders (Braun *et al.*, 1989). However, an acute intramuscular injection of 1 mg SCH 23390 to a single patient with Huntington's disease induced a rapid reduction in involuntary movements that was not seen following comparable administration of placebo; the patient yawned repeatedly following administration of SCH 23390 and fell asleep 40 min later (Gessa *et al.*, 1991). The possible capacity of acute SCH 23390 to suppress such involuntary movements is thus in urgent need of further investigation in comparison with the known partial effectiveness of selective D_2 antagonists, so as to clarify the substance or otherwise of this provocative finding and any basis in terms of $D_1 : D_2$ interactions.

Even more speculatively, species differences in the density and laminar variability of cortical D_1 receptors, as revealed by autoradiography, have been interpreted as suggesting a greater involvement in the higher cortical processing of non-human primates than presumed previously (Richfield *et al.*, 1989); it has also been suggested that a significant decrease in the density of frontal cortex D_1 receptors with increasing age might contribute to the decline in cognitive abilities evident among elderly persons (De Keyser *et al.*, 1990b). *In vivo* studies have sustained and elaborated these notions, via evidence for the actions both of SCH 23390 and of SCH 39166 in disrupting prefrontally mediated cognitive function in the non-human primate (Sawagushi and Goldman-Rakic, 1991). The finding of a decreased ratio of high- to low-affinity agonist binding sites of the frontal cortex D_1 receptor in Alzheimer's disease might suggest a functional alteration of cortical cell membranes bearing D_1 receptors (De Keyser *et al.*, 1990c) that might indicate an alternative or adjunctive therapeutic approach to this disorder.

10.5   Conclusions

The complexities inherent in $D_1 : D_2$ interactions in rodents (Chapter 3) are heightened yet further on considering their clinical implications, because of evidence for prominent species differences between rodents and non-human primates and the dearth of studies in human subjects. However, the results of investigations in non-human primates, while engendering this state of 'creative tension' relative to those in rodents, are so intriguing as to clearly justify those clinical studies that are now either proceeding or else in the process of formulation. Particularly, the efficacy and side-effects of full-efficacy, selective D_1 agonists in Parkinson's disease and of selective D_1 antagonists in schizophrenia remain fundamental questions that demand answers. Should they prove efficacious, new and improved treatment modalities might follow; if they do not so prove, it would become necessary to re-evaluate fundamentally both a considerable number of preclinical models that have previously proved reliable in predicting therapeutic efficacy, and many of our current notions of $D_1 : D_2$ interactions. These are challenging times for contemporary DAergic neuroscience and psychopharmacology in relation to $D_1 : D_2$ interactions. We await expectantly the clinical feedback that is likely to exert some considerable influence on further studies in this field.

Acknowledgements

The author's studies are supported by the Health Research Board.

References

Abbott, B., Starr, B.S. & Starr, M.S. (1991) *Pharmacol. Biochem. Behav.* **38**, 259–263.
Arnt, J. (1987) In *Dopamine Receptors* (eds Creese, I. & Fraser, C.M.), pp 199–231. New York, Alan R. Liss.
Arnt, J., Hyttel, J. & Sanchez, C. (1992) *Eur. J. Pharmacol.* **213**, 259–267.
Bedard, P.J. & Boucher, R. (1989) *Neurosci. Lett.* **104**, 223–228.
Boyce, S., Rupniak, N.M.J., Steventon, M.J. & Iversen, S.D. (1990) *Neurology* **40**, 927–933.
Braun, A., Fabbrini, G., Mouradian, M.M., Serrati, C., Barone, P. & Chase, T.N. (1987) *J. Neural Transm.* **68**, 41–50.
Braun, A., Mouradian, M.M., Mohr, E., Fabrini, G. & Chase, T.N. (1989) *J. Neurol. Neurosurg. Psychiatry* **52**, 631–635.
Brent, P.J. (1991) *Psychopharmacology* **104**, 201–207.
Breese, G. & Creese, I. (1986) *Neurobiology of Central D₁ Dopamine Receptors.* New York, Plenum Press.
Brewster, W.K., Nichols, D.E., Riggs, R.M., Mottola, D.M., Lovenberg, T.W., Lewis, M.H. & Mailman, R.B. (1990) *J. Med. Chem.* **33**, 1756–1764.
Camps, M., Cortes, R., Gueye, B., Probst, A. & Palacios, J.M. (1989) *Neuroscience* **28**, 275–290.
Casey, D.E. (1991) *Lancet* **338**, 185.
Casey, D.E. (1992) *Psychopharmacology* **107**, 18–22.
Chipkin, R.E. (1990) *Trends Pharmacol. Sci.* **11**, 185.

Chipkin, R.E., Iorio, L.C., Coffin, V.L., McQuade, R.D., Berger, J.G. & Barnett, A. (1988) *J. Pharmacol. Exp. Ther.* **247**, 1093–1102.

Christensen, A.V. (1990) *Behav. Neurol.* **3**, 49–60.

Clark, D. & White, F.J. (1987) *Synapse* **1**, 347–388.

Close, S.P., Elliott, P.J., Hayes, A.G. & Mariott, A.S. (1990) *Psychopharmacology* **102**, 295–300.

Code, R.A. & Tang, H.A. (1991) *Eur. J. Pharmacol.* **201**, 235–238.

Coffin, V.L., Latranyi, M.B. & Chipkin, R.E. (1989) *J. Pharmacol. Exp. Ther.* **249**, 769–774.

Coffin, V.L., McHugh, D., Chipkin, R.E. & Barnett, A. (1992) *Neurochem. Int.* **20** (Supplement), S141–S146.

Cortes, R., Gueye, B., Pazos, A., Probst, A. & Palacios, J.M. (1989) *Neuroscience* **28**, 263–273.

Daly, S.A. & Waddington, J.L. (1991) *Br. J. Pharmacol.* **104** (Supplement), 60P.

Daly, S.A. & Waddington, J.L. (1992a) *J. Psychopharmacol.* **6**, 50–60.

Daly, S.A. & Waddington, J.L. (1992b) *Br. J. Pharmacol.* **105** (Supplement), 7P.

Daly, S.A. & Waddington, J.L. (1992c) *Eur. J. Pharmacol.* **213**, 251–258.

Daly, S.A. & Waddington, J.L. (1992d) *Br. J. Pharmacol.* **107** (Supplement), 65P.

Darney, K.J., Lewis, M.H., Brewster, W.K., Nichols, D.E. & Mailman, R.B. (1991) *Neuropsychopharmacology* **5**, 187–195.

De Keyser, J., Claeys, A., De Backer, J.P., Ebinger, G., Roels, F. & Vauquelin, G. (1988) *Neurosci. Lett.* **91**, 142–147.

De Keyser, J., Walraevens, H., Ebinger, G. & Vauquelin, G. (1989) *J. Neurochem.* **53**, 1096–1102.

De Keyser, J., Ebinger, G. & Vauquelin, G. (1990a) *Ann. Neurol.* **27**, 157–161.

De Keyser, J., De Backer, J.P., Vauquelin, G. & Ebinger, G. (1990b) *Brain Res.* **528**, 308–310.

De Keyser, J., Ebinger, G. & Vauquelin, G. (1990c) *Arch. Neurol.* **47**, 761–763.

DeNinno, M.P., Schoenleber, R., MacKenzie, R., Britton, D.R., Asin, K.E., Briggs, C., Trugman, J.M., Ackerman, M., Artman, L., Bednarz, L., Bhatt, R., Curzon, P., Gomez, E., Kang, C.H., Stittsworth, J. & Kebabian, J.W. (1991) *Eur. J. Pharmacol.* **199**, 209–219.

Dewar, K.M. & Reader, T.A. (1989) *Synapse* **4**, 378–386.

Dubach, M., Schmidt, R., Kunkel, D., Bowden, D.M., Martin, R. & German, D.C. (1987) *Neurosci. Lett.* **75**, 205–210.

Duffy, R.A., Kaminska, G., Chipkin, R.E. & McQuade, R.D. (1991) *Pharmacol. Biochem. Behav.* **41**, 235–238.

Ehmann, T.S., Delva, N.J. & Beninger, R.J. (1987) *J. Clin. Psychopharmacol.* **7**, 173–174.

Ellenbroek, B., Peeters, B., Honig, W. & Cools, A.R. (1987) *Psychopharmacology* **93**, 343–348.

Ellenbroek, B.A., Willemen, A.P.M. & Cools, A.R. (1989) *Neuropsychopharmacology* **2**, 191–199.

Ellenbroek, B.A., Artz, M.T. & Cools, A.R. (1991) *Eur. J. Pharmacol.* **196**, 103–108.

Elsworth, J.D., Lawrence, M.S., Roth, R.H., Taylor, J.R., Mailman, R.B., Nichols, D.E., Lewis, M.H. & Redmond, D.E. (1991) *J. Pharmacol. Exp. Ther.* **259**, 595–600.

Falardeau, P., Bouchard, S., Bedard, P.J., Boucher, R. & Di Paolo, T. (1988) *Eur. J. Pharmacol.* **150**, 59–66.

Farde, L. (1992) *Psychopharmacology* **107**, 23–29.

Farde, L., Halldin, C., Stone-Elander, S. & Sedvall, G. (1987) *Psychopharmacology* **92**, 278–284.

Farde, L., Wiesel, F.A., Nordstrom, A.-L. & Sedvall, G. (1989) *Psychopharmacology* **99** (supplement), S28–S31.

Gessa, G.L., Canu, A., Zompo, M.D., Burrai, C. & Serra, G. (1991) *Lancet* **337**, 854–855.

Gomez-Mancilla, B. & Bedard, P.J. (1991) *J. Pharmacol. Exp. Ther.* **259**, 409–413.

Hall, H., Farde, L. & Sedvall, G. (1988) *J. Neural Transm.* **73**, 7–21.

Hess, E.J., Bracha, H.S., Kleinman, J.E. & Creese, I. (1987) *Life Sci.* **40**, 1487–1497.

Hietala, J., Lappalainen, J., Koulu, M. & Syvalahti, E. (1990) *Trends Pharmacol. Sci.* **11**, 406–410.

Kane, J.M., Honigfeld, G., Singer, J., Meltzer, H.Y. & the Clozaril Collaborative Study Group (1988) *Arch. Gen. Psychiatry* **45**, 789–795.

Kebabian, J.W., Britton, D.R., DeNimo, M.P., Perner, R., Smith, L., Jenner, P., Schoenleber, R. & Williams, M. (1992) *Eur. J. Pharmacol.* **229**, 203–209.

Lawrence, M.S., Redmond, D.E., Elsworth, J.D., Taylor, J.R. & Roth, R.H. (1991) *Life Sci.* **49**, PL229–PL234.

Lidow, M.S., Goldman-Rakic, P.S., Gallagher, D.W. & Rakic, P. (1991) *Neuroscience* **40**, 657–671.

Loschmann, P.-A., Smith, L.A., Lange, K.W., Jaehnig, P., Jenner, P. & Marsden, C.D. (1991) *Psychopharmacology* **105**, 303–309.

Lovenberg, T.W., Brewster, W.K., Mottola, D.M., Lee, R.C., Riggs, R.M., Nichols, D.E., Lewis, M.H. & Mailman, R.B. (1989) *Eur. J. Pharmacol.* **166**, 111–113.

Lubin, H., Gerlach, J., Hagert, U., Meidahl, B., Molbjerg, C., Pedersen, V., Rendtorff, C. & Tolvanen, E. (1991) *Eur. J. Neuropsychopharmacol.* **1**, 541–548.

Madras, B.K., Fahey, M.A., Canfield, D.R. & Spealman, R.D. (1988) *J. Neurochem.* **51**, 934–943.

Markstein, R., Seiler, M.P., Vigouret, J.M., Urwyler, S., Eng, A. & Dixon, K. (1988) In *Progress in Catecholamine Research*. Part B: *Central Aspects* (Sandler, M., Dahlstrom, A. & Belmaker, R.), pp 59–64. New York, Alan R. Liss.

McHugh, D. & Coffin, V. (1991) *Eur. J. Pharmacol.* **202**, 133–134.

Murray, A.M. & Waddington, J.L. (1990a) *Pharmacol. Biochem. Behav.* **35**, 105–110.

Murray, A.M. & Waddington, J.L. (1990b) *Eur. J. Pharmacol.* **186**, 79–86.

Nomoto, M., Jenner, P. & Marsden, C.D. (1988) *Neurosci. Lett.* **275**, 275–280.

O'Boyle, K.M. & Waddington, J.L. (1987) *Neuropharmacology* **26**, 1807–1810.

Peacock, L., Lublin, H. & Gerlach, J. (1990) *Eur. J. Pharmacol.* **186**, 49–59.

Pifl, C., Reither, H. & Hornykiewicz, O. (1991) *Eur. J. Pharmacol.* **202**, 273–276.

Pifl, C., Nanoff, C., Schingnitz, G., Schutz, W. & Hornykiewicz, O. (1992a) *J. Neurochem.* **58**, 1997–2004.

Pifl, C., Reither, H. & Hornykiewicz, O. (1992b) *Brain Res.* **572**, 87–93.

Richfield, E.K., Young, A.B. & Penney, J.B. (1989) *J. Comp. Neurol.* **286**, 409–426.

Rinne, J.O., Lonnberg, P. & Marjamaki, P. (1990) *Brain Res.* **508**, 349–352.

Robertson, H.A. (1992) *Trends Neurosci.* **15**, 201–206.

Rosengarten, H., Schweitzer, J.W. & Friedhoff, A.J. (1991) In *Neuromethods,* Vol. 18: *Animal Models in Psychiatry 1* (eds Boulton, A., Baker, G. & Martin-Iverson, M.), pp 245–266. New York, Humana Press.

Rouillard, C., Bedard, P.J. & Di Paolo, T. (1990) *Eur. J. Pharmacol.* **185**, 209–215.

Sawaguchi, T. & Goldman-Rakic, P.S. (1991) *Synapse* **251**, 947–950.

Schachter, M., Bedard, P., Debono, A.G., Jenner, P., Marsden, C.D., Price, P., Parkes, J.D., Keenan, J., Smith, B., Rosenthaler, J., Horowski, R. & Dorow, R. (1980) *Nature* **286**, 157–159.

Sedvall, G., Farde, L., Barnett, A., Hall, H. & Halldin, C. (1991) *Psychopharmacology* **103**, 150–153.

Seeman, P. (1980) *Pharmacol. Rev.* **32**, 229–313.

Seeman, P., Niznik, H.B., Guan, H.-C., Booth, G. & Ulpian, C. (1989) *Proc. Natl Acad. Sci. USA* **86**, 10156–10160.

Sibley, D.R. & Monsma, F.J. (1992) *Trends Pharmacol. Sci.* **13**, 61–69.

289

Sweidan, S., Edinger, H. & Siegel, A. (1990) *Pharmacol. Biochem. Behav.* **36**, 491–499.

Taylor, J.R., Lawrence, M.S., Redmond, D.E., Elsworth, J.D., Roth, R.H., Nichols, D.E. & Mailman, R.B. (1991) *Eur. J. Pharmacol.* **199**, 389–391.

Temlett, J.A., Chong, P.N., Oertel, W.H., Jenner, P. & Marsden, C.D. (1988) *Eur. J. Pharmacol.* **156**, 197–206.

Temlett, J.A., Quinn, N.P., Jenner, P.G., Marsden, C.D., Pourcher, E., Bonnet, A.-M., Agid, Y., Markstein, R. & Lataste, X. (1989) *Mov. Disord.* **4**, 261–265.

Tsui, J.K.C., Wolters, E.C., Peppard, R.F. & Calne, D.B. (1989) *Neurology* **39**, 856–858.

Venturini, G., Stocchi, F., Margotta, V., Ruggieri, S., Bravi, D., Bellantuono, P. & Palladini, G. (1989) *Neuropharmacology* **28**, 1377–1382.

Waddington, J.L. (1986) *Biochem. Pharmacol.* **35**, 3661–3667.

Waddington, J.L. (1988) *Gen. Pharmacol.* **19**, 55–60.

Waddington, J.L. (1989a) *J. Psychopharmacol.* **3**, 54–63.

Waddington, J.L. (1989b) *Current Opinion Psychiatry* **2**, 89–92.

Waddington, J.L. (1989c) *Int. Rev. Neurobiol.* **31**, 297–353.

Waddington, J.L. (1990) *Psychopharmacology* **101**, 431–447.

Waddington, J.L. (1992) In *Adverse Effects of Psychotropic Drugs* (eds Kane, J.M. & Lieberman, J.A.), pp 246–265. New York, Guildford Press.

Waddington, J.L. (1993a) In *Antipsychotic Drugs and their Side Effects* (ed. Barnes, T.R.E.). London, Academic Press (in press).

Waddington, J.L. (1993b) *Schiz. Bull.* **19**, 55–69.

Waddington, J.L. & Daly, S.A. (1992) In *Novel Antipsychotic Drugs* (ed Meltzer, H.Y.), pp 109–115. New York, Raven Press.

Waddington, J.L. & O'Boyle, K.M. (1987) *Rev. Neurosci.* **1**, 157–184.

Waddington, J.L. & O'Boyle, K.M. (1989) *Pharmacol. Ther.* **43**, 1–52.

Zarrindast, M.R. & Amin, R. (1992) *Psychopharmacology* **106**, 67–70.

Index

NEUROSCIENCE PERSPECTIVES

Editor: Peter Jenner
   Pharmacology Group
   Biomedical Sciences Division
   King's College London
   Manresa Road
   London SW3 6LX

Titles in this series:

Roger Horton and Cornelius Katona (eds), Biological Aspects of Affective
 Disorders
Trevor Stone (ed), Adenosine in the Nervous System
Judith Pratt (ed), The Biological Bases of Drug Tolerance and
 Dependence
Michel Hamon (ed), Central and Peripheral 5-HT_3 Receptors
John Waddington (ed), D_1:D_2 Dopamine Receptor Interactions
Thomas Barnes (ed), Antipsychotic Drugs and Their Side
 Effects (forthcoming)
Eva Giesen-Crouse (ed), Peripheral Benzodiazepine
 Receptors
David Nicholson (ed), Anti-Dementia Agents (forthcoming)
Alan Harvey (ed), Natural and Synthetic Neurotoxins